THE
HONEST
LIFE

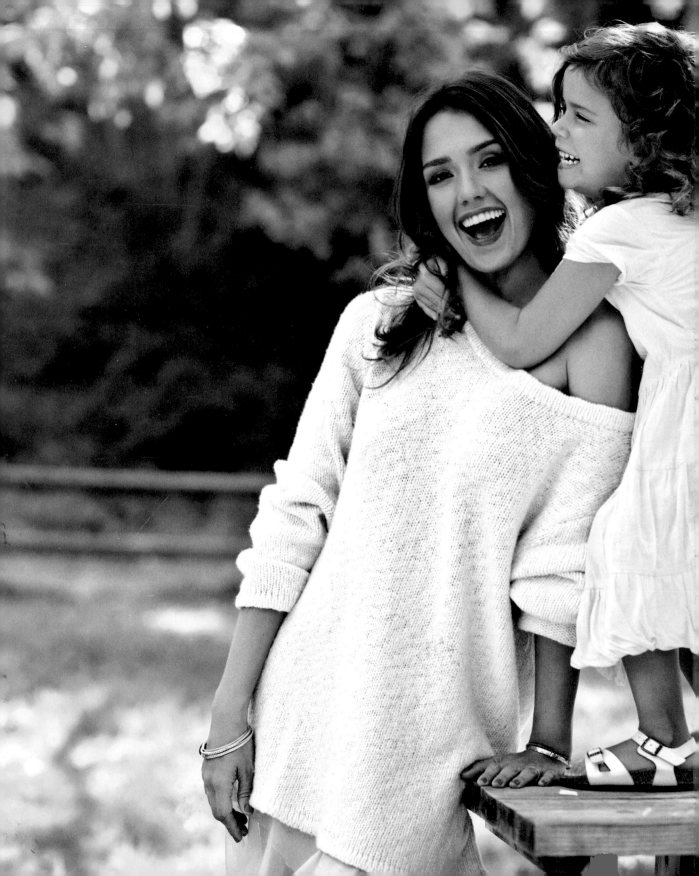

Jessica Alba

THE
HONEST
LIFE

LIVING NATURALLY
AND TRUE TO YOU

RODALE.

Rodale books may be purchased for business or promotional use or for special sales. For information, please write to: Special Markets Department, Rodale Inc., 733 Third Avenue, New York, NY 10017.

Printed in the United States of America

Rodale Inc. makes every effort to use acid-free ♾, recycled paper ♻.

Art direction by George Karabotsos and Kara Plikaitis

Book design by Kara Plikaitis

"Dirty Dozen Plus and Clean 15" copyright © 2013 Environmental Working Group, www.ewg.org. Reprinted with permission.

"Environmental Defense Fund Seafood Selector Chart" copyright © 2013 Environmental Defense Fund, www.EDF.org/seafood. Reprinted with permission.

"Make Your Own Cleaners" recipe copyright © 2013 Rodale Inc., www.rodale. com. *Penny Pincher* series, feature by Leah Zerbe. Reprinted with permission.

"Grains and Beans chart" © copyright 2009 Rodale Inc. Reprinted with permission from *The Rodale Whole Foods Cookbook*.

Library of Congress Cataloging-in-Publication Data is on file with the publisher.

ISBN-13: 978-1-60961-911-4 paperback

Distributed to the trade by Macmillan

4   6   8   10   9   7   5   3   paperback

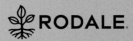

We inspire and enable people to improve their lives and the world around them.
rodalebooks.com

Photo Credits

All photos by Justin Coit, with the exception of the following:

© Andrew Arthur: 91

© Lesley Bryce: xvi

© Getty Images: 78 (all), 87 (Claire Danes, Jane Birkin), 105 (all)

© Mitch Mandel/Rodale: 31

© Walter McBride/Corbis: 87 (Diane Keaton)

© Nick Onken: 122–123, 158–159, and 206

© Superstock: 87 (Audrey Hepburn)

© The Honest Company blog: 201 (Christopher Gavigan, Ashley King, Sarah Reisert, Melissa Williams)

Jessica Alba's family photos: courtesy of Jessica Alba

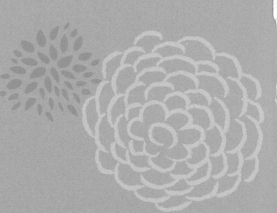

This book is dedicated to everyone out there who's trying
to make the world a better place for generations to come.

And to my sweet little angel pies, Honor and Haven.
Being your mom has been the greatest gift in life.

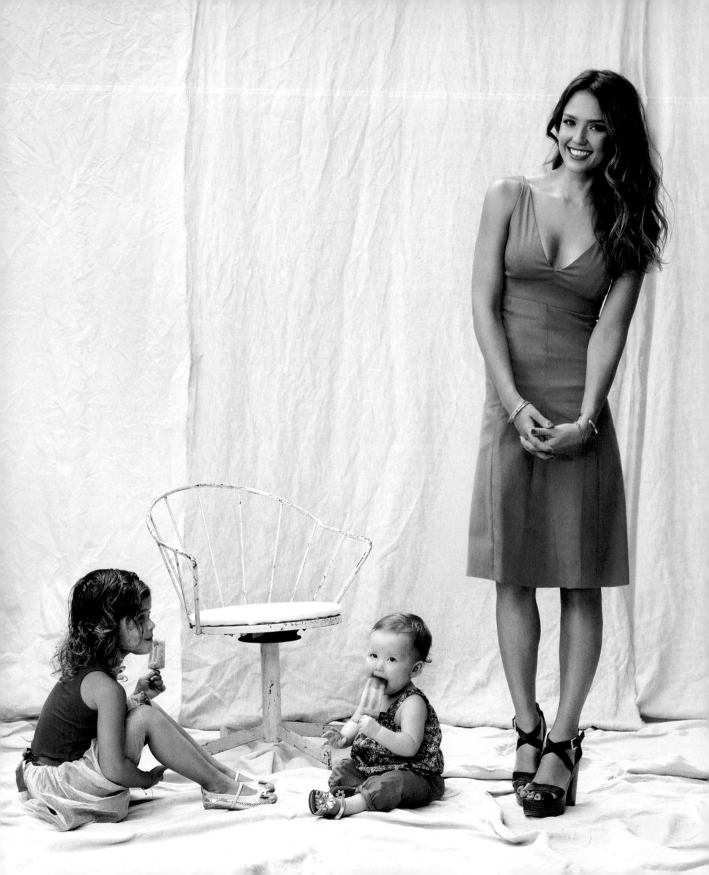

Contents

foreword

by Christopher Gavigan

Becoming a parent is not only a defining moment in most people's lives—it can be unexpectedly motivating. When I first met Jessica Alba, she was seven months pregnant with her first daughter, Honor. She came to the launch party for my book, *Healthy Child Healthy World*—named for the nonprofit where I was then the CEO—and introduced herself. I know most people admire her as an actress, but the person I met that night was a concerned parent who wanted nothing more than to create the healthiest and best possible life for her baby.

There she was, on the verge of this big moment, asking me where she could find the safest crib mattress or worry-free laundry detergents because she had done her research and realized regulations weren't necessarily in place to keep her baby or home free from questionable chemicals. I'm pretty sure I didn't give her the answers she wanted to hear—that unfortunately one still had to verify whether eco-products were actually safe—because she kept knocking on my door (i.e., "stalking me") to brainstorm solutions. As a father, I too felt her frustration. Jessica kept searching the world for the highest quality and purest products, and she kept running into walls. She'd ask, "What diaper is free from nasty chemicals but will hold my baby's business?" or "Flame-retardants on pajamas—really?!?" I'm glad she kept asking questions, searching for better solutions, and imagining a safer world for her children, because from that initial encounter and many subsequent conversations—ones we are still having to this day—The Honest Company was born.

Since first meeting Jessica, I've always been impressed by her thorough knowledge of the health risks of toxic chemicals and her instinctive scrutiny of claims made by supposedly safer or eco-friendly products. But I'm most moved by her passion—for always learning and growing, for striving to make better choices everyday, and for seeking solutions (affordable ones!) that help all families and people everywhere. In reading *The Honest Life*, I hope you'll get to know Jessica the way I do. You'll see that she's a dreamer, but also a doer. She's inspired by her friends, family, and community, by her childhood and motherhood, and by what's practical, beautiful, and fairly priced. And she really likes thinking (and cooking) outside of the box.

Once I stopped by her house for a dinner only to find her whipping up a four-course, or-ganic meal (this is a treat for her guests that she pulls off regularly, by the way). Between chatting with friends and sipping her wine, she somehow made an awesome dinner that we all devoured. She's such a talented cook—more like an amateur chef—that I can promise you'll enjoy the recipes she's included in this book. But my point is this: Jessica really does do it all herself.

She knows that busy moms don't have time to make multiple trips to the store for food and diapers, research which pacifier or paint is safe and which isn't, or dash away from the bath when the shampoo has run out. Drawing on inspiration from her everyday life and channeling her boundless determination to identify what's accessible and truly do-able with a parent's hectic reality, Jessica has become a savvy entrepreneur who speaks for a new generation of women and families who don't want to make compromises between what's healthy, what works, and what's fashionable and fun.

I think most people think of celebrities as normal people living extraordinary lives, but Jessica is an extraordinary person living a normal life—one that is relatable, attainable, and rooted in family. Which is why I know that *The Honest Life* will serve as great guide to help you make healthier choices when it comes to the food you eat, the products you bring into your home, and the purity of what you put on your and your baby's skin. Ultimately, though, I believe that Jessica's example can motivate many more of us to transform our family's health and happiness in ways that suit each of us best.

I'll be honest:

This is a book about how you can live a healthier and more sustainable lifestyle. But at the same time, it's really not about that at all—because this book is not about why you need to become a vegan, use cloth diapers, or grow all your own food.

> I eat (organic) meat.
>
> I don't have time to wash cloth diapers.
>
> I have a total black thumb—if I had to grow our food, we'd starve.

I DECIDED TO WRITE this book because I was sick of being told that "healthy," "safe," and "eco" means "boring," "beige," and "blah"—not to mention, crazy expensive and hard to find. Which really doesn't add up, right? So let me explain. Over the past five years (ever since I got pregnant with Honor), I've been on a quest to create a healthy environment for my family and myself. But I also want our life to be authentic, stylish, and fun, because that's who we are. The problem was that whether I was decorating Honor's nursery, testing out eco-friendly disposable diapers, or shopping for the perfect red lipstick, everything felt like a compromise. Somehow, it was a given that you had to sacrifice performance—and style—to be healthy.

You could either have stuff that looked and worked great but was filled with toxic chemicals, or you could have the not-so-cute, more-expensive eco-alternative that didn't get the job done . . . not both. I found this very frustrating. I'm a busy person—even more so since I became a mom—and I'm betting you are, too. We don't have time to waste on products that don't work.

I knew there had to be a better way—doable, more fun, no compromises—and figuring out how to do this has become my mission. It's one of the main things I talk about with my friends (both single and with families)—we're all working to make healthier choices without an extreme lifestyle overhaul, and we share tips and strategies. It's the reason I created The Honest

Company, so we could all have a single, trustworthy destination for nontoxic household essentials that are also extremely effective (and super cute). It's also the reason I wrote this book. Because with the help of friends, family, and experts, I've figured out a few things along the way. I wanted to share *my* version of a healthy, natural lifestyle—I call it Honest Living—with you.

But First, the Back Story

So HOW DID I get so passionate about Honest Living in the first place?

Well, it all started with a load of laundry.

It was the spring of 2008. I was pregnant with Honor—which is to say, I was hot and exhausted, had swollen ankles and an enormous belly, and (of course) was feeling excited, terrified, and a million other emotions all at once. I couldn't wait to be a mom, but I also was completely overwhelmed by how much we had to learn about being parents and creating a safe and nurturing environment for our child to thrive in.

Like any mom-to-be, I called my mother for advice. A lot.

My mom has raised two kids, and I have a lot of cousins, so she really knows babies. If you want to know what to do about colic or how to make the best lasagna to feed 40, seriously, just call my mom and she'll tell you. Which is why,

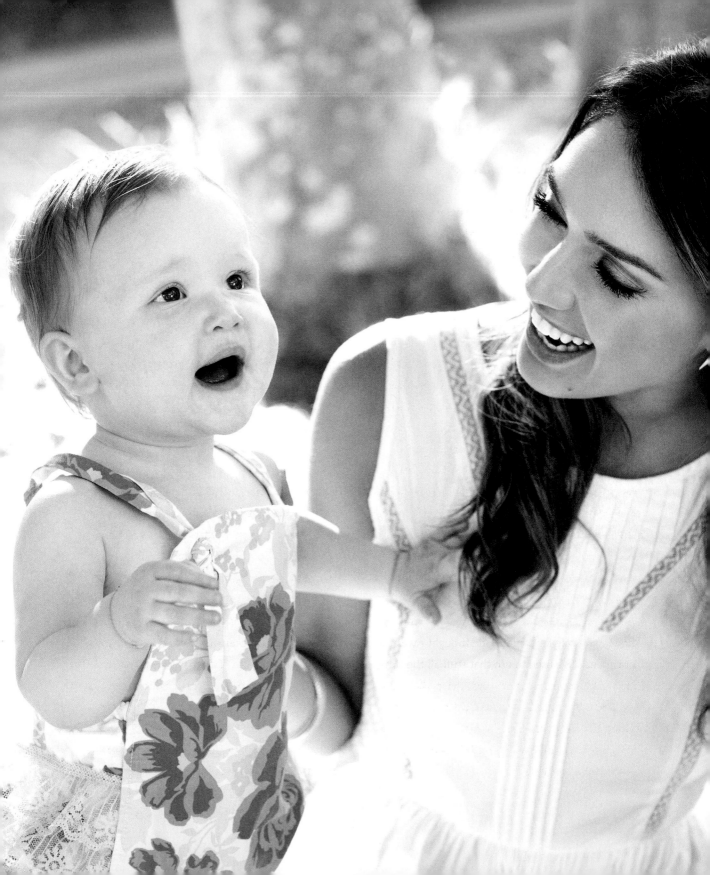

when she told me that I had to use a special brand of baby detergent to wash all of the onesies and little outfits I got at my baby shower, I didn't question it. Sure, this particular brand of baby detergent comes in a super-small box and costs a fortune (frankly, I couldn't believe my parents had sprung for it when we were little, because we were always on a budget), but my mom insisted it was worth every penny! "Everyone uses this detergent," she reassured me. "It's what I used for *your* baby clothes. It costs so much because it's the best stuff out there."

So I loaded up the washer with my first round of baby stuff and the recommended dose of that fancy detergent. I noticed the fragrance and thought it was kind of strong. In fact, I started sneezing uncontrollably. I was used to my fragrance-free "eco" detergent, but my mom said this was the bees' knees of detergents, so I kept it moving.

Until I folded the first load of clothes—and my hands broke out with itchy red welts. Meanwhile, the sneezing hadn't subsided.

I mean, my poor mom. I called her immediately and started ranting: "Are you crazy? I can't believe you wanted me to use this stuff—there's no way it's safe for babies!" She thought *I* was the crazy one. "We used to use that stuff all the time," she said. "If you don't want my advice, then don't ask for it. But don't call me and get mad at me when I'm just trying to help you."

I took a moment, realized she was right, and resolved to Google it.

I figured that would be the end of the story.

Except, as it turns out, that was just the beginning.

Why I Ask Questions

Maybe someone a little less . . . curious (my husband, Cash, might say obsessive!) would have just shelved the fancy baby detergent and called it a day. But that's not me. I know you probably know me from *Fantastic Four* or *Sin City*, and you might already be thinking, "Why is this chick so worked up about a laundry detergent?"

But being an actress hasn't always been my life. I didn't grow up with a lot of money. My parents were young and just starting out when I was born. Things were definitely tight. We moved around a lot while my dad was in the military, and then after he got out, we moved into one of my grandparents' homes so we could live in a better house than my parents could afford at the time. My mom and dad each worked about three jobs during certain periods, and we had to do a lot of coupon cutting and sometimes thrift-store shopping to get by. On top of all that, I was constantly sick. I had kidney surgery, tonsils taken out, cysts removed, and was diagnosed with severe asthma and allergies—all before I was eight years old!

Anytime I got a cold, it went straight to pneumonia. I was hospitalized several times for

Today there are more than 80,000 chemicals on the market that have never been properly studied to see if they're toxic to our health.

my asthma or related illnesses, which meant missing a lot of school and always being sort of out of sync with my classmates and teachers. The hospital where I stayed most often was a 2-hour drive from home, so I spent a lot of time hanging out with my mom and nurses in the hospital rooms, where reading and playing make-believe were my escape. When I did go back to school, I had usually already finished the assigned reading while the rest of the class was still on chapter 3. This meant I would get bored . . . and talk. A lot.

I guess being immersed in a more adult world at such a young age and being aware of my family's financial struggles caused me to grow up kind of fast. I always thought of adults as my equals, and I wasn't afraid to voice my opinions. Which isn't

always a good thing as a kid . . . but it is what influenced my questioning of everything around me. I didn't like seeing social injustice of any kind, especially if it impacted women and children.

Later, in my teens and twenties, I started working with nonprofits that help families in need, like Step Up Women's Network, V-Day, the Children's Defense Fund, ONE, March of Dimes, and Safer Chemicals, Healthy Families. Today, I'm on the board of Baby2Baby, a charity that collects new and gently used baby gear (i.e., diapers, wipes, cribs, car seats, and clothing—basically everything a parent needs) to distribute to 40 nonprofit partners, who then deliver it to families in need in and around Los Angeles. These are people dealing with homelessness, domestic violence, and poverty, making their struggles as parents unimaginable to most of us. We also bring truckloads of supplies to the pregnant and parenting teenagers who attend LA's McAlister High School. Spending time with those girls reinforces my mission to challenge the status quo and do anything I can to help moms in need, who are just trying to do what's best for their babies. It brings me back to my core values and, really, to my authentic self—that's another part of Honest Living.

So back to that expensive box of baby

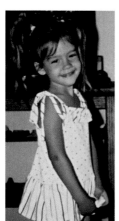

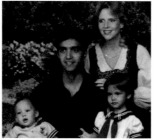

Me at four when I was first diagnosed with asthma; my mom Cathy, dad Mark, and brother Joshua.

detergent: I couldn't stop thinking about how I was going to be a mom with a baby to nurture and protect. Yet here I was trying to do something so simple—wash her clothes!—and it didn't feel safe. That wasn't right. And when I thought about how that detergent was so successful at marketing itself as the most pure, responsible choice for your baby—so they could charge moms *more*? Well, that made me really mad.

When I get mad, I ask questions, just like I did as a little kid: Why should safer products only be available to those who can afford them? Why would a laundry detergent sold today be different from the same brand of laundry detergent that my mom used 30 years ago? Just what was in this stuff anyway—and why would it make me break out in a rash?

The more I learned, the more questions I had.

Getting Honest(ly Disturbing) Answers

IT TURNS OUT that my mom wasn't crazy when she told me to use that special brand of baby detergent. The detergents—and cleaning supplies and baby clothes and toiletries and so on—that we buy today really *are* different from what our moms used to buy. Eventually I learned by listening to experts such as Dr. Philip J. Landrigan, the director of the Children's Environmental Health Center at Mount Sinai School of Medicine

in New York City, that there are more than 80,000 chemicals on the market that have never been properly studied to see if they're toxic to our health—almost 30 percent more than were in our laundry detergent and other consumer goods when President Gerald Ford signed the Toxic Substances Control Act (TSCA) in 1976. That special baby detergent? It may have been okay when my mom washed our baby clothes in the early 1980s, but today it contains synthetic fragrances and a chemical called propylene glycol, both of which can cause the skin rashes and other allergic reactions I experienced. It's also made with diethylene glycol, which is a known neurotoxin—that means it can mess with your neurological system and cause learning delays and even brain damage. (See page 220 for a super-easy-to-understand guide to the unpronounceable words in this book!)

And here's where things get bananas: The whole point of the Toxic Substances Control Act was to regulate the chemicals used in everyday products and *make things safer*—but instead, it's done almost the exact opposite. The government doesn't require any of these chemicals to be tested for safety before new products hit store shelves. The Food and Drug Administration can't require a recall even if a product does start making people sick (although they can request one), while the Environmental Protection Agency has no recall power—and those are the government agencies in charge of making sure our consumer goods are safe.

Why is this situation so ridiculously messed up? The chemical industries have powerful lobbyists in Washington, DC, and their whole job is to find gaping loopholes in the TSCA and make sure those holes stay there. Plus the chemical corporations have huge marketing budgets and can afford to put together ad campaigns that will make you think their products are safe and even environmentally friendly, when that couldn't be further from the truth. That's called "greenwashing," and it Makes. Me. Crazy. It's so dishonest! These companies don't care about people, let alone babies, who are the most vulnerable of all to these toxic chemical exposures—they care about protecting their profit margins. And that has to change. In 2011, I partnered with the Safer Chemicals, Healthy Families coalition to visit Washington, DC, and advocate for TSCA reform, because I don't think a parent should need a chemistry degree to have a safe home. This is a totally nonpartisan issue, and it won't cost taxpayers a dime—all it will do is put responsibility on the chemical companies to test their products for safety before we buy them. We're still facing an uphill battle to close all those loopholes in the TSCA and put a regulatory system in place that truly protects American families—but every day, more moms and dads are joining the fight.

In the past 35 years, the EPA has restricted only 5 toxic substances and the FDA has banned 11. Meanwhile, the European Union has banned more than 1,100 chemicals that it considers unsafe in personal care products alone!

The Honest Story

SOON AFTER my itchy brush with the baby detergent, I went to a launch party for a book called *Healthy Child Healthy World: Creating a Cleaner, Greener, Safer Home* by Christopher Gavigan. The timing couldn't have been better—I was $7\frac{1}{2}$ months pregnant and freaking out about the laundry and everything in our house. Christopher's book gave me a thorough education on what, exactly, I needed to worry about and why.

I pretty much cornered Christopher at his party and said, "I'm losing my mind here. Please tell me that there's a company I can trust, that makes products that really work and are safe for me to use around my baby!" But while he could point me to some very credible brands making safe, environmentally friendly products, all too often they were expensive, didn't work so well, or were still toxic despite the eco-packaging. Plus I was still overwhelmed by the amount of research I had to do on every brand to figure out if they were the real deal or just greenwashing me with a lot of eco-promises that didn't pan out.

That's when I decided that if this company didn't exist, I had to make it happen. After Christopher and I got to know each other, we thought: "Let's create a family brand that offers products that work tremendously well and are affordable, beautiful—*and* don't contain any of these chemicals."

I knew it was a big dream. Plenty of people told me that I should launch with just *one* product, like a perfume or a body lotion. Or that I'd be better off licensing my name and putting it on a line of clothing or home goods, like a lot of celebrities do. But that wasn't my passion. What I believe is that we need to make a safer environment for families, starting with the most vulnerable.

I also knew that parents today are way too busy to do tons of research and shop around. So the idea of one trusted company that met all of these needs and saved us a trip to the store was incredibly appealing.

It took us more than three years and a ton of hard work to go from that original aha! moment to the official launch of Honest.com in 2012. After all, I'm just a mom and an actress—not a toxicologist, a tech guru, or a businessperson. I had to surround myself with people who had the expertise I lacked. So with my cofounder and chief product officer Christopher Gavigan, who brings a ton of environmental health knowledge and branding experience from his time as the CEO of the national nonprofit Healthy Child Healthy World, we pitched Brian Lee, an e-commerce guru who cofounded ShoeDazzle.com and Legal-Zoom.com, to be our partner and CEO. Once Brian was on board, we got lucky and found Sean Kane, a master of managing and oversight, to be our COO. We decided that The Honest Company should offer customizable "bundles" of products so you get exactly what you need, delivered straight

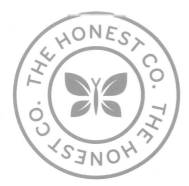

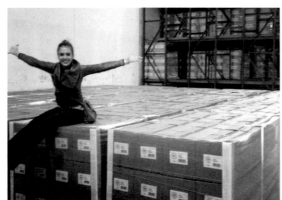

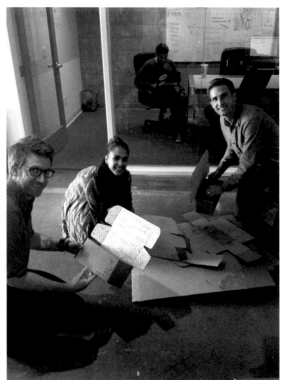

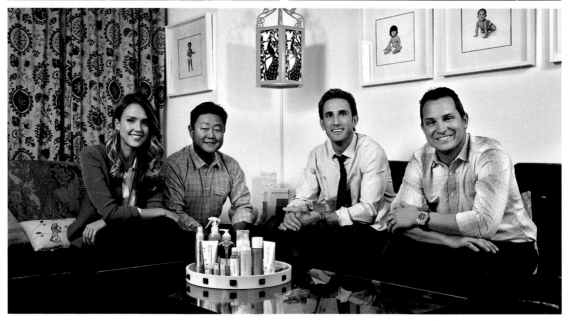

from us every month. This lowers our carbon footprint (since we don't need to ship through wasteful distribution systems) and keeps our prices lower because we don't have retail markups.

We also drew on the expertise of a number of environmental health and manufacturing experts to create our products. But the funny thing about being "just a mom"? It turns out that sometimes, we actually *do* know best—or at least, quite a lot about what makes a great diaper or cleaning product! Christopher and I road-tested every prototype on our own families (he's got three kids under age six), so if a diaper leaked or a laundry detergent didn't get stains out, we lived it—and sent it back to be improved. That often meant pushing manufacturers to think outside the box—like, I knew that hip moms would love a little skulls print diaper pattern (paying homage to Alexander McQueen). "Eco" does not have to mean putting your kid in a diaper that looks like a brown paper bag.

Fast-forward one year, and we're now sending bundles of diapers, wipes, cleaning supplies, and personal care products out every month to tens of thousands of customers. At home, I use everything on my two girls, Honor and Haven, and I love knowing that I'm giving them the safest, highest-quality products without compromising on style or function. But the best part is hearing from other moms who are using our products and loving them. After all, moms can be the toughest critics—and kids are even harder to please! But I hear from so many parents who were frustrated by the lack of options just like I was and are so happy with Honest.

We're also realizing that it's not just moms who want safer products—plenty of people without kids have reached out and asked when we're going to bring out more cleaning supplies, or personal care products like toothpaste, deodorant, and so on, because they love our message and want affordable, high-quality products that also happen to be better for their health and the planet. Well, we're on it. And we're proving that you don't need toxic chemicals to have a better-performing, affordable, beautiful product.

Clockwise from top left: Our very first pallet of products—Honest Hand Soap—arrives in our warehouse; putting together our first box with Tim Hankins, our head designer (left), and CPO Christopher Gavigan; the Honest partners, president (me), CEO Brian Lee, CPO Gavigan, and COO Sean Kane.

How to Use This Book

IF YOU'RE LEARNING about toxic chemicals in consumer goods for the first time, you're probably feeling frustrated and confused right now. I get it. I've been there. All that big-picture talk about lawmakers in Washington can be hard to wrap your head around—after all, what the heck are you supposed to do until we get the laws fixed?

That's where this book comes in. I've spent tons of time researching this stuff, talking to experts, trying things out, and figuring out what works, what doesn't, and what *really* suits our busy lives—and now I've downloaded everything I've learned into this handy guidebook. We're going to cover it all: how to eat seasonally, healthfully, and deliciously; how to clean and decorate your home with healthy, nontoxic materials and one-of-a-kind vintage pieces; how to put together a safe, fun, and functional nursery (and figure out what other baby gear you do and *don't* need); plus how to choose the purest and most-effective personal care products. And because *The Honest Life* is about so much more than making healthy choices, we'll explore how to edit your personal style (whether you're pregnant, post-baby, or simply need to break out of a beauty and fashion rut). I'm also going to share my strategies for staying organized in just about every area of your life—because honestly, if you can't find your car keys when you need them, not much else matters! I've got tons of inspiration to offer on ways to connect and engage as a family—as well as thoughts on what living "an honest life" really means.

Hopefully you'll be inspired by these tips and find yourself feeling healthier, happier, and more energetic. You'll spend less time stressing over the mundane things, freeing up more time to spend on what really matters: working on projects that feed your soul; enjoying quality time with your family and friends; being the kind of person you envision yourself to be . . . and living in a way that's true to that mission every day.

You can read this book cover to cover,
jump around to the topics that interest you most,
or just stick it in your tote bag and pull it out
whenever you have a question about
the best lead-free lipstick or kid-friendly recipe.

I'VE ALSO MADE this book super easy to navigate by coming up with icons that will help you spot some crucial information at a glance. They include:

DISHONEST INGREDIENT

Anything toxic, greenwashed, or otherwise not so good for you. (You can find a full list of these on pages 220 to 225.)

HONEST TIP

Any strategy or trick that I (or my girls or my Honest partners) swear by.

KEEPING IT REAL

My honest confessions of the not-so-natural compromises I make when I'm too busy or can't find an eco-friendly option that works or looks great—because nobody's perfect. This is all a work in progress!

You can read this book cover to cover, jump around to the topics that interest you most, or just stick it in your tote bag and pull it out whenever you have a question about the best lead-free lipstick or an easy, nutritious, kid-friendly recipe or dinner party idea. There are no impossible-to-pronounce ingredients to memorize and no dense science to wade through. Everything I suggest works the way you'd want it to work *and* looks fantastic doing it—the fact that it's all nontoxic

A NOTE TO NONPARENTS

Since my journey began as a mom trying to create a healthy environment for her babies, I knew any book of mine just wouldn't be complete without chapters devoted to those topics.

But that doesn't mean there isn't good info for nonparents in here, too. I'm also a girl—flip to page 99 to see my wall of shoes, and you'll see what I mean. And at The Honest Company, we're hearing every day from people who don't have kids but nevertheless want to make healthier choices. So you'll totally be able to use all of the information in the food, beauty, style, and home chapters—and pass the kid-focused tips along to your mom and dad friends!

and way healthier for you is just the icing on the cake.

So yes, this is sort of an eco-lifestyle book. But here's what this book really is: a fun, practical handbook for people like you and me. It's realistic, a little bit irreverent, and 100 percent authentic.

No lectures.
No judgment.
No guilt.

Just tons and tons of useful tips, stylish ideas, and inspiration that you can incorporate—easily and affordably!—to live a healthier, more organized, joyful, and, above all, *honest* life . . . that's true to you.

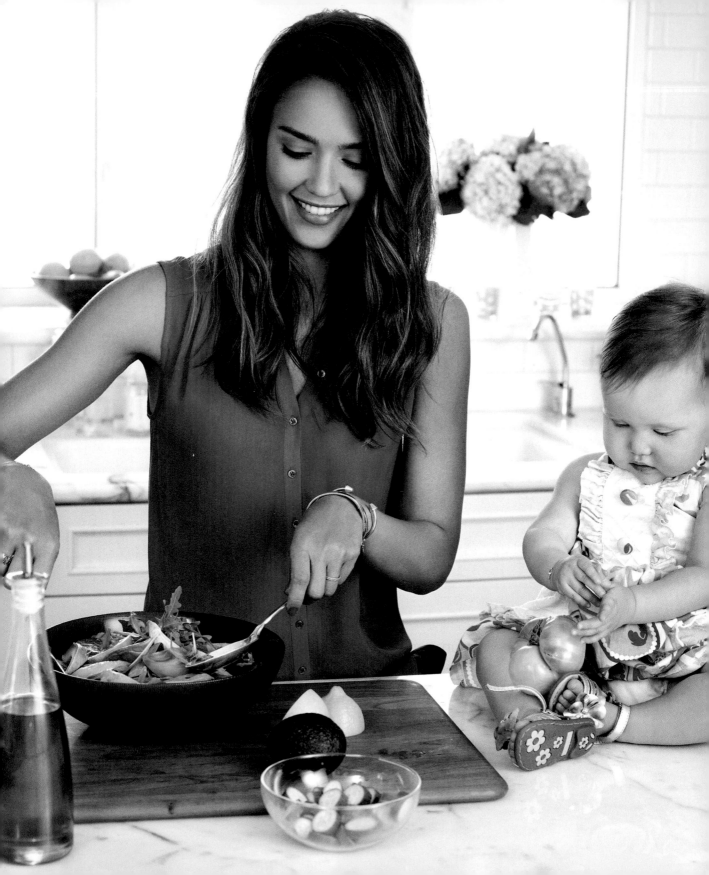

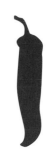

chapter 1

HONEST
food

FRESH, WHOLE,
FLAVORFUL—AND
MADE WITH LOVE

HERE'S A FACT ABOUT ME THAT MIGHT SURPRISE YOU (unless you've seen my Twitter or Instagram feeds): I'm crazy about food. Nothing makes me happier than cooking an amazing meal for my family or good friends. Even if it's a hectic Tuesday night and I've had back-to-back meetings at The Honest Company offices and then came home to deal with end-of-day meltdowns—you know, one of *those* days—I'll still spend 2 hours making a homemade dinner of Cornish game hens and roasted butternut squash and invite over six friends. I swear it's how I unwind. (For me, a bit of vino and a nice playlist while cooking are pure bliss.)

Okay, yes, it's a ridiculous amount of work and I can be a mental case, finding recipes on my laptop, and racing outside to grab another handful of rosemary from my wall garden. But when everyone sits down to the table, I'm so happy. There is no better way to spend an evening than with great food, great wine, and great conversation.

When I was growing up, dinner was the time of day when, no matter what, my family came together.

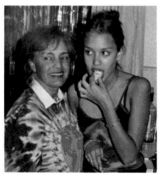

Growing up, I loved hanging out in my grandmother's kitchen. There was always something delicious simmering on the stove—homemade chicken soup was a mainstay.

My grandmother always had *carnitas* (that's a Mexican braised pork dish, and it is the bomb) simmering all day in the slow cooker for tacos or snacks. And my mom made everything from fried chicken, biscuits, and gravy to pork chops, lasagna, and steak dinners. I'm not sure she even knows how to cook for, say, four people because we always had enough to feed 10 or 20. I loved helping them out in the kitchen from a pretty young age, and what I remember best was the sense of connection and comfort. We were the kind of family who prayed before meals, and whatever your religious beliefs, I love taking that moment to be grateful for what you have and who you get to share it with. There's something

about the love and time you put into making food for your family—I think people are nourished by that energy as much as by the meal itself.

So that's the foundation of my love for food. Honor is already an awesome sous chef, so I encourage her to participate in food prep whenever possible—it's such a cool way to talk to her about where food comes from and to develop her taste for fresh ingredients. Yes, kids make a mess in the kitchen and slow you down, but they also make the whole process way more fun! I want my girls to love food and respect how much effort goes into growing and preparing it.

Some Honest Challenges

UNFORTUNATELY, WE'RE ALL so busy today that it's easy to lose that connection to our food. We're eating in our cars, at our desks, out of our handbags . . . no judgment, I'm right there with you. On any given week, I might be in the Honest office, on location for a film, or traveling. Believe me, you have to fight hard to create any kind of stability, let alone a regular meal schedule for yourself, when life is that erratic. Even at home in LA, some days are so hectic I'm lucky if lunch is one of my coworkers' half-eaten sandwiches left in the fridge.

Whether you're eating on the go or shopping to cook at home, it's often an ordeal to find fresh, healthy food, because frankly, a lot of what

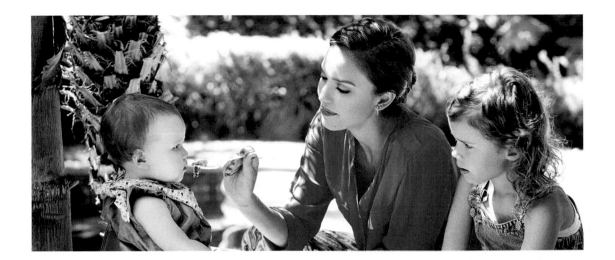

ends up on restaurant menus and grocery store shelves can't even be called food in the first place. As we've seen in the past year alone, with the outrage over pink slime additives in ground beef and the use of antibiotics in chicken, the quality of our food has declined now that most of it is raised on enormous factory farms. Many of these chemicals and additives weren't used in food production 30 years ago, so we're just beginning to understand what they can do to our health. But science is showing links between the industrialization of our food and the rise in obesity and the earlier onset of puberty in girls, as well as medical conditions like diabetes, heart disease, and cancer. I can't say that I'm surprised. How could we have thought these chemical exposures weren't going to affect our health? We are what we eat.

It can be so overwhelming to sift through the claims on food packaging and try to figure out what will nourish your family and what's a "health halo" designed to trick you into thinking some processed, additive-laden food is a smart choice. My personal strategy is to avoid foods that come in packages as much as possible. I call my food philosophy Honest Eating, and it means feeding my family whole, fresh foods that look as close as possible to the way they did on the farm. But it's also about a lot more than that—and I don't mean a diet. Honest Eating is an attitude, not a prescription. And it's darn tasty. Let me explain.

Why I Eat Honestly

MY FOOD PHILOSOPHY has been evolving in this direction ever since I announced I was going vegan at age 12. As you might imagine, with all the carnivores in my house, that decision wasn't too popular! My grandmother was all about her

Eating tons of fruit, veggies, and whole grains makes your skin amazing and gives you way more energy.

coffee can full of bacon grease—she used it to cook everything!—so when I said I wasn't eating any meals with meat, dairy, or fish, I was out of luck.

At the time, I thought giving up animal products was the sole key to healthy eating. Plus I was really concerned about animal welfare and creeped out about killing anything. I stuck with a vegan diet until I was 15, and since I couldn't eat almost any meal my family was eating, I had to learn to get creative in the kitchen. I started experimenting with putting fruit, nuts, and avocado in my salads and making my own soups using beans or lentils flavored with cumin, sage, and garlic. I discovered so many amazing foods that weren't prepared the way I grew up eating.

The more I explored vegan cooking, the more I realized how much healthier I felt eating a mostly plant-based diet. I've suffered from allergies my whole life, and I found that I was sneezing and wheezing way less without dairy and foods with highly processed ingredients. This makes sense: Cow's milk is one of the eight foods most responsible for allergic reactions. While cow's milk allergies are most common in babies and little kids and are often outgrown, dairy may continue to play a role in allergies and other health problems as we get older. Plus eating tons of fruits, vegetables, and whole grains, while reducing sugar and processed foods, makes your skin completely

amazing and gives you way more energy. It's also super important for long-term health stuff like preventing cancer, diabetes, and heart disease. And—isn't this a lovely coincidence?—it's better for the planet, especially if you eat organic.

You'll notice that I said *mostly* plant based. Unfortunately, a 100 percent vegan diet just didn't work for my body in the long term. I struggled to get enough protein and ultimately became anemic without *any* meat in my diet. Plus I really disliked how many processed and packaged foods seem to be marketed at vegetarians or other *blank*-free diets—whether you give up dairy, gluten, or any other food group, it seems like food marketers will figure out a way to slap that label all over to lure you in. Usually, those products are pretty devoid of nutrients and often contain *more* calories, additives, and other crap. No, thank you.

Bottom line, I like beef, poultry, seafood, and cheese (preferably unpasteurized)! My body feels and works best when I'm eating a varied diet with plenty of lean protein. The more I educate myself on these issues, the more I believe that if you purchase and consume animal foods thoughtfully, you can be just as healthy and environmentally conscious as your average vegan—if not more so. I promised no lectures, though, so if being vegetarian or vegan makes sense for your body and your lifestyle, rock on.

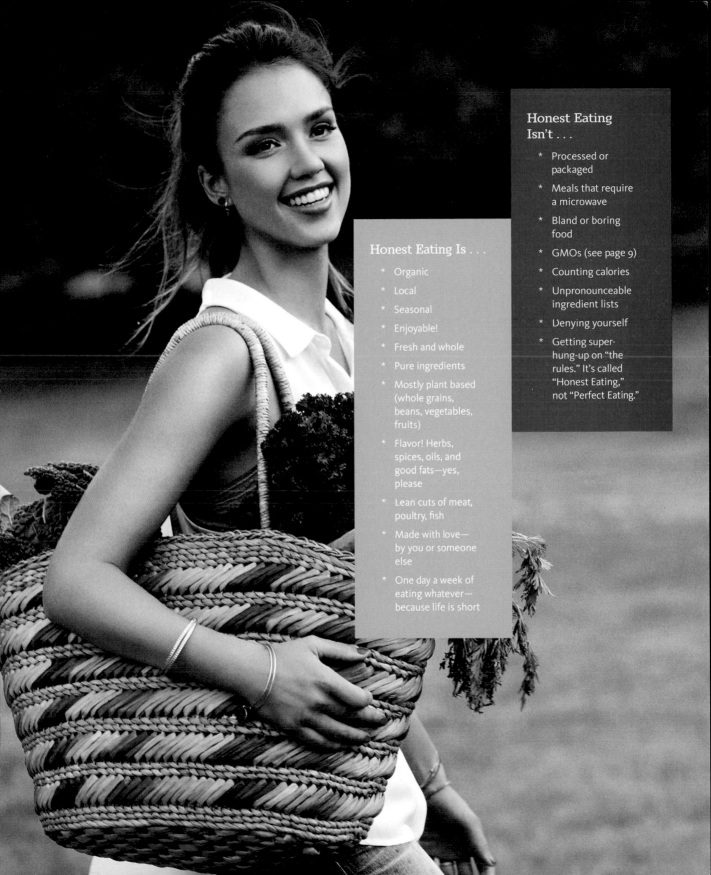

Honest Eating Is . . .

* Organic
* Local
* Seasonal
* Enjoyable!
* Fresh and whole
* Pure ingredients
* Mostly plant based (whole grains, beans, vegetables, fruits)
* Flavor! Herbs, spices, oils, and good fats—yes, please
* Lean cuts of meat, poultry, fish
* Made with love— by you or someone else
* One day a week of eating whatever— because life is short

Honest Eating Isn't . . .

* Processed or packaged
* Meals that require a microwave
* Bland or boring food
* GMOs (see page 9)
* Counting calories
* Unpronounceable ingredient lists
* Denying yourself
* Getting super- hung-up on "the rules." It's called "Honest Eating," not "Perfect Eating."

Honest Eating: My Definition

HERE'S A QUICK overview of what this whole Honest Eating thing means to me, and how to incorporate these strategies into your own life.

Organic

WHETHER I'M BUYING produce, meat, or dairy, the USDA "Certified Organic" label is a must for me. It's the hands-down biggest deal, whether you're worried about your health, the environment, or animal welfare—or, like me, you think all three are important and intersecting. When you see the organic label on a whole, fresh food, you can relax, because you know you've covered your bases. If it's a fruit or vegetable, it wasn't sprayed with toxic pesticides or fertilizers, and the farmers couldn't use genetically modified (GMO) seeds (see page 9 for more on what that term means). If it's meat or dairy, the animals weren't given antibiotics or growth hormones, and they were fed a 100 percent organic diet and given access to the outdoors. The USDA regulates how food brands can use the organic label and checks to make sure they're upholding all of these standards.

Organic isn't a perfect label—some advocates believe regulations should be even tighter. But it's the best protection we have right now, so I always buy organic—the more we support this label, the more the food industry and the government will realize how important it is to us.

Local

THIS IS MY second priority when food shopping. Most of the food on your supermarket shelves traveled an average of 1,500 miles to get there— even farther if it's, say, February and you're buying strawberries in New York. They cannot grow anything in New York when there's snow on the ground—so the grocers ship that fruit in from Chile or China. And forget about fresh. It takes four to seven days for those strawberries to reach you—that's almost a week of being packed on smelly trucks, ships, and freight trains. This is a huge waste of energy, yes, but it's also bad for you. Produce starts to lose its nutritional value and its flavor the minute it's picked, so a bunch of week-old carrots aren't nearly as nutritious or delicious as the just-dug version for sale at your farmers' market. Bonus: The more we support local farms practicing sustainable agriculture, the more our local soil quality improves.

KEEPING IT REAL

EASY DOES IT

You'd go bananas if you tried to make sure every food you purchased was local. Also, you'd be the saddest person, living on nothing but root vegetables and good intentions all winter. So don't try to turn your entire grocery list local right away—get to know your neighborhood farmers' market, start picking up a couple favorite foods there, and gradually incorporate more local foods into your life in a fun and stress-free way.

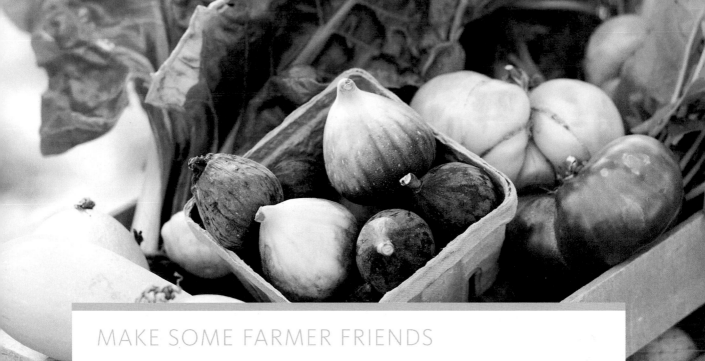

MAKE SOME FARMER FRIENDS

"Local, seasonal, organic—sounds delish," you're thinking. "Now where do I find all of this amazing food?" Here's how I get more farm-fresh goodness into our kitchen every week:

❋ SHOP YOUR FARMERS' MARKET. The number of farmers' markets has doubled in the past decade, so odds are good there's one happening in your neighborhood. And most offer more than just produce—think meats, cheese, eggs, even honey and flowers. **Find yours by plugging in your ZIP code to www.localharvest. org/farmers-markets.**

❋ JOIN A CSA. CSA stands for "community supported agriculture." You typically pay upfront for a "share" of the farm's harvest and then collect your bounty weekly throughout the season. **Find a CSA at www.localharvest.org/csa.**

❋ SIGN UP FOR A DELIVERY SERVICE. We get a box of organic veggies delivered weekly to our home and even to my office from a local farm, and it's been such a game changer! I love knowing I'll always have fresh ingredients on hand, and Honor loves seeing what comes in the box each week. These services aren't available everywhere, but they are becoming increasingly popular: **Search www.localharvest.org.**

❋ VISIT A U-PICK FARM. Try picking your own berries, apples, or pumpkins (depending on the season). **Find a farm at www.rodaleinstitute. org/farm_locator.**

❋ STOP AT ROADSIDE STANDS. Whether you're running errands or taking a road trip, if you see local farm goodies for sale, pull over! Especially if it's late in the day, these mini–farmers' markets may give you an awesome deal on a dozen ears of corn or sell you a giant watermelon for a song.

❋ GROW YOUR OWN. I wish I could say we had a fantastic vegetable garden—I'm all black thumbs. But I have started venturing into the world of herb gardening and think it's such an amazing way to teach my girls about caring for living things.

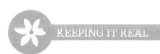

THE DIRTY DOZEN

Synthetic pesticides, which are sprayed on most conventional produce, are among the top 10 chemicals associated with an increased risk for autism and learning disabilities. Pound for pound, kids ingest four to five times more fruits and veggies than adults and are more vulnerable to smaller doses of pesticides because their brains and bodies are still developing. I try to buy certified organic when I can, but it's impossible to find (or afford!) organic produce all the time. So don't sweat it; just use this handy guide to make sure you're at least eating clean for those grown with the highest pesticide levels.

Dirty Dozen Plus	Clean 15
(Highest in pesticides; buy these organic!)	*(Lowest in pesticides)*
* Apples	* Onions
* Celery	* Sweet corn
* Sweet bell peppers	* Pineapples
* Peaches	* Avocado
* Strawberries	* Cabbage
* Nectarines (imported)	* Sweet peas
* Grapes	* Asparagus
* Spinach	* Mangoes
* Lettuce	* Eggplant
* Cucumbers	* Kiwifruit
* Blueberries (domestic)	* Cantaloupe (domestic)
* Potatoes	* Sweet potatoes
* Green beans	* Grapefruit
* Kale/greens	* Watermelon
	* Mushrooms

Source: Environmental Working Group, 2012

Seasonal

WHEN YOU START eating more locally grown food, you also have to eat with the seasons. At first, it sounds like such a bummer—no tomatoes in December? Why would anyone live like that? Well, here's the thing—that December tomato? It tastes terrible. You know it does. It's watery and bland, and you're just eating it because it's there. Forget nutrients. Forget flavor. But the tomatoes you eat in July and August? They are the best things ever—change-your-life delicious.

So seeking out more local foods means eating more of what's in season—aka actually fresh and tasty—around you. That means you're changing up your diet every few months, bringing in new foods right when you might otherwise start getting bored of eating the same old things all the time. And those new foods bring new nutrients, often just when our bodies need them most. There's a very cool synergistic thing that happens between health and flavor when you start eating seasonally—try it out and you'll see what I mean. Of course, what's in season near you might be totally different from what's in season for me. **Find out what's freshest right now by plugging in your state and season at www.sustainabletable. org/shop/seasonal.**

Enjoyable!

THERE'S ABSOLUTELY NO POINT in trying to change your eating habits if you can't also enjoy your food. You won't stick with it, you'll feel gross, and everyone who has to eat what you eat will be miserable right along with you. With Honest Eating, there's no emphasis on calorie counting or nibbling sad little portions of prepackaged diet foods, because that takes all the joy out of cooking and sharing meals with loved ones. By skipping processed, toxin-laden foods, you're going to remove some empty calories off your plate from the get-go. Losing or maintaining your weight becomes effortless, freeing you up to focus on how *good* your meals taste.

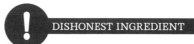

DISHONEST INGREDIENT

GMOs

FOUND IN: Canola, soybeans, and corn. These are the main ingredients in animal feed—and key grains in tons of processed foods, although the label won't indicate if GMOs are present.

WHAT IS IT? "Genetically modified organisms" are engineered into food crops to make them hardier—usually a toxic chemical pesticide is bred right into the grain!

WHY IS IT SKETCHY? The health consequences of GMOs are largely unknown, but they've been banned throughout Europe. Personally, I'd rather be safe than sorry. GMOs are not allowed in organic food, so if you're eating mostly organic, you're already limiting your exposure.

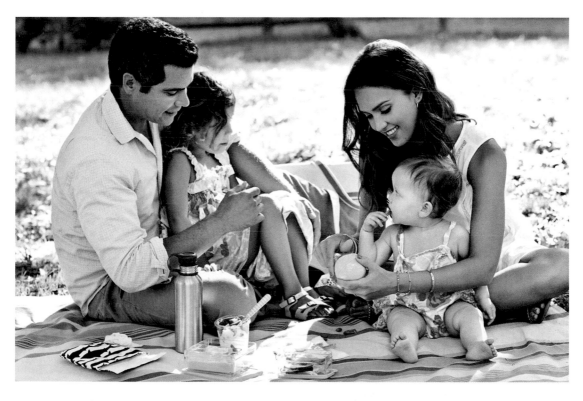

Good, Honest Food

So NOW, LET'S get to the fun part: What to eat! These are my family's favorite foods—and are all pulled from the actual list I use to stock our fridge and pantry week to week so we always have delicious, fresh ingredients on hand to whip up snacks and meals.

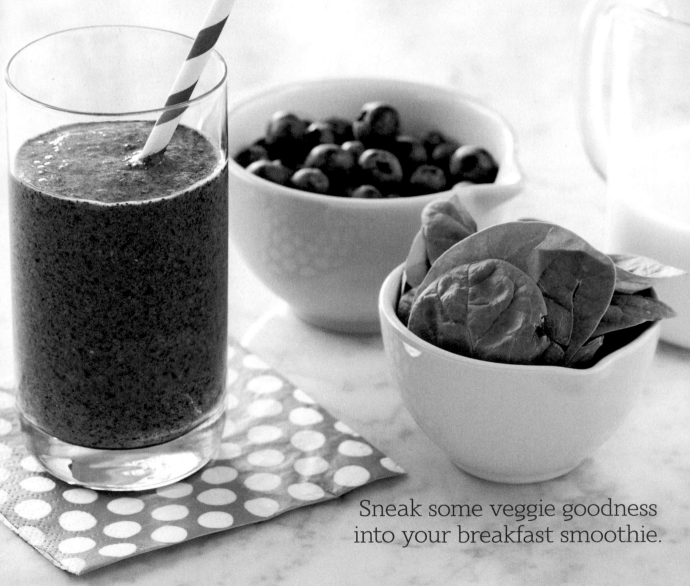

Sneak some veggie goodness into your breakfast smoothie.

Pure & Simple: Produce

SINCE WE EAT SEASONALLY, the fruits and veggies we bring home vary a lot—although in California, we're fortunate to have such a long growing season that many kinds of produce are available all year long. Here are some favorite ways to use them up. I'm a "pinch of this" and "dash of that" kind of girl, so play with your own proportions.

Spring
This season's all about tender, earthy flavors.

ASPARAGUS
Roast it! Just drizzle trimmed asparagus with olive oil, sprinkle with salt, and roast at 450°F for 10 to 15 minutes.

AVOCADOS
Full of "good" fats that are great for your brain, these are the staple of Honor's diet—but they make Haven gag!

✳ ### BABY SPINACH
I like to slip some into Honor's sandwiches and smoothies. Here's a quick smoothie recipe: Blend a cup each of raw spinach, frozen blueberries (raw are okay, too), and unsweetened vanilla almond milk. Great for breakfast; definitely tastes best cold.

BEETS
Roast or boil these, then dice them and throw into a salad with goat cheese.

BOK CHOY
Steam, then lightly drizzle with sesame oil and black sesame seeds.

BROCCOLI
Roast florets tossed with a little bit of olive oil and a clove of minced garlic at 400°F for 15 minutes, or until they start to brown.

CARROTS
Shred a bunch of carrots; mix with a diced avocado, slivered almonds, and raisins; and dress with lemon juice and olive oil.

CELERY
It's a natural diuretic! Juice it with apples for a baby's first drink (I do 80 percent celery and 20 percent apple juice for my girls).

GRAPEFRUIT
Toss mixed greens, sliced avocado, sectioned grapefruit, and ribboned jicama with a simple lemon salad dressing; top with pepita seeds.

LETTUCES
The darker the leaf, the healthier it is (romaine and red leaf top the list).

ONIONS
My familiy loves them in everything! Great in stir-fries, sauces, and especially roasted.

ORANGES
In my house, a healthy alternative to dessert.

PEAS
Haven's obsessed—she loves to roll them around on her highchair tray.

RADISHES
A spicy but delicious addition to crudité.

RHUBARB
I'm a little scared of cooking rhubarb except when it comes to pie.

STRAWBERRIES
Strawberry shortcake for sure!

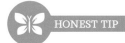

HONEST TIP

WASH YOUR PRODUCE

It may be tempting to skip this step, particularly if you're buying organic or prewashed produce. But all sorts of yuckiness, from pesticide residue (as a result of pesticide drift) to other chemicals and pathogens (like *E. coli*) can hitch a ride on your salad. Just give a quick cold rinse to all fruits and veggies (I use a liberal squirt of Honest Fruit + Veggie Wash, or you can DIY with a 1:4 vinegar-to-water solution) and soak leafy greens for a minute, separating the leaves.

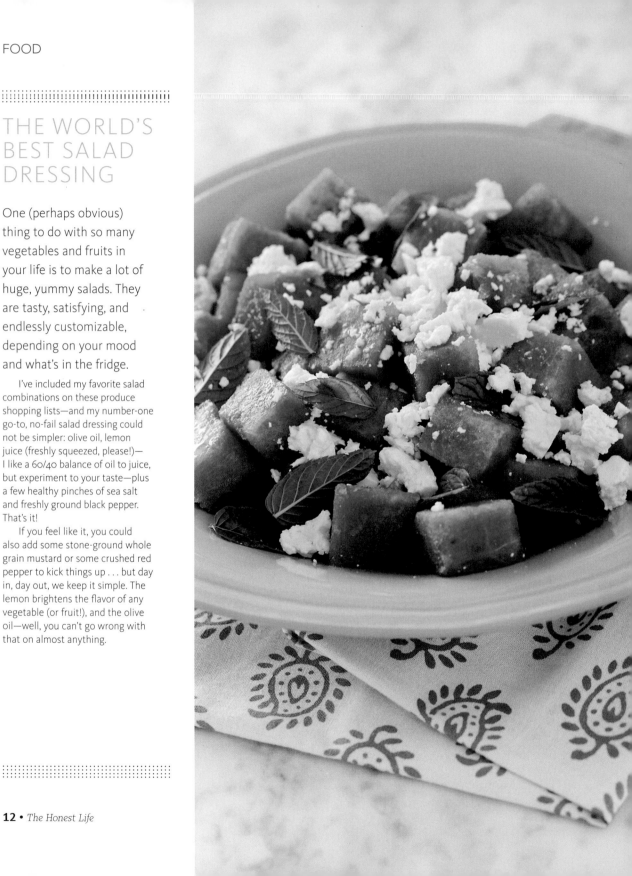

THE WORLD'S BEST SALAD DRESSING

One (perhaps obvious) thing to do with so many vegetables and fruits in your life is to make a lot of huge, yummy salads. They are tasty, satisfying, and endlessly customizable, depending on your mood and what's in the fridge.

I've included my favorite salad combinations on these produce shopping lists—and my number-one go-to, no-fail salad dressing could not be simpler: olive oil, lemon juice (freshly squeezed, please!)— I like a 60/40 balance of oil to juice, but experiment to your taste—plus a few healthy pinches of sea salt and freshly ground black pepper. That's it!

If you feel like it, you could also add some stone-ground whole grain mustard or some crushed red pepper to kick things up . . . but day in, day out, we keep it simple. The lemon brightens the flavor of any vegetable (or fruit!), and the olive oil—well, you can't go wrong with that on almost anything.

Summer

We love a bumper crop of the season's juiciest produce!

APRICOTS
Roast and slice them and add to a scoop of vanilla gelato.

BERRIES
Blackberries, blueberries, raspberries . . . a berry medley with yogurt and honey is the best.

CHERRIES
No prep required—we devour them right out of the bag!

CUCUMBERS
With ranch dressing for kids, or with olive oil, lemon, salt, and ground red pepper for us.

EGGPLANT
Amazing sliced thin, brushed with olive oil and sea salt, then broiled or grilled.

KALE
Thinly slice a bunch of kale and toss with dried cranberries, pine nuts, olive oil, and balsamic vinegar.

MUSTARD GREENS
Love 'em steamed with lemon and olive oil or stir-fried with spicy sausage, vinegar, onions, and garlic.

PEACHES
Roast slices, chill, and add to a green salad with feta and pine nuts. Or peach pie, of course!

PEPPERS
Roast and puree with a little fresh garlic, salt, olive oil, and pepper for a ketchup alternative.

SNAP PEAS
I'm allergic to them raw, but Honor loves them with her crudité of carrots, celery, and jicama with ranch dressing to dip.

SWISS CHARD
I'll mix chard with kale and/or mustard greens in any salad or stir-fry.

TOMATOES
DIY tomato sauce: Simmer 2 pounds of chopped tomatoes with a couple sliced garlic cloves, olive oil, salt, and a pinch of oregano and sugar for 30 minutes; puree.

✳ **WATERMELON**
Toss cubed watermelon with a little arugula, mint, and crumbled feta. Dress with olive oil and red wine vinegar.

ZUCCHINI
I love a ribboned zucchini salad with pine nuts and Parmesan—see page 186 for my recipe.

 KEEPING IT REAL

MY BLACK THUMB

I wish I was the kind of eco-mama who grew all her own vegetables and canned jam . . . but it's not in the cards between my busy work schedule and my natural black thumb. Don't beat yourself up if you, too, can't keep a cactus alive. I've found simple ways to teach Honor and Haven about where their food comes from. For example, we're lucky that rosemary grows like a weed in our hot, sunny California climate and that there are a couple of orange and lemon trees in our backyard that are amazingly maintenance free.

We also recently planted an herb wall garden (see page 200 for the how-to)—Honor helped pack the plants into the pockets, and she can pop out to pick a bunch of basil or parsley when we need it.

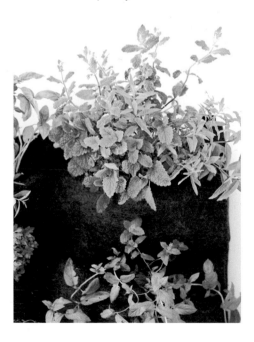

Autumn

We still enjoy all of our late-summer favorites, plus:

APPLES

I love making my own applesauce. Just peel, core, and chop about 10 apples (Gala work great), then cover with water in a big pot. Bring to a boil, reduce to simmer, and cook 30 to 45 minutes until saucy. Add cinnamon (and a bit of sweetener if the apples are tart) and grab a spoon!

CABBAGE

Shred half a head and sauté with a glug of olive oil for a couple minutes. Then toss in raisins, a little white vinegar, and a bit of salt; sauté for 15 to 20 minutes. (I learned this from a caterer on a set when I was 14.)

CAULIFLOWER

I'll roast a head of it, chopped and tossed with olive oil, salt, and a bit of rosemary and chopped garlic for 30 to 45 minutes at 400°F. Puree it with up to 1 cup chicken stock as an alternative to mashed potatoes for the kids.

GRAPES

I love, love, love frozen seedless grapes!

PEARS

Add a delicious crunch to sandwiches and salads.

SQUASH

A fantastic alternative to pasta—we love it with marinara sauce and/or turkey meatballs.

Winter

We hang on to as much fall produce as can be found at the grocery store, but frozen organic fruit and veggies are a great way to get through the winter months.

❋ **BRUSSELS SPROUTS**

Roast 1 pound with chopped candied walnuts, 2 cloves garlic, and a couple pieces of diced thick-cut bacon. Oh, god . . .

LEEKS

A no-fail soup staple.

❋ **SWEET POTATOES**

Oven fries! Peel, slice, toss in olive oil and sea salt, and roast at 400°F for 35 minutes.

TURNIPS

Excellent in a tray of roasted mixed veggies— see the opposite page for how to perfect it.

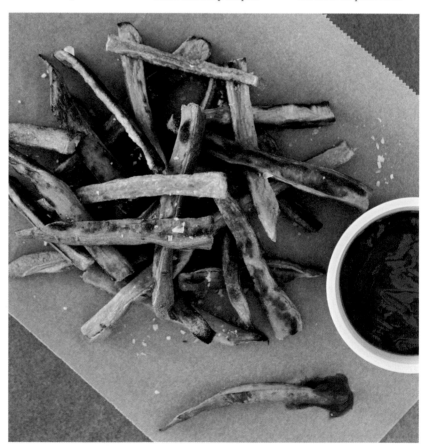

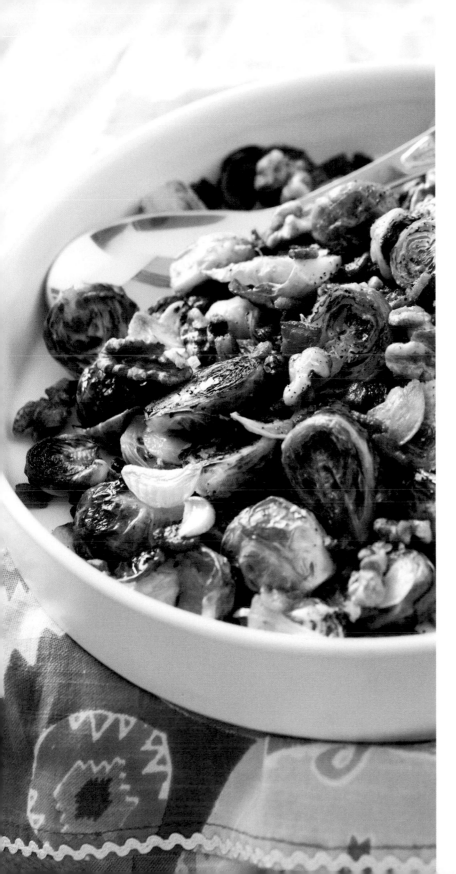

WHEN IN DOUBT, ROAST IT

If you're looking at that long list of veggies and wondering how on earth you'd ever find time to cook them all—let alone persuade your family to eat them—I have one word for you: roasting.

I honestly don't know why anyone would even boil a vegetable again once they discover how great any produce becomes when you cut it up, sprinkle it with olive oil and salt, and stick it in the oven. Suddenly, Brussels sprouts taste better than potato chips!

WHAT TO DO:

1. Preheat your oven to 400°F.

2. Spread cut-up vegetables in a thin layer on a rimmed baking sheet; toss with olive oil, sea salt, and any other herbs or spices of your choice. (I love garlic and lemon; fresh rosemary, thyme, or crushed red pepper are also fantastic.)

3. Roast until everything is nice and crispy (probably 20 to 40 minutes, depending on the quantity and type of vegetable), stirring the vegetables every 10 minutes so they don't stick to the pan. Serve!

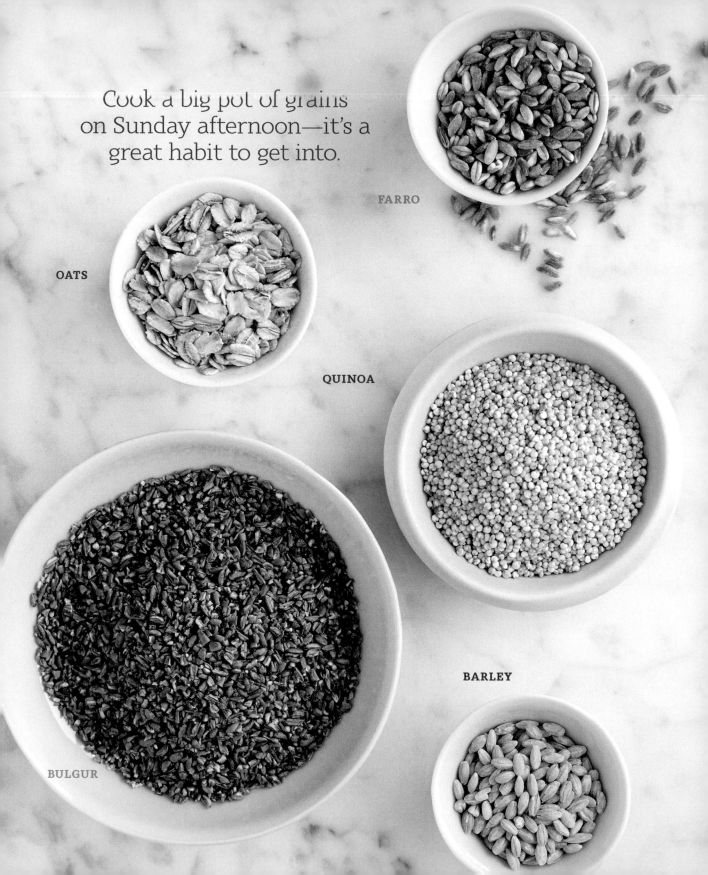

Cook a big pot of grains on Sunday afternoon—it's a great habit to get into.

FARRO

OATS

QUINOA

BULGUR

BARLEY

Pure & Simple: Whole Grains

A LOT OF PEOPLE freak out about whole grains. They have weird names and weird textures— why can't we just stick with bread, pasta, and rice, right? I know, but here's the good news: You *can* eat those things—just switch to 100 percent whole grain breads and pastas, and brown or wild rice. Done! Even better, most whole grains are actually way easier to cook and more delicious than we give them credit for. Just grab a handful whenever you want to add some whole grain goodness to your stir-fries, soups, or salads. (**For a complete guide to cooking grains, see page 209.**)

BULGUR

Bulgur is a fancy name for cracked whole wheat kernels. It has a crunchy, nutty taste and is essential in tabbouleh (a Middle Eastern salad made with parsley, tomatoes, cucumbers, garlic, and lemon). You don't even need to cook it—just soak it in hot water for half an hour. Also great served hot for breakfast with almond milk and maple syrup or honey.

BARLEY

Barley is a good alternative for al dente pasta lovers—it's got the same satisfying chew but so much more protein and fiber. Both hulled and pearled barley (which cooks faster in a pinch) are super satisfying in winter soups and stews—I also love barley in a grain salad with goat cheese, a little nitrate-free bacon or salami (Cash's favorite!), diced spring onions, and, of course, olive oil with lemon.

OATS

We went through a serious oatmeal phase in our house because for ages, it was all Honor would eat for breakfast. Look for rolled or steel cut: Both are made from oat groats, the edible kernels milled from whole grain oats. They cook in 10 (rolled) to 45 (steel cut) minutes and can be cooked like oatmeal or fluffy like rice. Don't bother with instant oats—they're lower in fiber and taste like cardboard.

FARRO

This is a wheatlike berry (but higher in fiber and much lower in gluten!) used in traditional Tuscan cooking, so it's big with pasta lovers and good with almost any rustic tomato sauce or pesto. It has a tasty, almost grassy flavor and cooks in 30 minutes.

QUINOA

This might be the best gateway grain for a skeptic. In addition to packing plenty of the fiber and complex carbs that make whole grains so satisfying, quinoa is a complete source of protein. Plus it cooks in just 15 minutes and is great for risottos or pilafs.

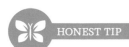

HONEST TIP

QUINOA FOR KIDS

I got in the habit of making quinoa instead of rice for Honor as a way to sneak her some extra protein. She loves it cooked in chicken broth with a little olive oil, salt, and Italian herbs; I use the leftovers for a salad with cranberries and pine nuts. It's fluffy and fun—kids are really into it!

Pure & Simple: Clean Protein

I'M COMBINING plant and animal protein here because meat doesn't have to be at the center of every meal—there are lots of delicious ways to get your protein fix! I do find that I feel better and have more energy when I include a good source of lean protein in every meal, especially breakfast. That sustains me so I'm not tempted to just snack idly on foods I don't need.

ORGANIC BEEF

I always choose cuts labeled "lean" and "extra-lean," like sirloin steak, top round, and bottom round roast. This is so I know I'm minimizing saturated fat and cholesterol, which is a good idea for everyone—but is super important if you're pregnant or breast-feeding. That's because nasty cancer-causing chemicals called dioxins can pile up in animal fat and, once you eat them, make their way to your baby. You should also opt for grass-fed beef whenever possible—cows raised out in the pasture have much less saturated fat and higher levels of omega-3 fatty acids (a good fat!) than grain-fed cattle. Purchasing grass-fed, organic, and local beef also helps ensure you avoid added hormones—which many farmers add to promote rapid growth—as well as that nasty pink slime business (the mess of animal by-products, trimmings, ammonia, and other gunk used as filler in much commercial ground beef). Enough said.

ORGANIC LAMB

One great thing about lamb (and goat, for that matter) is that the USDA doesn't allow the use of growth hormones on these animals. Lamb also happens to be delicious—I love grilling it in kebabs with peppers, onions, and rosemary in the summer (which makes it very kid friendly, too). Look for lean cuts and grass-fed when possible.

ORGANIC CHICKEN

Conventionally farmed chickens are pumped full of antibiotics—to prevent diseases from spreading—and garbage like animal by-products, which helps them grow super fast, until they're barely able to move (not that there's anywhere to go in those tiny cages). For those reasons, "Certified Organic" or "Certified Humane Raised and Handled" is really the only way to go with chicken these days. The CHRH label is monitored by the nonprofit Humane Farm Animal Care to make sure conditions aren't disgusting. That being said, once you start buying one of these better kinds of chicken—you'll never go back. The flavor and freshness are worth it!

ORGANIC, CERTIFIED HUMANE, AND/OR CAGE-FREE EGGS

Fresh, local eggs are great, and most grocery stores nowadays are stocking an organic, cage-free option. Check to see if your grocer carries a local farm's eggs or opt for a certified organic, certified humane, and/or certified cage-free brand. All of these terms are pretty trustworthy and at least ensure that the chickens were spared that brutal caged life, not to mention the heaping doses of antibiotics that are doing us no favors. "Pasture Raised," "Free Farmed," and "Biodynamic" are also good signs.

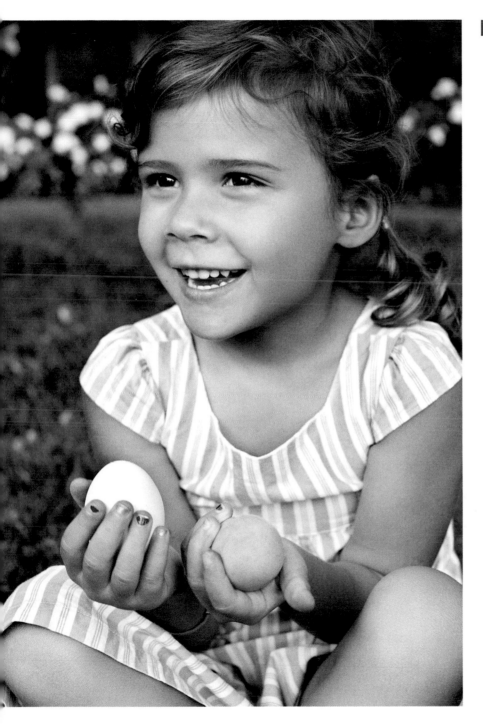

ANTIBIOTICS

FOUND IN: Most commercially raised animals—cattle, hogs, sheep, and poultry

WHAT IS IT? A drug fed to livestock to prevent or treat diseases, particularly because animals that live in confined spaces tend to be more susceptible

WHY IS IT SKETCHY? This practice contributes to the growing problem of antibiotic-resistant bacteria, which you definitely want to avoid (it increases the odds of picking up a food-borne illness—or worse, when people really get sick, doctors won't have drugs that work). Look for the words "no antibiotics added" to be sure your dinner hasn't been raised on medication.

LENTILS, PEAS, AND BEANS

Whenever people say that healthy eating is just too expensive, I want to take them to the grocery store and show them the possibilities. You can get a 1-pound bag of any kind of bean—red lentils, green lentils, black beans, cannellini beans, you name it!—for about a dollar. Add on a bag of brown rice for maybe another $2, cook them both in some chicken broth, and toss with olive oil, onions, garlic, tomatoes—any combination of flavors you love and happen to have in the house. You'll have rice and beans, the classic or a remix version. Legumes are a great side dish with almost any meal; as with whole grains, you can make a pot on the weekend and keep it in the fridge to use as the foundation of many meals for the rest of the week.

These days, I'm a big fan of lentils and love to make them with cumin, coriander, and other Indian spices. But I encourage you to try lots of different beans (and forget everything you thought you knew about hating them when you were a kid) to figure out what you love. We'll make a pot of black beans to use as a side dish for Honor for several days—and I'll warm them up for myself when I need a snack. They are cheapest to buy dried (from the grocery store or health food store bulk bins) and quicker to cook than you might think. But canned is okay, too, if you're time pressed. Just be sure to choose a brand like Eden Organic, whose cans are free of BPA, a hormone-disrupting chemical (see page 159), and rinse the beans well; about 30 seconds under the tap will help clear away a lot of the excess sodium and other additives that can sneak into canned beans. **For a chart on how to cook beans to the right consistency, see page 210.**

ORGANIC TOFU

This is totally optional—but I do find it comes in handy every now and then as a quick breakfast or stir-fry dinner option. It can be difficult to find organic beef chuck hot dogs—so we buy veggie Smart Dogs sometimes. Soyrizo (meatless soy chorizo sausage) has changed my life. It's fantastic in beans—just the right amount of spicy. If possible, make sure that any tofu or soy meat alternative you buy is made with certified organic or non-GMO soybeans. Otherwise, you may be defeating the point of making a healthier choice with soy-based options.

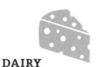

DAIRY

We use dairy pretty sparingly in my house because both Honor and I find it aggravates our allergies. If you have kids, going organic is a must in this category, since many conventional dairy farmers boost milk production by injecting herds with recombinant bovine growth hormones (rBGH), which can interfere with hormone function (they also may use antibiotics to curb disease). But low-fat dairy can be a tasty source of calcium and protein—and here are some that work for us.

* **Low-fat Greek yogurt.** It's higher in protein than regular yogurt. I like to sweeten it with a little fruit or honey.

* **Parmesan cheese.** It has less lactose than most cheeses, so it's a better choice if dairy gives you GI trouble—plus a little bit goes a long way toward pumping up flavor.

* **Goat cheese.** Usually okay for folks with milk allergies or lactose issues, and tastes so decadent and creamy while being pretty low calorie.

* **Faux dairy.** If you are lactose intolerant, try cashew or almond milk cheese. Honor won't drink regular milk, but she loves a comforting glass of almond milk.

SMART SEAFOOD

On the one hand, fish is the greatest: It's way lower in saturated fat and cholesterol than other animal sources of protein and way higher in omega-3 fatty acids. These are amazing for our health for all sorts of reasons (think great hair, great skin, strong heart—and omega-3s may even help improve brain function).

On the other hand, some fish can be really bad for you. Because our oceans are so polluted, many species are very high in mercury and other toxic chemicals; we've also overfished and depleted some populations almost to the point of extinction.

To help you make good choices, use the **Environmental Defense Funds' Seafood Selector chart on page 211** when shopping or ordering fish in restaurants. They also have a Sushi Eco-Ratings List worth checking out at eat.org/oceans, which we use a lot now that Honor has started to like sushi.

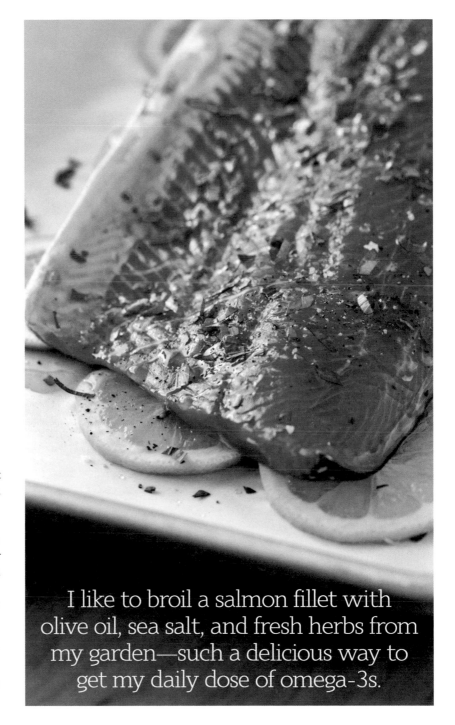

I like to broil a salmon fillet with olive oil, sea salt, and fresh herbs from my garden—such a delicious way to get my daily dose of omega-3s.

Pure & Simple: In the Pantry

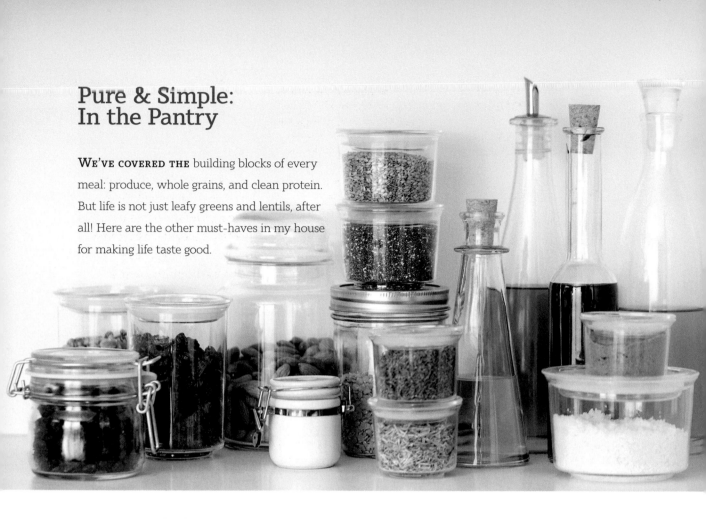

WE'VE COVERED THE building blocks of every meal: produce, whole grains, and clean protein. But life is not just leafy greens and lentils, after all! Here are the other must-haves in my house for making life taste good.

PANTRY STAPLES

Keep these natural ingredients on hand for cooking; that way, you can whip up quick, healthy meals without having to floor it to the grocery store. (Remember to buy certified organic whenever you can!)

* OILS: Olive, coconut, and grapeseed are my go-tos.

* CHICKEN, BEEF, AND VEGGIE BROTH. Great for sautéing with lots of flavor but not a lot of calories. Look for no-MSG, low-sodium varieties (or make your own! See "Stock Up," opposite).

* VINEGARS: Apple cider, balsamic, rice, and white wine vinegars are my faves.

* SALTS: I sprinkle Celtic sea salt and Himalayan pink salt on almost everything.

* HERBS AND SPICES: I live for cumin, coriander, rosemary, sage, basil, oregano, thyme . . . really, I have yet to meet an herb or spice I dislike!

* DRIED AND CANNED BEANS: Red, black, pinto, lentils, broad beans . . . they're all good.

* WHOLE GRAINS: I keep everything on the previous list in steady supply (barley, bulgur, farro, oats, and quinoa) plus wheatberries.

* ORGANIC FLAXSEEDS. Add to meatballs, smoothies, muffins, pancakes, or pretty much anything that can use a boost of fiber and antioxidants.

* CHIA SEEDS. Runners swear by these—you have to soak them, and they form a kind of paste, but, like flax, they add fiber and antioxidants to smoothies, muffins, and pancakes.

* GLUTEN-FREE PANCAKE MIX. The pancakes taste normal, I swear—Cash loves to make pan-

cakes or waffles and bacon on the weekend, so the King Arthur brand is a good go-to.

* ORGANIC MAPLE SYRUP. For pancakes, obviously, but also great for baking or drizzled on ice cream or oatmeal.

* WHOLE GRAIN FLOURS. I use organic wheat flour, rice flour, and tapioca flour for baking.

* ORGANIC SUGARS. We use brown or raw cane sugar for cakes and pies, and powdered for icing.

* ORGANIC HONEY. Raw honey is a great sugar substitute—it is crazy high in antioxidants! Be sure it's 100 percent organic, because some industrial farmers feed their bees—get this—high-fructose corn syrup. No thanks.

* ORGANIC PASTA SAUCES. Great over spaghetti squash, quinoa, or farro.

* ORGANIC JARRED TOMATOES. Toss in anything from soups to sauces. In a jar, they're BPA free.

FOR SNACKS AND QUICK MEALS
(Again, organic is best for kids!)

* WHOLE GRAIN BREAD. Look for at least 3 grams of fiber per serving and no added sugars or additives.

* WHOLE GRAIN CEREALS. Watch the added sugar!

* NATURAL PEANUT BUTTER AND ALMOND BUTTER

* JAMS AND SPREADS. Look for no-sugar-added brands—I try to buy homemade preserves from the farmers' market.

* ALMONDS. Honor is obsessed with all things almond!

* RAISINS, DRIED BLUEBERRIES, CRANBERRIES, AND APPLES. Great with the almonds; we also like freeze-dried fruit, which concentrates the antioxidants.

* GLUTEN-FREE PRETZELS. Honor adores Glutino's pretzels because they're so buttery tasting—and while she's not gluten intolerant, I find her digestion works better when I minimize gluten in her diet.

* ORGANIC BABY FOOD. I love Plum Organics when we're traveling and can't do the homemade thing for Haven.

* GLUTEN-FREE WAFFLES. These frozen treats are great for weekends—or weekdays, for that matter! Van's makes a good one.

* GLUTEN-FREE PIZZA CRUST. Honor loses her mind when we have pizza night, and this is the best way to cheat when you're not going to do the full pizza oven experience. Glutino makes a crust with brown rice.

* ANNIE'S ORGANIC MAC & CHEESE. A favorite standby.

* GREEN & BLACK'S ORGANIC CHOCOLATE. Because, obviously.

STOCK UP

Whenever you roast a chicken (or a leg of lamb or any other big-boned cut of meat), save the bones (even better if they still have some meat on them!) to make your own stock. It's so much more delicious and healthier than store bought (which can have too much salt and other additives). Plus you get points for wasting nothing.

WHAT TO DO:

1. Place the leftover bones from 1 chicken into a large stockpot, along with a bunch of leftover veggies (say, a quartered onion and a couple roughly chopped carrots and celery ribs).

2. Over medium heat, cook the contents for 3 to 5 minutes. Once the veggies begin to sweat, add 2 whole cloves garlic, plus 1 tablespoon salt and 2 teaspoons whole peppercorns.

3. Add in enough water to cover the contents with an inch or so of water on top. Bring to a simmer for 45 minutes to an hour, or more. The longer you simmer, the more flavor you'll get. Strain and store in an airtight container; can be frozen for up to six months.

Life isn't just leafy greens and lentils. Here are other must-haves for making life taste good.

Honest Little Eaters

So NOW THAT YOU KNOW what to eat—how do you get your family to eat it, too? I see so many kids whose parents are always having to pack them special snacks with the rationale, "That's just how my kid eats." But in my house, we don't have discussions or give the girls tons of options. It's "Here's what you're eating." If that sounds kind of old school, it is—that's how my mom raised my brother Joshua and me, and I think she got this so right. There was no special children's meal versus the adults' meal. Whatever my mom made, we all ate it—and questioning it wasn't an option.

The fact is, kids don't need alternatives to what the adults are eating. With too much choice, they can get overwhelmed, and that makes them cranky and more prone to putting up a fight. In contrast, since Honor has been eating what we eat almost from day one (just age-appropriate versions, of course!), she's pretty open to trying new things. When we go out for a family dinner, we don't have to worry about the type of restaurant or what we'll find on the menu for her. Of course, she's still a kid—not a food critic—but I truly appreciate the ease of having a kid who's not at all picky.

By showing the girls all the fun sides of cooking and trying new foods, we're ensuring that they grow up loving food for all the right reasons.

We've always made sure that Honor has a vegetable with every meal—now she's come to expect them!

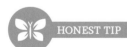

HONEST TIP

REDUCE THE JUICE

Pediatricians often warn that kids shouldn't drink too much juice—it's full of sugar, particularly the sweetened "juice drink" kind, and can fill them up quickly. In our house, we love some great organic juices that aren't too sweet, like Evolution Fresh cucumber and celery juice (try it with a splash of pear juice) or Honest Kids organic juices and teas. Soda is off-limits (except for Reed's Original Ginger Brew mixed with sparkling water on special occasions!), but kids love bubbles, so we also drink a lot of seltzer. A great way to DIY your own seltzer is a Sodastream maker, which lets you fizz up a bottle in just a minute: so much better for your health than regular soda, and better for the planet than buying tons of the bottled stuff.

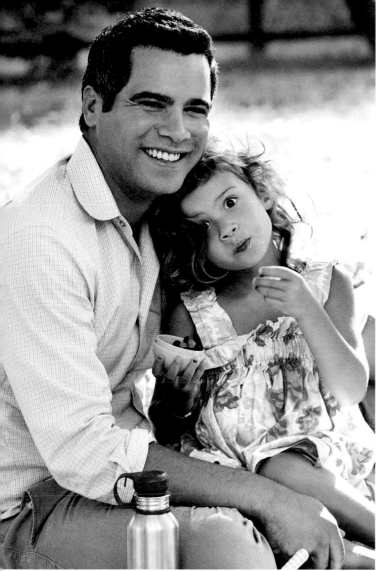

SNACKS TO GO

I like Honor's snacks to come from two different food groups: usually a fruit or vegetable plus some protein or a complex carb. This way, I know she's getting a good mix of nutrients—as well as a tasty flavor combination. Some good ones to try (that are also pretty portable):

❋ LOW-FAT GREEK YOGURT (6-ounce container) and fruit

❋ ALMONDS ($\frac{1}{4}$ cup) and preservative-free dried blueberries or other fruit (if you're a nice mom, you can also throw in chocolate chips or something gummy—I'm a "mean" mom, so it's just nuts and fruit!)

❋ CORN TORTILLA QUESADILLA with cheese and veggies

❋ CARROTS AND HUMMUS

❋ ANTS ON A LOG (celery with peanut butter and raisins)

❋ SMOOTHIE (milk or almond milk with $\frac{1}{2}$ banana and frozen berries)

❋ APPLE OR BANANA with a tablespoon of peanut butter

❋ AVOCADO ($\frac{1}{4}$ cup) and whole grain crackers

❋ TURKEY BREAST SLICES with sliced pear, apple, or peaches

❋ CUCUMBER with organic yogurt ranch dressing

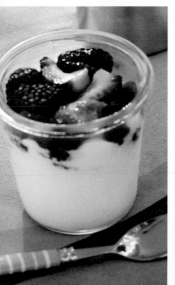

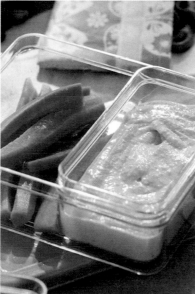

Feeding Babies

I **STARTED BOTH** my babies on an all-fruits-and-vegetables diet at about 6 months, per the advice of Jay Gordon, MD, a pediatric nutrition expert who is the author of *Good Food Today, Great Kids Tomorrow*, and a member of the teaching attending faculty of UCLA Medical Center.

Most weekends, I set aside a chunk of time to make all of Haven's baby food for the week ahead. I get Honor to help, which makes it more fun and, again, is a great opportunity to talk to her about how healthy food makes babies grow. I always blend savory with sweet in a ratio of three-to-one. I think we work too hard to make food "kid friendly" with lots of sweet flavors—all that does is make them want sugary things later on when they start getting picky. I usually use what I have around the house, but Haven's favorite combinations are squash, cauliflower, and banana; carrots, peas, and apples; green lentils and broccoli.

Adding Protein

A **COUPLE OF MONTHS** into both of my girls' transitions into solid foods, I began adding finely chopped lean animal protein like chicken, beef, or leftovers from a weekend barbecue to their veggie mixes. For example, I blend broccoli, sweet potato, chicken, and apple—or beef, broccoli, and cauliflower. Beans are another good source of protein, and they puree so well. We like chickpeas, black beans, or lentils in almost anything!

Adding Grains

DR. GORDON SUGGESTS holding off on introducing whole grains until your child is 7 or 8 months because they can be hard on babies' digestion—and he recommends skipping the refined grains (all those baby cereals!) altogether. Once your baby is old enough, the doc's all about an organic quinoa and/or organic oatmeal cereal. I soak the grains before boiling, and add a handful to whatever blend of veggies, legumes, and meats I'm making, with a bit of olive oil, salt, onion, and garlic for flavor.

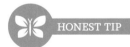 HONEST TIP

DON'T HEAT YOUR FOOD IN PLASTIC!

This can cause toxic chemicals to leach out of some plastic containers into your food. The big one to avoid is bisphenol A (BPA), a chemical that strengthens plastic but is also an endocrine disruptor—which means it messes with healthy hormonal development.

Look for glass food storage containers (I like Pyrex, Ball mason jars, or Wean Green Cubes for Haven's food). At the very least, ditch old, scratched plastic for BPA-free replacements. To be sure you're not getting anything sketchy, check the number usually stamped on the bottom of a container in a little triangle. **And remember the mantra: "4, 5, 1, and 2—all the rest are bad for you!"**

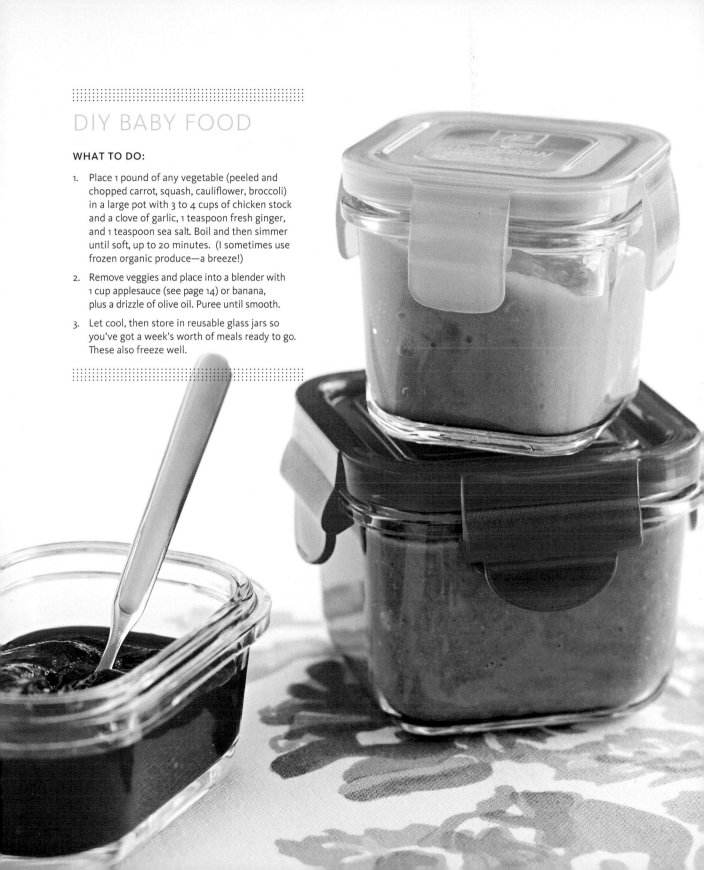

DIY BABY FOOD

WHAT TO DO:

1. Place 1 pound of any vegetable (peeled and chopped carrot, squash, cauliflower, broccoli) in a large pot with 3 to 4 cups of chicken stock and a clove of garlic, 1 teaspoon fresh ginger, and 1 teaspoon sea salt. Boil and then simmer until soft, up to 20 minutes. (I sometimes use frozen organic produce—a breeze!)

2. Remove veggies and place into a blender with 1 cup applesauce (see page 14) or banana, plus a drizzle of olive oil. Puree until smooth.

3. Let cool, then store in reusable glass jars so you've got a week's worth of meals ready to go. These also freeze well.

Honestly Worth Avoiding

You'll notice that most of this chapter focuses on what you *can* and *should* eat, instead of what *not* to eat. That's because the whole beauty of Honest Eating is that you don't have to sit around memorizing lists of off-limits foods. You simply focus on enjoying whole, fresh foods (and educating yourself a bit on how to make the best choices) and you automatically avoid the junk. But since we're so inundated with misleading food marketing and junk food pretty much everywhere we go, I thought it might help if I also explained a little more about what I don't eat and don't buy for my family—because I honestly don't want these non-foods in our lives. Period.

REFINED SUGAR

This is a hard one. I'm not going to lie and say, *Oh, I never even miss sugar*. I absolutely have a sweet tooth—if you put a plate of red velvet cupcakes with butter cream frosting in front of me, I'll eat the entire thing. Because that's how sugar works: The more you eat, the more you want. I find it easiest to minimize our intake as much as possible by saving baked goods for special occasions and skipping all the packaged foods that are loaded with extra sugar we just don't need day to day.

REFINED FLOUR

This ingredient is in the same camp as sugar—because as far as your body is concerned, it *is* sugar. Refined flour (like the kind you find in white bread, regular pasta, muffins, pies, and so on) breaks down into glucose almost as soon as you eat it, which causes a quick spike of your blood sugar and then a terrible crash. When that happens, you feel like death, and then you're hungry again in about 5 minutes anyway. Swapping all the refined flour foods in your diet for their whole grain equivalents is probably the easiest way to incorporate a little Honest Eating into your life—and reap huge rewards in terms of fewer mood swings, more sustained energy, and fewer crazy, overpowering food cravings, too.

ARTIFICIAL SWEETENERS

These are bad news. Like regular sugar, they overdevelop our palate for sweet things and make us want more, more, more all the time. And kids' foods are loaded with them, which I'll never understand. Little kids' taste buds are already way stronger than the average adult's, so why do they need foods to be so sweet? Answer: They don't. The worst part about these sweeteners is the slew of health problems associated with them. Check it out:

* ASPARTAME: May trigger migraines, increase your risk for diabetes, and break down into formaldehyde. Next!

* SPLENDA (SUCRALOSE): We don't have adequate research to draw conclusions about how it impacts our health.

TRANS FATS

This fake food ingredient is found in lots of chips, crackers, icing, microwave popcorn, and other snack foods. Trans fats increase a product's shelf life and do only bad things to your health. The good news is that a lot of companies have gotten the message about the dangers of this type of fat. So be sure to look for "no trans fats" on the label when you're shopping and double-check ingredient labels; trans fats may be lurking as "partially hydrogenated oils."

ARTIFICIAL COLORS

This one is kind of a no-brainer. If it can make yogurt blue, it's probably not good for your kid. In particular, avoid FD&C Blue No. 1 and 2, Green No. 3, and Yellow No. 5 and 6.

SODIUM NITRATES

These keep hot dogs and bacon looking tasty and red—and can trigger migraines, may be linked to cancer, and are bad news for pregnant women. Steer clear of cured and processed meats unless they are labeled "nitrate free."

MSG

Monosodium glutamate is a flavor enhancer used in lots of canned soups, salad dressings, shake-on seasonings, and fast food. Some people are really sensitive to it, and it makes them sick; it's probably not doing the rest of us much good either. If you're eating clean, you're already cutting a lot of MSG out, so it should be a nonissue. But double-check for "no MSG" and no hydrolyzed protein on ingredient lists.

* HIGH-FRUCTOSE CORN SYRUP: This sweetener is practically on America's Most Wanted List at this point, so you don't need me to rehash the discussion. But bottom line: It's super caloric and a cheap way for food manufacturers to make things very sweet (and it's linked to childhood obesity).

* AGAVE: Okay, technically, this one is a "natural" sweetener, which means it's healthy, right? Not quite—many brands consist of 70 to 80 percent fructose—more than what's found in high-fructose corn syrup! If you do use agave, at least hunt for types that contain no more than 30 to 40 percent fructose. And make sure it's organic and 100 percent pure.

KEEPING IT REAL

WE CAN'T LIVE WITHOUT . . .

Cash's biggest weakness is bacon—he'll put it on anything, and he loves to make us all waffles or pancakes and bacon for breakfast. These days, I limit that to a weekend treat—most of the baby weight I put on during my pregnancy with Honor was thanks to bacon every morning! I love wine and cheese and the aforementioned red velvet cupcakes . . . dinner parties with friends are definitely my favorite time to indulge!

Honest Eating for Weight Loss

THE MORE YOU INCORPORATE the idea of Honest Eating, the less you'll need to worry about your weight. My mother-in-law lives in the south of France, and whenever we visit, I eat more bread, cheese, oil, salt—and drink more wine!—than I do probably the rest of the year combined . . . but I never gain a pound. I believe it's a combination of two things: France's total lack of genetically modified foods and their smaller portion sizes. Even if you're not in France, when you practice Honest Eating, you might find that your body weight and size are at a place where you are pretty happy and comfortable in your skin.

Of course, there are times when life gets in the way and it's more difficult to eat the way we want. Or if you've just had a baby, you're probably dying to get your pre-baby body back! If that's the case, focus on filling up with a serving of clean protein and unlimited produce at every meal— think a big salad topped with a serving (no bigger than the palm of your hand) of grilled organic chicken breast, salmon, or legumes.

When I was leaning out after both of my pregnancies (I gained nearly 70 pounds with Honor), I basically lived on that menu of salad and lean protein. While you may feel kind of hungry as your body adjusts to this new way of eating, you should never feel miserable or crazy deprived. Drinking tons of water helps, too—yes, you'll be

peeing constantly (which is so annoying), but it's essential for losing the water weight associated with pregnancy, and being well hydrated will make you feel better.

Sipping on my green drink (opposite) throughout the day helps fill you up as well, and it's packed with nutrients. I have a great blender that can puree the skin of a lemon, but any juicer or blender should do the trick.

PS. Even when you're in full-on weight-loss mode, don't forget to include some indulgences so you don't lose your mind. I like to take a day a week to eat whatever I want; the rest of the time, nondairy frozen fruit or fudge ice pops give me my sweet fix. (We love organic FrütStix and Sweet Nothings!) The key is to have just one, not the entire box.

PPS. New mommies: If you're breast-feeding, *don't* try to diet right after birth. In fact, give yourself a few months before you really reduce your calorie count. The most important thing is to stay well hydrated and stress free. When you feel ready to shed a few pounds, be kind to yourself and patient: Every body is different. After Honor, it took me a year to get to a weight where I felt good in my skin. I know I'll never be the weight I was before I had my kiddos, but I'm cool with that; I love my body more post-babies than I ever did!

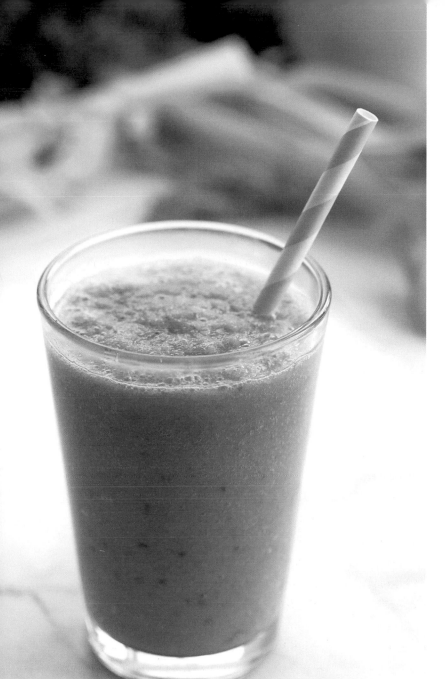

MY GO-TO GREEN DRINK

This became my best friend when I was trying to lose the baby weight, but it's great anytime you feel like you've overindulged. It fills you up and is completely packed with nutrients.

1 whole cucumber, peeled and roughly chopped

2 handfuls chopped kale

2 celery sticks, chopped

2 lemons, juiced

2 apples, cored and seeded

1 teaspoon fresh ginger, finely diced

Frozen watermelon or a dash of the natural sweetener stevia or Truvía for sweetness

WHAT TO DO:

Blend well; refrigerate what you don't drink immediately (makes about 2 servings).

Even when you're in full-on weight-loss mode, don't forget to include some indulgences so you don't lose your mind.

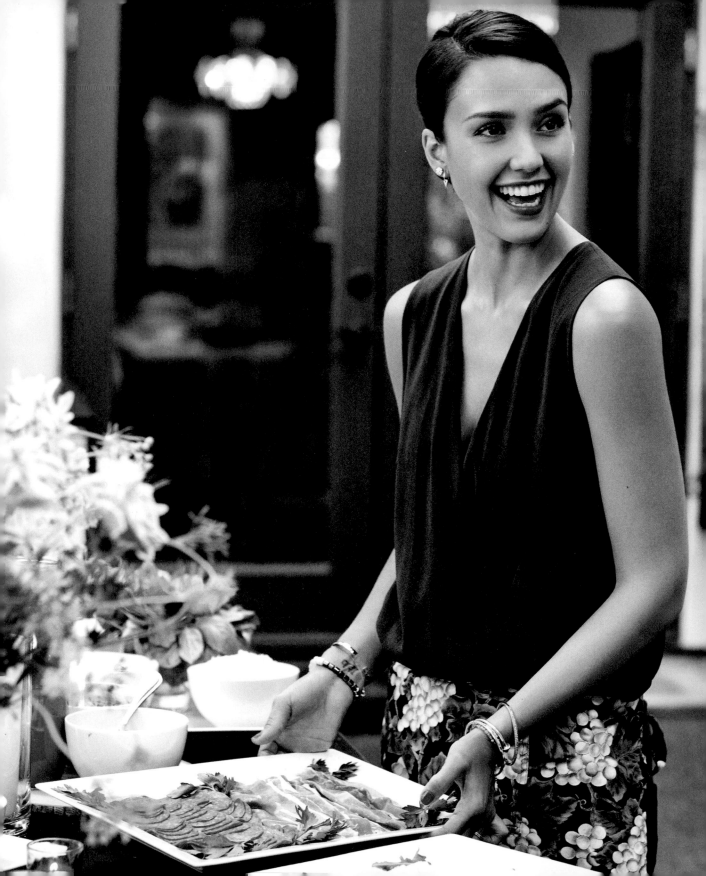

Honest Entertaining

IN CASE you can't tell by now, for me, food is all about sharing the love. And that means I love throwing parties. I go nuts for my girls' birthday parties, but I also love a grown-up moment—having our friends over for a relaxed, stylish dinner party after all the kiddos are tucked into bed.

I think a lot of people get so panicked that their social lives are dead and over once they have kids—and yes, some stuff changes. But it's so important to Cash and me to carve out this time with our friends, because they are still such a big part of our lives. And so I love lighting candles, picking the right music, and pulling out my pretty serving dishes to make a beautiful table. I love catching up with my girlfriends over wine and cheese in the kitchen while Cash and the guys man the grill. And then, when everyone sits down to eat and talk for hours—well, I love that most of all.

What I don't love: stressing over needlessly complex recipes, seating charts, or other fussy details. Here are my secrets for chic, easy entertaining, Honest-style:

PICK QUICK RECIPES

I like to make lots of dishes so everyone will find something they love no matter what their meat-eating status or special diet. But if everything involves 10 ingredients and lots of complicated steps, you're going to be an unhappy camper. Look for salads that showcase one special, in-season vegetable, and cuts of meat that can be roasted with just a little olive oil and sea salt to bring out the flavor.

FUSS OVER FOOD, NOT WHAT YOU'RE WEARING

I always want to look polished—I am hosting, after all!—but at the same time, I think it's important to be dressed down so your guests feel relaxed and at home. I'll do a great top, jeans, and ballet flats or a simple dress with my hair in a topknot. And go easy on the jewelry—your amazing food is your best accessory tonight!

INVOLVE YOUR GUESTS

One of my favorite things about our kitchen is that it's big and open to the rest of our house, so guests can easily congregate and talk to me while I'm cooking . . . and that means I can put them to work! Nobody minds chopping something or minding a sauce on the stove if you give them a glass of wine. In fact, one of our favorite ways to entertain is to throw a pizza party where everybody basically makes their own dinner.

MY FAVORITE PARTY IDEAS

Planning a menu is truly an art—you need flavor, texture, color, and balance (a heavy stew shouldn't be followed by an overly decadent dessert unless you want your guests slipping into food comas by 9:00 p.m.). I usually like to pick a theme, because it can be a great way to simplify and unify the menu. Here are a few favorites:

* PIZZA PARTY: We have a wood-burning pizza oven in the backyard and love to fire it up and have friends over to mix their own toppings. You can do it on a regular oven; see page 183 for my how-to.

* WEEKNIGHT MEDITERRA-NEAN: Think cozy, traditional, and healthy. I mean roast chicken with olives and lemon, grilled lamb chops, plus raw zucchini and kale salads.

* SATURDAY NIGHT INDIAN: Crowd-pleasers are saag paneer, chicken tikka, and cauliflower roasted with olive oil and cumin. The trick with any Indian recipe is to sauté spices in oil before you add other ingredients. That makes them nice and aromatic!

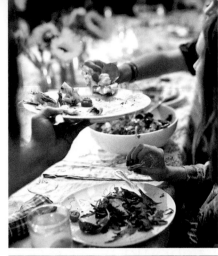
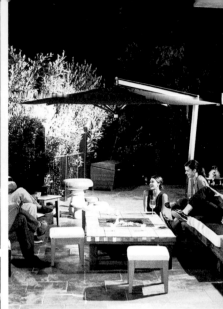
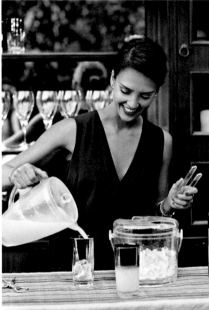
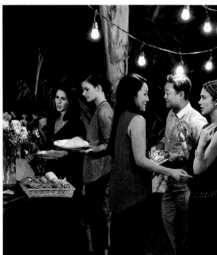
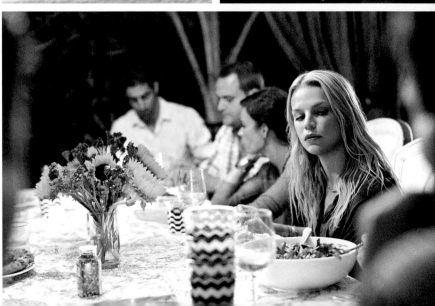

One of my weeknight dinner party tricks is
to never waste time making appetizers
or dessert. Store-bought cheese, nuts, and olives
make a great starter, and you can
ask guests to bring a favorite dessert.
This frees you up to focus on the main course,
which really should be the star of the show.

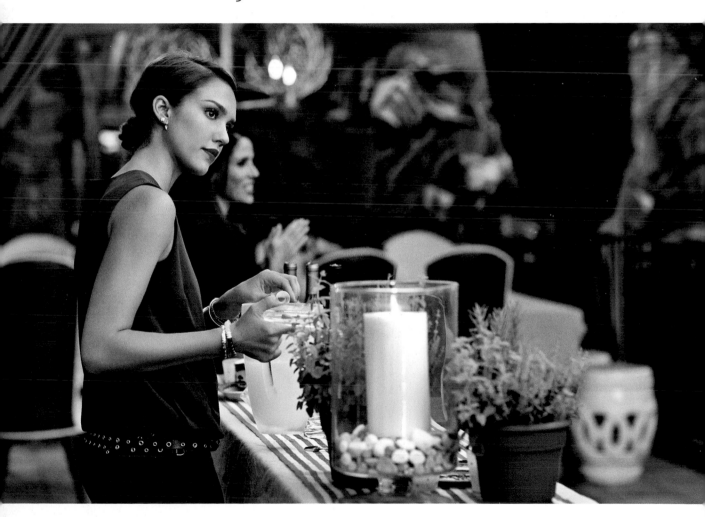

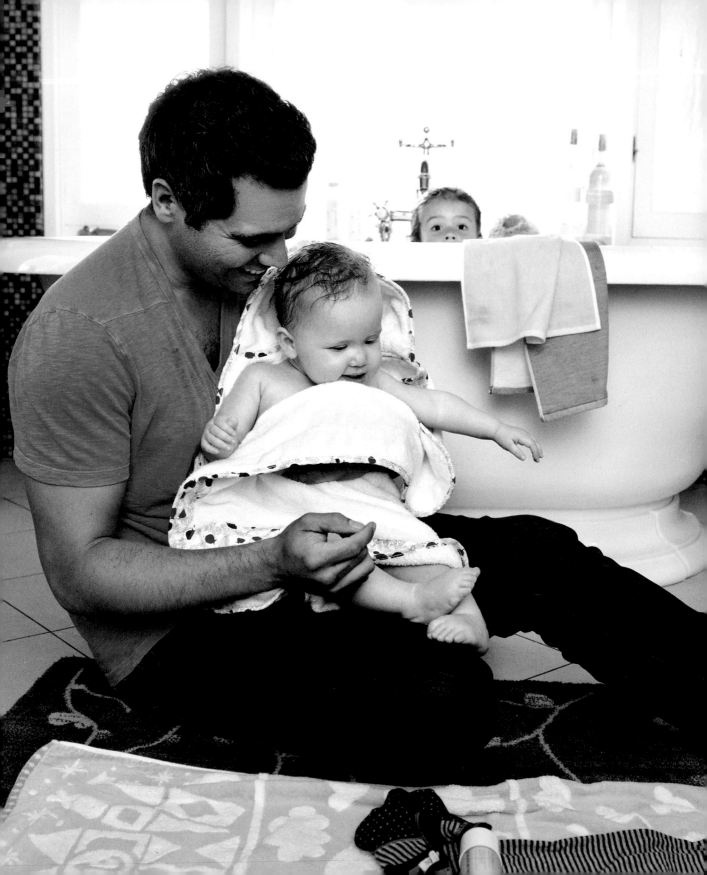

chapter 2

HONEST
clean

YOUR SKIN IS
YOUR LARGEST
ORGAN—FEED IT
NATURALLY

IS THERE ANYTHING MORE DELICIOUS THAN CUDDLING with a squeaky-clean baby fresh out of the tub? I don't think so. Cash and I adore bath time with our girls because it's a such a sweet part of our busy days: Honor makes up hilarious stories while she plays with her tub toys, Haven's cute pink cheeks get even pinker after a bath, and then we get to wrap them both up in snuggly, fluffy towels.

Yum!

Unfortunately, sometimes, cleaning your kids feels like cleaning the house—yet another chore—like when the water isn't perfect or the soap stings the crap out of their sensitive little eyes, and suddenly, everyone switches into melt-down mode. Or when you realize why most "tearless" shampoos and soaps *don't* sting their eyes—because of chemicals that numb the eyes instead. But I'm getting ahead of myself. The main reason bath time is fun, not frustrating, at my house? Because *I'm* so much more relaxed now that I know that all of the personal care products we're using are safe and healthy.

Among other parenting duties, my mom became my home health expert due to my various medical conditions.

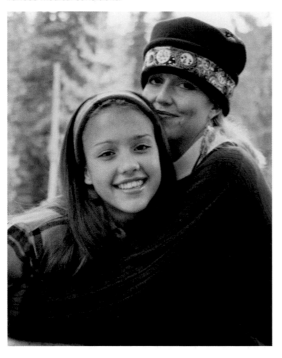

Just Call Me Allergy Girl

I spent most of my life holding my breath every time I soaped up or slathered on a new lotion, because I never knew what was going to give me an itchy rash or, worse, trigger an asthma attack.

It all goes back to when I was a kid and my mom and I started figuring out that I was allergic to what felt like the entire world: latex (Band-Aids = welts for me), synthetic fragrances (every great-smelling shampoo, conditioner, body wash . . .), and any product that's super heavy in petrochemicals, like petroleum jelly, which is a common ingredient in everything from antibacterial ointments to lotions. Not to mention: dander, dust, hay, grass, and whatever they put in most conventional cleaning supplies. Sneezing, watery eyes, and an itchy nose were just part of my day-to-day existence growing up.

Having all of these allergies made it hard for me to fit in with other girls at school. I was a tomboy to begin with, and then, whenever I did try to be girly at somebody's sleepover when we were playing beauty parlor, I was the weird kid who would start sneezing 50 times in a row. I had to bring my nebulizer and inhaler with me everywhere I went—it was such a bummer. But since I had to learn which ingredients in products were likely to give me a rash, I also started to learn pretty early on about what those ingredients in your personal care products actually *do*—so I could figure out what's necessary in a moisturizer or a cleanser, for example, and what's just the filler stuff that's likely to trigger a bad reaction. And, by the way, we aren't *just* talking about allergies—these chemicals are associated with all kinds of problems that can make even the healthiest person sick, as you'll see in a minute. Since this was all around the same time that I became vegan and started experimenting more in the kitchen, I began to learn how food could benefit my skin and how to come up with my own fresh beauty concoctions. There were definitely some missteps here. Eggs might do wonders for your hair (assuming you aren't allergic), but trust me—you do not want to leave a bottle of homemade egg shampoo in a steamy bathroom for 2 days! But I also hit on some pretty amazing homemade beauty treatments that I still swear by. (See pages 188 to 189 for some of my favorite recipes.)

Once I started working as an actress, I began to realize that there were other products out there and that it might be possible for me to stop living on allergy medicines. But I also faced new challenges. When I'm working on movie and television sets and forever on the road for press tours, I'm constantly subjecting my skin to an onslaught of abuse from all the bright lights and heavy makeup. Especially in the beginning, I didn't get much of a say in what products got used or which chemicals they contained. Working long hours (read: never getting enough sleep!) doesn't help matters. At this point, I go back and forth between New York and Los Angeles so often, I don't even feel jet lag—but if I'm not careful to take good care of myself, I won't realize I've been going too hard until a couple of weeks later when I'll suddenly hit a wall and get super sick.

By the time I reached my early twenties, I was caught in this vicious cycle: Use personal care products and cosmetics that aggravate my health and wreck my skin. Work too hard, stress out my body and my skin even more—and reach for more lotions, scrubs, and concealers in an effort to combat the problem . . . which, instead, make everything worse. I knew there had to be a better way.

I started asking every makeup artist I met on set for advice on the best brands that wouldn't clog my pores. Again, I started experimenting and found I got fewer breakouts if I made a point to wash my face during the middle of a 16-hour shoot, as well as before bed. I also discovered that adding a drop of tea tree oil to a gentler cleanser

Sneezing, watery eyes, and an itchy nose were just part of my day-to-day existence growing up.

left me less prone to breakouts—naturally! Then I tried mineral makeup, which is completely oil free (so it can't clog your pores), and that was another major breakthrough. Bottom line: I realized that finding skin care that works is a huge trial-and-error process, but you shouldn't settle for anything that irritates your skin, causes breakouts, contains toxins, or just plain isn't working for *you*.

Once I got a handle on my own personal care products, it was a no-brainer that as soon as I found out I was pregnant, I would start trying to find the safest and healthiest products for my baby. But again, this was so much harder than I expected. That's why the whole experience with the Fancy Baby Detergent was so upsetting—and eye-opening. Before I had kids, I assumed that our government would have all kinds of strict standards in place for any consumer goods marketed to children, particularly infants. As it turns out, this isn't the case, especially when we're talking bath time. Children's soaps and lotions are as unregulated and untested as their grown-up equivalents, despite the fact that big corporations spend millions marketing them as "safe," "pure," and "natural." (See "Liar Labels,"

opposite, for why these words don't mean what you think.)

When Christopher Gavigan and I started planning The Honest Company, I knew that soap, shampoo, conditioner, lotion, and sunscreen would be on our product list from the get-go, purely due to the difficulty I'd had navigating the world of safer personal care products for me and my babies. We've since expanded the line to bug spray, conditioning mist, and many others. I'll admit, once I got on the other side and started actually trying to make safer versions of these products, I had a *little* more sympathy for all the other personal care brands out there. We went through dozens of prototypes before we hit on a shampoo/shower gel formulation that didn't sting children's eyes—I know, because I tested every last one of them on myself and Honor, and she fussed at me every time yet another nontoxic-but-still-too-harsh drop of soap got in her eyes. Most personal care companies have an easier job because their priority is profit—the health ramifications of their ingredients don't concern them. My priorities are the opposite, which makes my job a lot tougher—but way more rewarding.

One hundred percent of women of childbearing age have detectable levels of phthalates (fragrance ingredients that may be reproductive toxins) in their bodies, probably because of cosmetic use.

The amazing chemists we hired finally cracked the nontoxic-*and*-effective code, and I'm so proud of the Honest personal care line. But don't worry, because this isn't an infomercial. While we've been doing our homework, a bunch of other awesome companies have been doing the same—some small and scrappy and a few pretty giant (or at least, owned by giants who seem content to let these brands keep doing things their way). So there are tons of new options on the market now for healthy, safe products that will keep you and your kids clean and happy, whether you're prone to allergies, have sensitive skin, or you just want fewer toxins in your morning shower.

The Inside Dirt on Clean

THERE'S A GOOD CHANCE that right about now you're thinking, "Good for you, Jess, but I don't have allergies. So excuse me while I go off on my merry way." Fair enough—but remember: This is about a lot more than skin rashes. Regular, low-dose exposure to many of the chemicals used in mainstream personal care products may contribute to your risk for cancer, asthma, and other serious health complications. You can't always trust what you read on a product label, because companies have gotten very good at trying to convince you that their products are as clean and green as possible—take a look at this "Liar Labels" chart.

LIAR LABELS

These marketing claims sure sound healthy—but don't fall for their greenwashing.

Hypoallergenic

WHAT YOU THINK IT MEANS: That somebody has tested the product to make sure it won't cause any allergic reactions.

WHAT IT REALLY MEANS: Nothing—there are no government regulations around the term "hypoallergenic," so companies are free to define it however they like.

Natural

WHAT YOU THINK IT MEANS: That a product was made with all-natural, plant-based ingredients.

WHAT IT REALLY MEANS: Who knows? The government doesn't regulate the term "natural," so it can mean just about anything.

Organic

WHAT YOU THINK IT MEANS: That every ingredient in a product comes from a USDA Certified Organic farm.

WHAT IT REALLY MEANS: That *some* of the ingredients in your product are certified organic—but the rest can be anything at all. Opt for brands that tell you *what percent* of the product's ingredients are *USDA Certified Organic*—the higher, the better.

Unscented

WHAT YOU THINK IT MEANS: Hooray! No allergy-triggering, sketchy synthetic fragrances.

WHAT IT REALLY MEANS: The product may contain a fragrance—you just can't smell it because it's formulated with masking agents that block the smell of all the other ingredients. But these masking agents can still cause allergies and other problems. Look for *"fragrance free"* instead.

A Safer Clean, Every Day

BY NOW, I bet you're ready to start swapping out at least a few items in your bathroom cabinet. But maybe you're super sensitive, like me, and worried that testing a bunch of new products will mean freaking your skin out for weeks while it adjusts to a new routine. Or maybe you used to break out all the time and your skin is finally behaving itself (this is one of my favorite things about being over 30), so you're hyperventilating at the thought of parting with your current skin care regimen. Or it just seems wasteful to ditch everything and buy a bunch of new stuff just because it might be better for your health.

But listen, nobody is suggesting that you should grab a garbage bag and throw out everything in your bathroom cabinets at once. If you're going to adopt that mentality, you might as well also start unplugging from the grid and inflating your new bubble home, because the sad truth is we're exposed to most of these chemicals every day in all kinds of ways—the problems with our chemical industry run way deeper than toxic soap. But unlike, say, air pollution, which you can't avoid because you pretty much have to breathe, polluted personal care products are an exposure source that we *can* control, since we're the ones slathering up our faces and bodies every day.

To be clear: This doesn't mean you *must* control every last possible source of exposure.

Because—I promised—no lectures! Also, I can't always do this completely myself—and I'll be letting you know it anytime you see one of those "Keeping It Real" boxes. Whether or not your shampoo contains a potential carcinogen is not going to be the sole deciding factor in whether you (or your kids) get cancer someday. It just doesn't work that way—and even if it did, it's not practical or reasonable to make the absolute safest and healthiest choice every single time. Sometimes, you just need the shampoo that makes your hair shiny. Or the wrinkle cream that ensures you still get carded every time you order a cocktail. Or whatever.

But when there's a safer option that also works and costs about the same? Well, why wouldn't you use that? No good reason. I'm not just obsessed with avoiding allergic reactions and toxic chemicals—I'm also a beauty product junkie. So I've road-tested hundreds of products on my friends, my husband, my kids, and myself in order to find the very best. There are certain things I cannot resist splurging on (like eye cream and tinted moisturizer) and others where I go pretty basic (anything bubbly—cleanser, body wash, bubble bath—because I know I can doctor it up with my own blend of essential oils). But regardless of the price point, I need them to work *and* be clean and healthy.

What follows are a few pointers and product suggestions for taking the very best care of your skin.

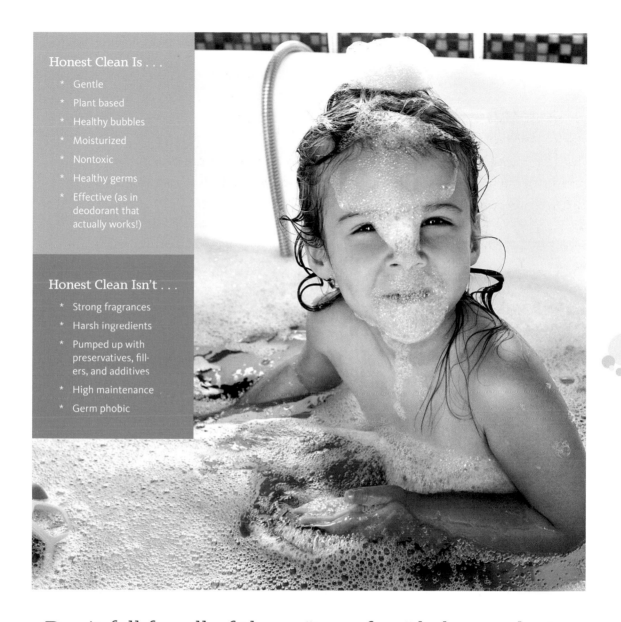

Honest Clean Is . . .

* Gentle
* Plant based
* Healthy bubbles
* Moisturized
* Nontoxic
* Healthy germs
* Effective (as in deodorant that actually works!)

Honest Clean Isn't . . .

* Strong fragrances
* Harsh ingredients
* Pumped up with preservatives, fillers, and additives
* High maintenance
* Germ phobic

Don't fall for all of those "tear-free" baby products. They contain a special mix of toxic chemicals that work by numbing your baby's eyes so she can't feel all the other harsh chemicals stinging!

Pure & Simple: Face

I'm *very* PICKY about what goes on my face. After all, there's so much pressure in our society today to look as young as possible, and it can mess with your head. Plus, like any working mom, I'm never getting enough sleep, and nothing shows up on your skin faster than exhaustion. To deal, I get facials monthly (or whenever I can) with my amazing aesthetician, Shani Darden (shanidarden.com). The rest of the time, I focus on drinking plenty of water and taking excellent care of my skin. It's working!

CLEANSER

Here's my cardinal rule of skin care: Always, always wash your face before bed—you have to remove the grime of the day, and I'm not just talking dirt. Your skin absorbs a ton of pollutants, like volatile organic compounds (VOCs), which can damage the skin's epidermis layer and exacerbate eczema. A good cleanser won't wash away every trace of toxin, but it's your first line of defense. I also wash my face when I wake up, but if your skin is very dry, you might want to skip this—it's not like it gets crazy dirty while you're sleeping!

In terms of what type of cleanser to use, I look for hydrating formulas designed for dry skin—Suki Moisture Rich Cleansing Lotion is the bomb. But I do notice that I break out a lot more whenever I'm working on a movie. We're logging incredibly long hours, wearing tons of makeup, short-changing on sleep . . . all of these things can really take their toll. When that happens, I'll step up from my usual gentle cleanser to the Burt's Bees Natural Acne Solutions line—it's intense, but it works! Sometimes I also like to use a cleansing brush (100% Pure makes a nice one), which cleanses and exfoliates in one go.

MASKS

Shani Darden suggests using masks at home weekly or biweekly. If you're prone to dryness, a mask can help you hydrate; look for cream-based masks if you're super dry or a gel-based product if you have combination skin. They can also do wonders for preventing and clearing up breakouts, so if you're oily, get yourself a good clay mask (John Masters Organics and Dr. Hauschka make lovely ones). It will absorb all that excess oil and clear out your pores like nobody's business. And they can help with anti-aging concerns. (Tata Harper's Resurfacing Mask is really nice for that.)

TONER

I like to follow my cleanser with a toner, but they aren't for everyone. Be careful of overstripping your skin if you're oily, because too many astringent ingredients will make your skin produce even more oil in response. Hydrating mists are nice if you're dry or need to reapply makeup during the day but don't want to wash your whole face off. I find my skin can withstand the long days on film sets much better if I wash my face midway through the day and reapply my makeup—but sometimes it's just too much work to take off everything. So I'll leave my eyes done but take off my foundation, concealer, and such, then use a hydrating mist before I reapply.

MOISTURIZER & CREAMS

One of the biggest skin care misconceptions is that you don't need to moisturize if you have oily skin. False! Dermatologists say that your skin might actually be producing *too much* oil because you're overdrying it with lots of harsh, astringent products in your quest to de-grime and shine. At the very least, moisturize with a light, water-based formula before bed. It will help bring things back into balance.

If your skin is dry like mine, you really can't skimp on the moisturizer. Make sure you put it on in the morning (your makeup will adhere so much better—no flakiness!) and use a rich night cream before bed, too. I also like an eye cream to prevent those dark circles—no one needs to know how little sleep I got! And bedtime is usually the best time to layer on any serums you like. Don't freak if they are über-pricey—a few drops of an antioxidant serum or eye serum will go a long way when added to your night cream.

LIP BALM

I pretty much die if I don't have a lip balm handy in my purse. But this is a tricky category because so many are made with petrochemicals, which will just dry out your lips even more in the long run (see box, right). My go-to these days is Honest Organic Lip Balm —or, if I'm really chapped, Honest Healing Balm—they're petroleum free and so hydrating. (Yes, that's the same stuff I use to diaper Haven—busy moms need products that multitask!) But I also like something tinted like Korres Lip Butters when I want a bit more color.

SUNSCREEN

Last thing, before I start my makeup, I always put a thin layer of sunscreen all over my face and neck. Everyone hates wearing sunscreen—but these days, you just have to:

DISHONEST INGREDIENT

PETROCHEMICALS

*Includes mineral oil, petroleum jelly, propylene glycol, and paraffin

FOUND IN: Foundations, lotions, cleansers, lipsticks, lip balms—unless they say "oil free"

WHAT IS IT? A moisturizer

WHY IS IT SKETCHY? Using a lot of petroleum-filled products can cause breakouts because they block your pores; dermatologists recommend an oil-free, water-based formulation if your skin is sensitive or acne prone (shea butter and jojoba are great plant-derived alternatives).

Long-term, we don't totally understand how petrochemicals in personal care products affect our health, but petroleum distillates may cause cancer—and anyway, this stuff is used in paint, antifreeze, and gasoline. Does that sound like something that should go on your face?

It prevents skin cancer and it's anti-aging. The key is to find one that actually feels good on your skin—and this is finally possible with new formulations. Shani suggests looking for an oil-free formula if your skin is oily or a hydrating moisturizing one if you have normal or dry skin (layer it on top of your regular moisturizer if you're super dry). I love Cell-Ceuticals PhotoDefense Anti-PhotoAging Daily Skin Protector because it doubles as my tinted moisturizer on super-sunny days. You also

The average personal care product contains around 126 ingredients. The government doesn't require pre-market safety testing on any of them.

Make sure a product is scented with natural fragrances or is specifically labeled "fragrance free."

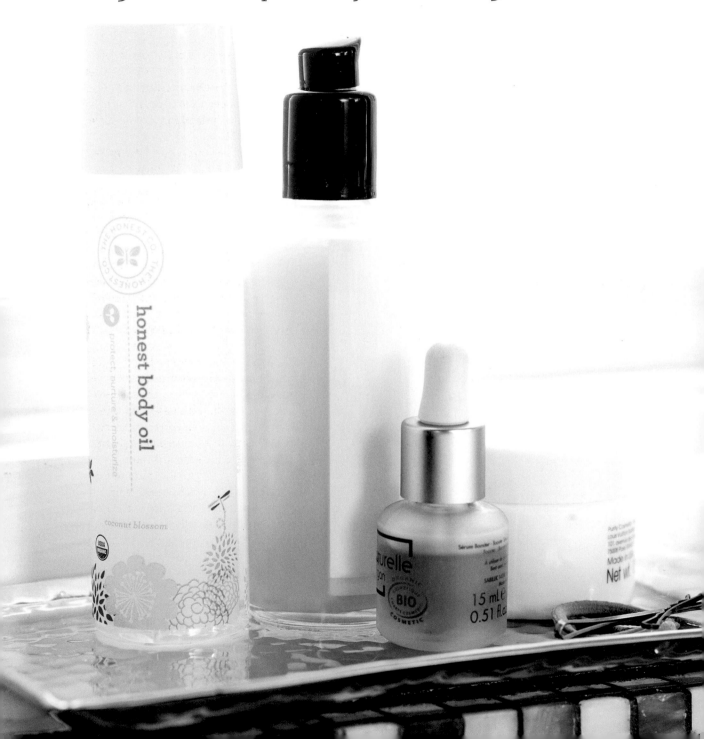

can't go wrong with a dab of our basic Honest Sunscreen with a dime-size squirt of your foundation—it's completely nongreasy and absorbs easily so you can wear it on your face without looking like a lifeguard.

TOOTHPASTE

Most regular toothpastes are packed with—irony alert!—artificial sweeteners, plus preservatives, dyes and artificial flavors that you just don't want in your mouth. And while we do need fluoride every day to help fight cavities, we don't need a lot of it. There is also some concern about the long-term health effects of fluoride, so if you know your community fluoridates your drinking water (like ours does), you may want to choose a fluoride-free toothpaste—Honest now makes one—to avoid overload, which can lead to white spots on your teeth. Otherwise, fluoride toothpaste is a good bet because we all need some for cavity prevention.

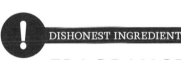

DISHONEST INGREDIENT

FRAGRANCE

FOUND IN: Almost everything—unless a product is specifically labeled "fragrance free"

WHAT IS IT? Synthetic perfume components (parfum, dyes, and synthetic musks) that give a product its scent (or mask the smell of other ingredients, so the product can be billed as "unscented")

WHY IS IT SKETCHY? Product manufacturers don't have to tell you what's in their fragrance formulas because they're considered "trade secrets." But many do, in fact, contain phthalates, which can interfere with hormone function, plus synthetic fragrances are one of the top-five known allergens.

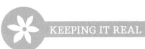

KEEPING IT REAL

MY LOVE AFFAIR WITH RETINOL

While I steer clear of a lot of Hollywood beauty trends, there is one that I pretty much can't get enough of: retinol or retinoids, which are compounds derived from retinoic acid, a form of vitamin A. What's the big deal? Vitamins come from nature, right?

Well . . . the retinol products on the market today, whether prescription (Retin-A, Renova, Atralin, etc.) or over the counter, are made in a lab, not squeezed out of carrots. And retinoic acid is on California's Proposition 65 list of known human toxins because some research suggests it can harm our reproductive health and cause birth defects, so pregnant women—even those who think they might be pregnant—should *absolutely* avoid it. Additionally, retinol works by exfoliating your skin, so it can make you extremely sensitive and prone to sunburn.

But here's the thing: Retinol works better than anything else I've tried—it prevents signs of aging and can even help minimize the wrinkles you already have. Plus it erases acne. So for me, this is a case where the trade-offs are so worth the benefits. I use ReSurface by Shani Darden Retinol Reform serum every night and think it makes my pores and dark spots look smaller while also making my skin all smooth and soft. Her formula is pretty gentle and doesn't give me the redness and irritation I've experienced with other retinol products—though I do also always wear my sunscreen in the day, to be safe.

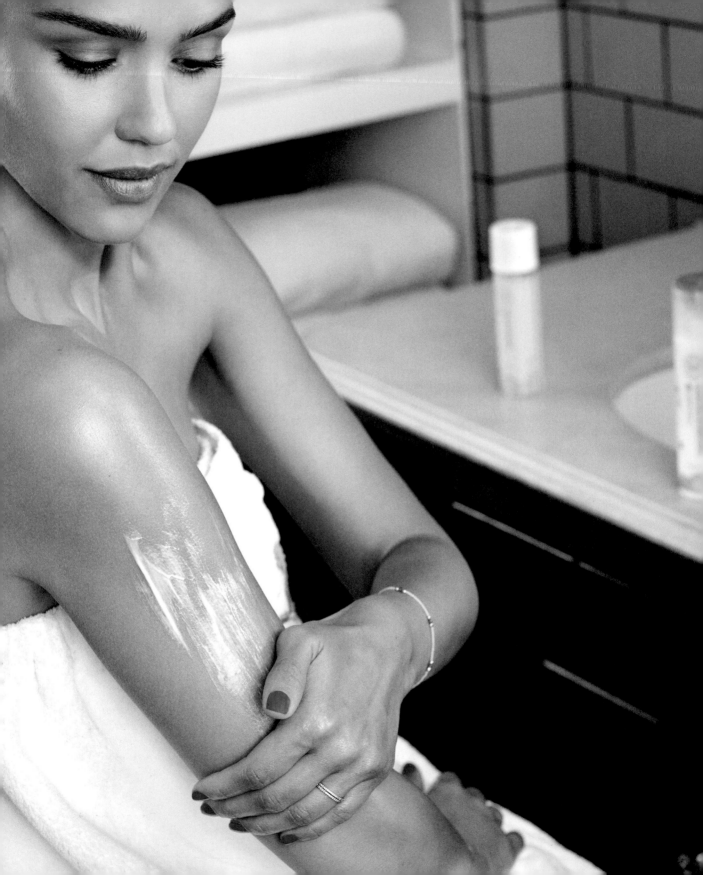

Pure & Simple: Body

WHEN IT COMES to cleaning up your personal care products, body care is a great place to start because it's a such a huge win: You'll be covering a lot of surface area (i.e., most of you!) with cleaner products, significantly reducing your chemical exposure in one fell swoop. But there are definitely some challenging categories here (see: deodorant!). Remember, the goal isn't to do everything perfectly. If you can swap out a couple of products for cleaner versions, I think that's an awesome start.

SOAP & SHOWER GEL

This is a category where I'm happy to go with something basic and effective—it's just getting you clean, after all. But most conventional soaps are way too harsh for my dry skin, and it's amazing how many sketchy chemicals end up in the average body wash! I prefer liquid shower gel, but I'm not opposed to a nice simple clean bar either—look for some kind of plant-based moisturizing ingredients. If my skin is feeling particularly rough or flaky, I'll follow up washing with a homemade scrub to exfoliate (see pages 188 to 189 for some easy recipes).

BODY BALM

Balms are amazing. I'm always slathering some on my lips and nose (because my beloved retinol can cause some peeling here and there), and using one to keep dry heels at bay and make my pedicures last longer and look better.

As with lip balm, it's important to avoid the petrochemical-based balms—they don't really do your skin any favors, no matter what your mom told you about the giant jar of petroleum jelly that most of us grew up with! Look for balms made with plant oils and glycerin instead.

LOTION

Because I have such dry skin, moisturizers are a big deal to me. I always try to slather some on while my skin is still a little damp from the shower—this helps trap moisture on your skin so it's extra hydrating. Again, you want to avoid the added fragrances and other synthetics that can be irritating to your skin and choose plant-based ingredients (they'll make your skin smell great naturally!). I'm a big fan of mixing our Honest Face and Body Lotion with a few drops of our Honest Body Oil to make it even creamier and more luxe.

HONEST TIP

NATURAL HEALING

Kids get boo-boos all the time (and sometimes grownups do, too). I like treating our scrapes and bruises naturally, if possible, instead of piling on the chemicals. We use a concoction of tea tree oil and purified water on minor wounds because it's a natural antiseptic—and you really don't need that triple antibacterial gel on a tiny cut. Arnica gel is a natural alternative to synthetic menthols for soothing bruises. And, of course, I love our Honest Healing Balm for rehydrating and protecting any chapped or scraped skin.

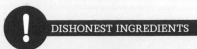

PARABENS

FOUND IN: Water-based products, like shampoo, conditioner, cleanser, shower gel, lotion—you name it

WHAT IS IT? A preservative

WHY IS IT SKETCHY? We can absorb parabens through our skin, blood, and digestive system, and they've even been found inside breast tumors (and, thus, linked to cancer). They may also be toxic to our reproductive, immune, and neurological systems and can cause skin rashes.

TRICLOSAN & TRICLOCARBAN

FOUND IN: Antibacterial soap, hand sanitizer, toothpaste, deodorants (plus some fabrics and plastics)

WHAT IS IT? Antimicrobial agents that kill bacteria and fungus and prevent odors

WHY IS IT SKETCHY? This stuff gets absorbed and piles up in our bodies, where it may disrupt our hormones. And because we use so much of it, it's also helping to create dangerous bacteria that are resistant to antibiotics. In 2005, the FDA found no evidence that antibacterial soaps are in any way superior to good old soap and water. So stick with that—and always lather hands for at least 20 seconds.

BODY OIL

Oils are nice when you want a lotion that will also give your legs a little shine, or during the winter when dry air and central heating makes our skin super thirsty. I also find that most plant-based body oils can double as a hair de-frizzer in a pinch (rub a few drops between your hands, then smooth over the ends of your hair). And I constantly rub a drop or two into my cuticles to keep them smooth.

One of the most popular plant oils right now is argan oil, which is derived from the kernels of the argan tree in Morocco. Fun fact: I used to think I was allergic to argan oil—until I tried some on a trip to France and realized that, actually, I'm allergic to the fillers and additives that go into so many salon and drugstore brands. It's always a good idea to do a patch test before you slather any new product all over your skin. Just because it's natural doesn't mean it won't disagree with you or cause a reaction.

DEODORANT & ANTIPERSPIRANT

I won't lie: If I have to walk a red carpet or give a big presentation, I'm reaching for that trustworthy but toxin-filled Big Name Super-Strong Antiperspirant. You can't risk pit stains in those high-pressure situations, and the non-toxic deodorant formulas just aren't there yet. Part of it is a chemical issue: Manufacturers are having a heck of a time finding something that stops sweat but doesn't contain nasty ingredients. And part of it is a health thing: Sweating is actually *good* for you, so you don't want to stop it altogether (at least, not all the time). For now, my strategy is to layer my conventional antiperspirant over a natural, nontoxic deodorant (Alba Organics—no relation!—is my current favorite). I figure that way I've got a layer of protection from the aluminum and triclosan in most mainstream brands. On regular days, it's natural all the way.

SUNSCREEN

Tanning is *sooo* dangerous—I've watched my mom deal with melanoma, so I know firsthand where it can lead. Not to mention, it makes you look way old before your time! I just don't get the obsession, and it makes me sad to see young girls baking at the beach or in tanning salons, just wrecking their skin.

The most important thing you can do for your skin health is to make sure you put on your sunscreen every day, no excuses. And for sure, your kids need to be wearing sunscreen. This is especially true if you and they are fair (like my little strawberry blonde, Haven!).

But it's important to make sure you're putting on a sunscreen that is really good for your skin, on every level. Lots of conventional sunscreens contain oxybenzone, a chemical that is an endocrine disruptor and notorious for its ability to screw with hormonal health and development in children. You shouldn't have to choose between skin cancer and developmental problems when you're picking a sunscreen for your kids!

Instead, opt for mineral sunscreens that are made with zinc or titanium dioxide; avobenzone and ecamsule (AKA Mexoryl SX) are good alternatives. While you're at it, skip the sunscreen sprays and powders, which are more likely to contain problematic ingredients. Instead, choose a cream formula that provides broad spectrum protection (from both UVA and UVB rays) and is water resistant for the beach, pool, or exercise. It should also contain a minimum of SPF 30, but keep in mind that the FDA doesn't regulate SPFs over 50, so a higher number may not offer much extra protection, especially if you think it means you can skimp on reapplying. Always slather on another coat if you've been outside swimming or sweating for a couple of hours.

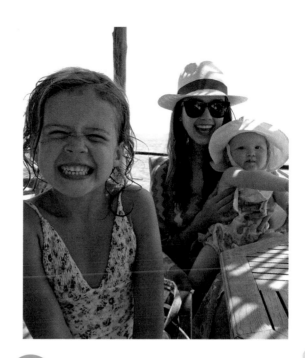

 HONEST TIP

BE A SHADE WORSHIPPER

Okay, not really. But when you're going to be in the sun, you need to play it smart. I always wear my UV-protectant sunglasses to shield my eyes, and I love a wide-brimmed straw hat (my current favorite is by Tory Burch) to cover my face, ears, and neck on sunny days. I also love sun hats for my girls. And when we're at the beach, I make sure we all have tunics or T-shirts on hand to throw over our swimsuits. You want something loose, not only because it will be cool and breezy but also because the closer fabric is to skin, the less sun protection it provides.

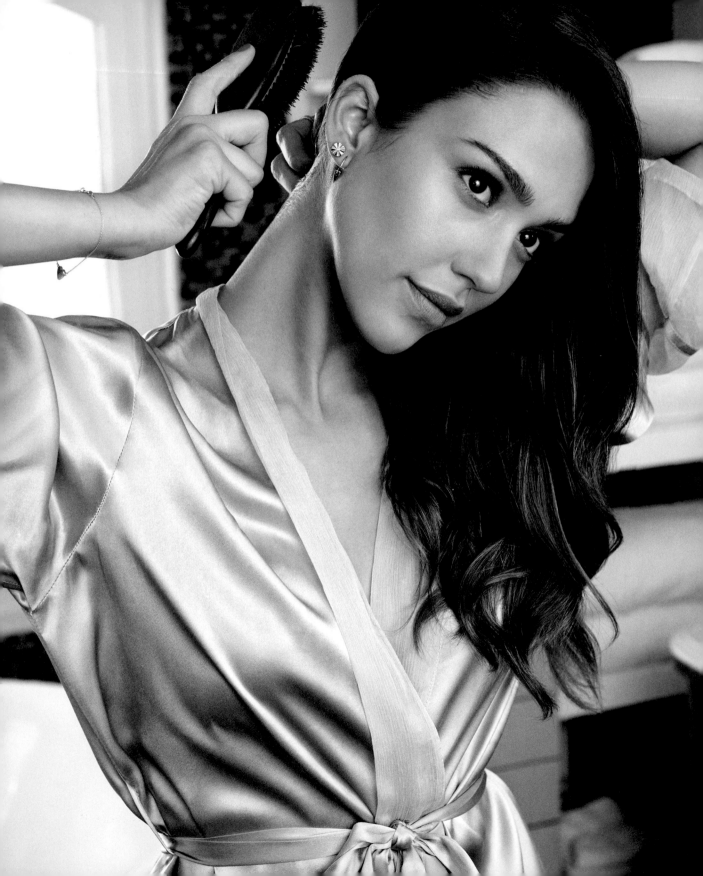

Pure & Simple: Hair

YOU KNOW ALL those bad hair days where your locks are totally flat and lifeless, or worse, frizzy and out of control? You weren't born that way, lovely. Mainstream hair care is tough on our heads. Heat styling and coloring dry out and damage the hair follicles, making us even more prone to frizz because the hair shaft is constantly roughed up and trying to suck up whatever little bit of moisture it can find in the air. Plus most of the products we use at home contain harsh detergents and more dehydrating ingredients like alcohol or silicones and gels that just weigh you down.

Since my hair is put through the ringer on most acting jobs, whenever I'm not shooting, I give it a chance to detox: no heat styling, just a gentle shampoo and a deep conditioner or a leave-in one. Sure, we'd all love blowout-perfect hair all the time, but these recovery days are so important—and I actually like that beachy, free-flowing, air-dried look, especially in the summer. And remember: Your next blowout will be even more awesome because you've given your hair this opportunity to bounce back.

SHAMPOO

How often you need to shampoo depends on your hair and scalp. I try really hard not to overwash my hair because it gets subjected to so much heat styling and such; I need to let it breathe when I can! But my hair is too fine to go for very long between shampoos (it just falls flat). Like my preferences for soap and shower gel, I like to stick with a pretty basic, plant-based formulation for gentle cleansing. If you're dealing with dandruff or buildup, try to avoid conventional dandruff shampoos—they're very harsh. Rinsing your scalp weekly with apple cider vinegar (see recipe on page 189) will help keep flakes at bay naturally. But do rinse well with water and follow up with a conditioner—otherwise you'll smell like a salad! For oily scalps, adding a bit of tea tree oil to your shampoo and only conditioning the ends will work best even if you have to shampoo daily.

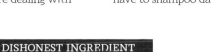

! DISHONEST INGREDIENT

FORMALDEHYDE

* Includes formaldehyde-releasing preservatives like DMDM hydantoin, imidazolindinyl urea, and quaternium-15

FOUND IN: Shampoos, body washes, nail polishes, polish removers, keratin hair straighteners, hair gels, and eyelash glues

WHAT IS IT? A preservative (or sometimes, a by-product released by other preservatives) that prevents bacteria growth and (weirdly) makes your hair silky smooth

WHY IS IT SKETCHY? Formaldehyde can cause cancer after chronic, long-term exposure, plus it can trigger allergic reactions, rashes, nosebleeds, asthma, and other respiratory issues.

::

TRY "NO-POO"

If you have coarse, frizzy, or curly hair, you'll need to be careful *not* to shampoo it too often. In fact, a lot of curly girls I know swear by the DevaCare No-Poo method—or rarely even shampoo their hair at all! Shampooing strips hair of the natural oils it needs to keep frizz at bay, so when you switch from shampoo to a cleanser, your curls will have more definition and fewer flyaway issues.

If you are used to daily shampooing, going No-Poo does require a serious level of commitment—I suggest starting on a vacation (like camping!) when you can rough it and not care how you look for a week, because there's definitely a detox period where your scalp sort of freaks out and gets mad oily, wondering why you aren't sudsing it up every day like usual. But after a week or two, this usually calms down and you start to see hair ah-mazingness.

Other curly girls find they really do need to wash a couple times a week—every two or three days, say—to keep the grease at bay. Experiment and figure out what works for you . . . and don't worry if it's not the beauty gospel you've read in fashion magazines or whatever! For more tips on how to ditch the suds, search "curly hair" on nomoredirtylooks.com; cofounder Alexandra Spunt has amazing curls and she hasn't shampooed her hair in I don't know how long.

::

embracing your natural wave!—are big again. This is especially helpful if you live in a humid climate; it's like, why fight it? Let your hair be free. So what's the key to happy (not fuzzy) curls? Making sure your hair is properly hydrated. Frizz is just your hair follicle's way of trying to suck up more moisture from the air—that's why it gets so much worse when it rains. A good, hydrating curl cream can combat this problem. Look for a lightweight, water-based formula and steer clear of gels containing alcohol, which can be super drying.

CONDITIONER

Conditioner is so important for keeping your hair soft and shiny. But remember that less is often more here. If you use gobs of product, you'll run out faster (which gets expensive!), and it can also weigh your hair down so it looks flat and dull. I like to comb conditioner through my ends in the shower but keep it off my scalp to prevent buildup. As usual, avoid lots of added fragrances and opt for plant-based moisturizing ingredients where you can.

STYLING—CURLS

As much as I enjoy a sleek blowout, I also love that curls—and

STYLING— STRAIGHT/ NO FRIZZ

After the Brazilian blowout made headlines a couple of years ago because it was found to release formaldehyde, I got a lot more careful about the kinds of products I

Since my hair is put through the ringer when I'm working, I like to give it a chance to detox.

use when I want sleek, straight hair. When it's not too humid, I find that a little dab of argan oil or another natural leave-in on my ends is enough to keep everything shiny and smooth. When you need something more hard core, you might want to steer clear of keratin-containing products—we're still trying to figure out which brands are safe and which are problematic. You're better off using a lightweight silicone gel (although, I know, the results won't last as long—such a bummer!). Divide damp hair into sections and blow it out a piece at a time using a big round brush. Then smooth everything over with a flat iron. All this heat can be tough on your hair, so I'd advise against making this your everyday style . . . but it will give you that sleek look without the toxicity.

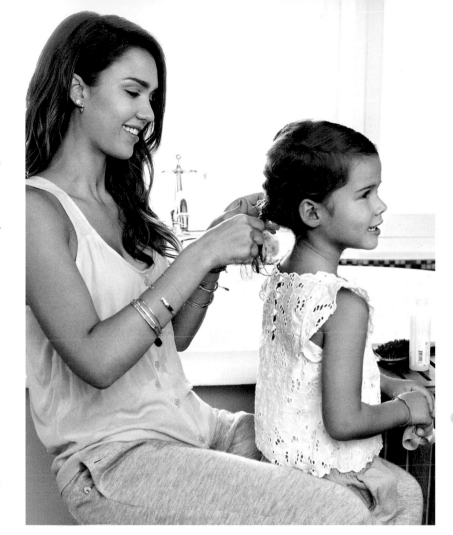

CARING FOR KIDS' HAIR

Honor has such fine, curly hair—it tangles easily and can become such a battle! I've learned that detangler (like Honest Conditioning Mist) is key. And so is gently combing out her hair with a wide-tooth comb while it's still wet—the snarls slide right out. If we're doing braids, I'll do those wet, too—they hold much better, and we make hair time fun by letting her choose clips or ribbons. I love my little girl's curls!

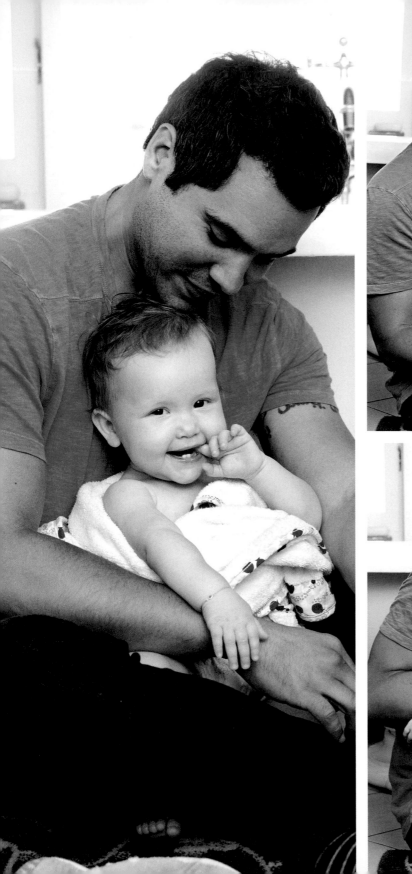
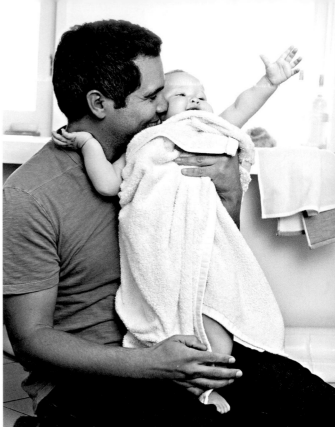
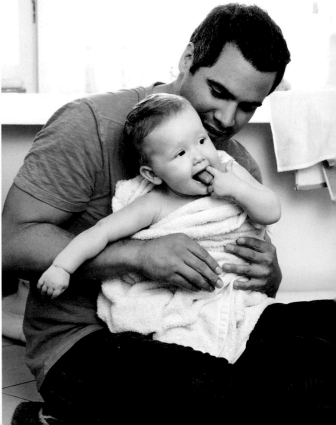

Pure & Simple: Babies

AND THIS IS what it's really all about: how to find safe, healthy stuff that you can slather all over your little ones. Of course, I firmly believe that while we need higher safety standards for children's products, in a perfect world, we'd use those same standards for everyone. After all, Haven spends a fair amount of time snuggled up to my skin . . . and now that Honor is a bit older, she's all about stealing Mommy's beauty products to use on herself. But there's no question that what you put directly on their skin needs to be the purest of all. Remember to check ingredient labels for all of the "Dishonest Ingredients" listed in this chapter (parabens, phthalates, and sodium lauryl sulfate are the top ones to avoid no matter what!) and always buy fragrance free unless the company tells you they only use plant-based fragrance ingredients (and they list what those are).

No-Crying Cleansing

MY HONEST TEAM and I tested dozens of formulations to find the perfect no-crying recipe for our Honest Shampoo & Body Wash. That's because most baby shampoos and shower gels are just as harsh as any others on the market—but manu-

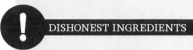

DISHONEST INGREDIENTS

SLS & "PEG"

FOUND IN: Baby shampoo, kids' bubble bath, regular shampoo, soap, and shower gel

WHAT IS IT? Sodium lauryl or sodium laureth sulfate and "PEG" are sudsing agents, which make things foamy. (Beware of any ingredients that include the terms "xynol," "ceteareath," and "oleth.")

WHY IS IT SKETCHY? When these chemicals are manufactured, they release a toxic by-product called **1,4-dioxane.** This chemical easily penetrates our skin and may cause cancer and birth defects. It may also be toxic to our kidneys, neurological system, and respiratory system.

facturers add a numbing agent so your baby's eyes don't sting. Not to mention, they also put in chemicals linked to cancer, allergies, and other health problems. I mean, come on. Do we really need to use chemicals linked to cancer to bathe our babies?

Plant-based actives are best here. Our product uses fruit extracts, essential oils, shea butter, and kukui nut oil, plus organic calendula and aloe, so it won't dry out baby's skin. It's also pH balanced so it's not as harsh as many other soaps and shampoos, and it won't irritate delicate eyes or skin.

Remember always to do a patch test when you try a new product on your baby.

BUBBLE BATH

Just like soap and shower gel, lots of conventional kids' bubble baths contain SLS, 1, 4-dioxane and other problematic ingredients —more than half of the kids' bath products tested by the Campaign for Safe Cosmetics have turned up formaldehyde and 1, 4-dioxane!

It's especially important to look for bubble baths that are formulated with hydrating ingredients, because as fun as it is, sitting in a tub full of bubbles can seriously dry out sensitive skin. (Honest Bubble Bath is made with organic aloe vera, calendula, and chamomile to soothe skin.) And be sure to follow up your kids' tub time with a good lotion or body oil (or a combination) to seal in moisture.

LOTIONS

A lot of kids hate putting on lotion, but it's important not to skip this step. Honor complains about it, but I remind her that we have to prevent her skin from getting all pruney, whether it's

BETTER BATH TOYS

Since I don't want to expose the girls to unnecessary doses of PVC, a harmful material used to make squishy plastics, we don't use rubber duckies or bath books. Instead, I give Haven some bowls and spoons made out of a safe silicone or plastic (remember: "4, 5, 1, and 2—all the rest are bad for you!"). She has a blast splashing and scooping water while I'm scrubbing up Honor, which is key when you've got two soapy kids in the tub!

summer and she's spending tons of time playing mermaids in the pool, or winter when we're all spending too many hours indoors with central heating (which can be very drying).

I also find that if I let Honor put it on herself, she gets more into it. And most key of all is to pick a lotion that absorbs quickly—kids hate to feel sticky, just like grown-ups do!

DIAPER CREAMS & BALMS

Again, this is a category where you want to avoid petroleum and look for plant-oil-based formulas instead. (Honest Healing Balm is formulated with organic sunflower, tamanu, chickweed, and olive and castor oils, which soothe and help prevent and treat diaper rash.) Using a good diaper cream should allow you to skip the baby powder, which is full of talc and other not-so-great stuff. Remember always to do a patch test when you put a new product on your baby, and wait 24 hours to make sure she doesn't have a reaction. If you're dealing with really aggressive diaper rash that doesn't resolve when you switch products, consult your pediatrician.

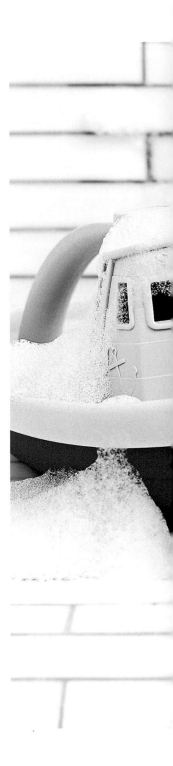

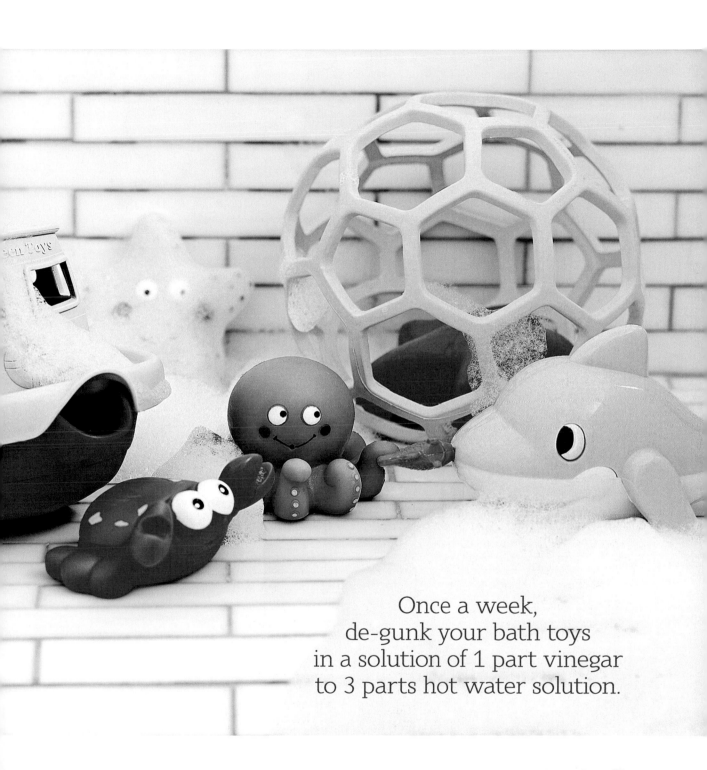

Once a week,
de-gunk your bath toys
in a solution of 1 part vinegar
to 3 parts hot water solution.

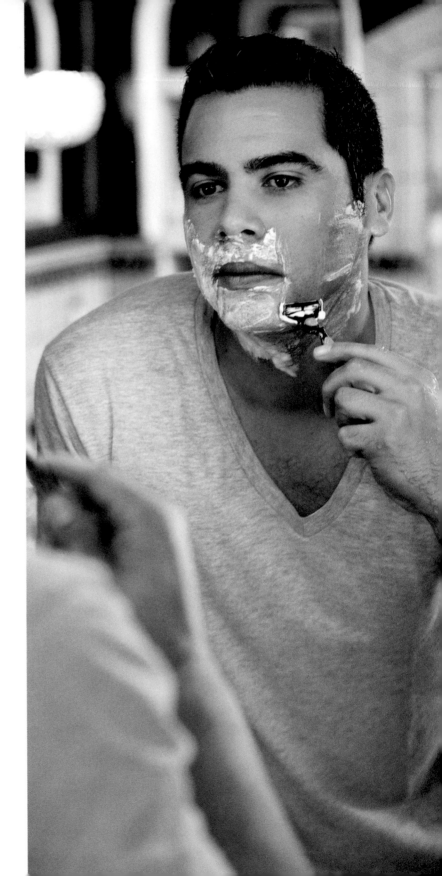

CLEANER GROOMING FOR GUYS

Ahem. Here's a kinda dirty secret about how my family gets clean: Even though I've had all these no-more-toxin epiphanies (and hello, launched a natural personal care products company!), I cannot get Cash to break up with his drugstore-brand soap. It costs about $3, and he's such a guy's guy, it's basically the only thing he uses. He just doesn't want to mess around with any other products. And you know what? It's fine . . . this is all about being honestly imperfect, right?

Fortunately, my business partner, Christopher Gavigan, is the Honest Company's chief product officer for a reason—he's all about experimenting and finding the cleanest stuff that really works. He loves all-in-one products, like our Honest Shampoo & Body Wash, or Dr. Bronner's Magic Soap (which you can use to wash your hair, your body, your dog, and your dishes . . .). And he turned me on to the Herban Cowboy line of guy's grooming products, which are super clean and effective (and I love that the company was founded in a log cabin in rural Montana). I'm sneaking as many as I can into Cash's side of the bathroom!

RESOURCES FOR MORE HONEST CLEAN

Use these lists as a starting point to help you learn more about finding the safest products out there. These are my go-to sources—but don't be afraid to do your own research.

❋ ENVIRONMENTAL WORK-
ING GROUP DATABASE
(ewg.org/skindeep) For this
online reference, researchers
have crunched safety data on
more than 74,000 personal care
products and given each a score
from 0 to 10 based on its level
of toxicity. I always check any
new purchase by searching for
it on this site. But it's not perfect: EWG is an underfunded
nonprofit organization, so they
don't have the manpower to
keep the database up to date
with every new product that
hits the market, and they don't
cover products released over-
seas. But for now, it's a tremen-
dous resource.

❋ GORGEOUSLY GREEN
(gorgeouslygreen.com) is
a fun and super useful Web
site. Sophie Uliano has tons of
great advice for every aspect
of your lifestyle and does solid
research on any product she
awards with her "Gorgeously
Green Seal of Approval."

❋ NO MORE DIRTY LOOKS
(nomoredirtylooks.com) is
another one of my favorite resources; it's a beauty and health
blog run by two cool girls, Siobhan O'Connor and Alexandra
Spunt, who wrote a book by
the same name and now keep
their readers up to date on all
the latest eco-health news and
offer tons of helpful reviews of
eco-beauty products. They're
my go-to when I want to find,
say, a nontoxic deodorant that
doesn't leave me stinky—because they're all about super-
safe products but they also
insist on stuff that *works*.

 HONEST TIP

DON'T BE A GERMOPHOBE

There's no evidence that washing your hands with antibacterial soap or spritzing on lots of antibacterial hand sanitizer is any better for you than good old soap and water—and we may be contributing to anti-biotic resistance and other problems by using them. (See "Triclosan," page 50.) So keep it simple—or if you do need some kind of sanitizer (after changing diapers, cleaning the cat litter, or riding the sub-way, for instance!), use an alcohol-based hand sanitizer that doesn't contain any triclosan, like, yes, Honest Hand Sanitizer.

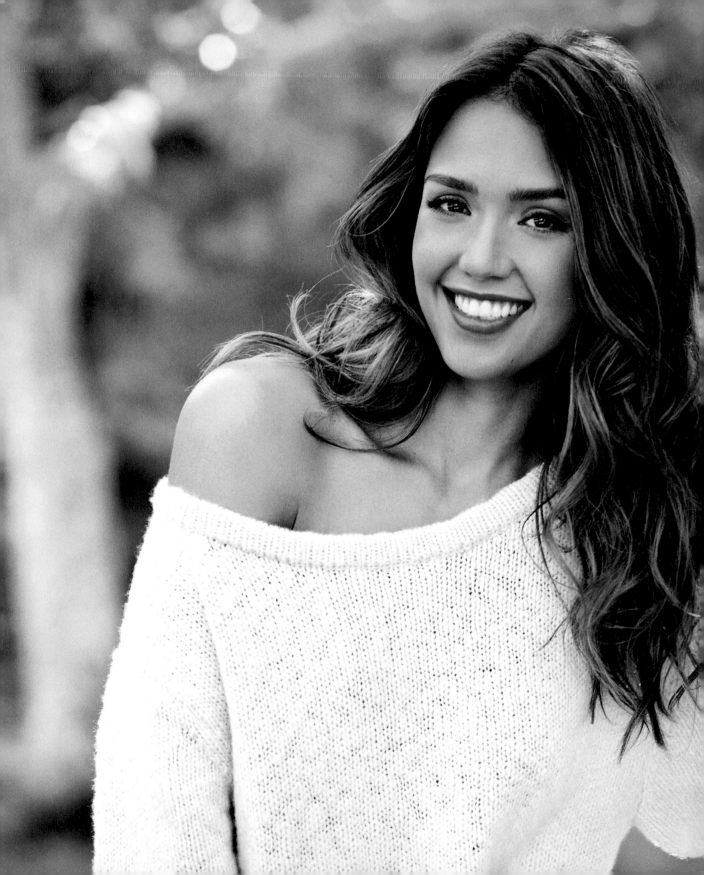

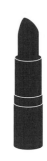

chapter 3
HONEST
beauty

LET YOUR NATURAL
BEAUTY SHINE
THROUGH

THERE ARE SOME DAYS WHERE I WAKE UP IN THE MORNING and I have to pinch myself. I'm 31 years old, and I get to play make-believe for a living! I feel so blessed that my creative outlet is also my career. I love acting because it's this space where dreams can be realized, fantasy comes to life, and there are no limitations on what's possible.

And makeup is a big part of that.

Because makeup can be pure fantasy—it can transform you into any kind of magical creature, whether that's a superhero or a retro Hollywood icon or just a more fun, fresher version of yourself. Looking like a stress-free, well-rested working mom? That's some kind of magic to me.

Growing up, my style icons were my grandmother and my mom—and they could not have had more different takes on beauty and makeup. My grandmother (who, by the way, could have been my identical twin) was a one-product woman. It was all about her matte orange-red lipstick. Before applying the one product all over thing was big, she was doing it. Every day, she'd do her lips with that lipstick, blot and dab the excess on her cheeks, and swipe it across her eyelids. And she looked so glamorous! She was also forever pinching her cheeks—and mine!— to bring the color in.

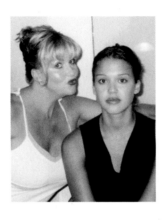

My mom serving her signature burgundy lip.

My mother, on the other hand, never left the house without her face on. I'm pretty sure that's still true to this day. She was raised in the South with a house full of women and went to cosmetology school while I was growing up, so we always had a lot of makeup around. Back then,

her daily look included two colors of eye shadow, an angled rouge on her cheeks, lip liner, and frosted lip color. Now her style is a bit simpler, but she's always hip to the "look of the moment" and loves to experiment, something I've always admired.

I'm a mixture of them both. I like an easy, convenient routine (see " My 10-Minute Face," page 79), and I don't do a full face of makeup every day. But I'm not a one-product woman either. I have boxes of cosmetics in my bathroom, all organized and labeled so I can play around and get creative when the mood strikes.

For me, makeup is about being your best self. If I wake up in a foul mood and have to deal with temper tantrums and an exploding diaper—I know taking 10 minutes to get my game face on will reset my stress levels. It's a chance to check in and remind myself, *you got this*—whatever your "this" happens to be. When I look good (and not tired), I feel good. It really is that simple.

But having been such a non–girly girl as a kid, I know that there's also a lot about makeup that can be super intimidating. When I was 12, my idea of makeup was some Bobbi Brown eyeliner— except I could never get it to go on smoothly, so I'd just smudge it everywhere (and I'm not talking, like, artfully smudged). Now, since I'm lucky enough to get my makeup done by some of the best professional makeup artists in the world, I'm constantly grilling them for their best tips and tricks. Like, how do you get mascara not to clump? How do you do a glam red lip . . . that doesn't end up on your teeth or bleeding beyond your lipline like a hot mess? How do you pull off a smoky eye . . . that doesn't look broke-down and tired? Why do some foundations cake and others flake?

I mean—these are the serious questions of our time, right? Or, at least, of our morning routine! And with the help of my dear friend and makeup artist Lauren Andersen (we've known each other since we were 14), I've uncovered the answers—but more on that in a

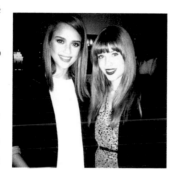

My sweet Lauren and me at a party (she did my makeup).

minute. Because first we need to talk about what, exactly, is *in* all of those waxy sticks and powdery cakes. As you might expect, all of this gets a little more complicated when you add the need for safe, healthy cosmetic formulations to the mix.

The Not So Pretty Face

IF YOU'VE BEEN FOLLOWING ALONG in Chapters 1 and 2, you know where this is going. A lot of the makeup we put on our faces every day is filled with toxic crap. It's pretty hard to argue that this is an unavoidable toxic exposure, like, say, air pollution—because there is no law that says you have to wear any makeup at all.

But what if you just want to, dammit? I honestly mean no offense to my friends in the environmental movement with what I'm about to say, but this is where they lose a lot of us—by acting like you're a bad person for getting a pedicure, when maybe you had a tough day and you need a treat. This shouldn't be about pointing fingers at each other for our personal decisions, though. The point is that wanting straight, shiny hair is not supposed to cause cancer. Period. End of story.

But until we get some decent chemical industry regulations passed in Washington, we consumers have to get educated and make some smarter shopping decisions. Just as I've done with my lotions and body washes, I've had to learn how to navigate the world of cosmetics to avoid allergic reactions. Once, when I was in Paris for Fashion Week, I had my makeup done for a party and woke up the next morning to find my eyes had crusted shut—disgusting! I had less than two days to get the situation under control before I was supposed to attend a Dior show, and it was a nightmare, trying to hunt down prescription eyedrops in a foreign city so I didn't look like a boxer who'd just been handled. To this day, if I use too much liquid liner or any shadow with a lot of red pigment, I get a serious rash.

Since so many brands of makeup irritate my skin, I've tried just about every eco- or natural line out there. When it comes to cosmetics, I'm here to tell you that this can be an epic pain. Think about everything we demand from something as simple as mascara—we want it to volumize, curl, lengthen, and, oh yeah, be waterproof—and that's only for our eyelashes! Now you want cosmetic companies to do all that *without* using any potentially toxic chemicals?

Well, of course you do, and so do I.

But a lot of the eco-friendly cosmetic brands I've tried have been . . . disappointing at best. Forget volume, curl, length—most natural mascaras clump. The lipsticks don't glide and the eye shadows rub off after about an hour. That's because it's hard to make color cosmetics without a whole jumble of synthetic ingredients. We can't just

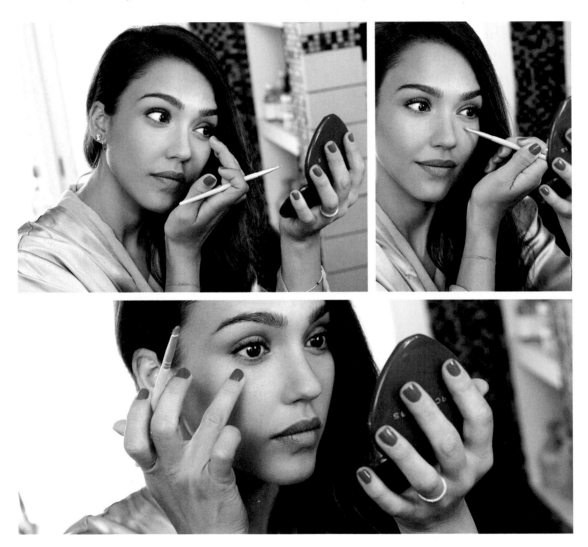

crush some organic berries on our lips and call it a day—we need chemicals that will hold the formula together, make it glide on nicely, prevent bacterial growth, and so on. There's a reason mascara today does about 50 million more things to your eyelashes than the mascara your mom used when she was our age—the beauty industry has added hundreds of new chemicals to all of their cosmetic formulations to improve performance. Now the pressure is on to find safer alternatives for the chemicals we know may work great—but aren't so great for our health.

The Honest Makeup Bag

Now the fun part! I'm going to give you all my beauty secrets and tips to help you achieve your own version of Honest Beauty.

The good news is that a lot of beauty brands are starting to get there. I've seen a huge improvement in the quality of products offered even in just the past couple of years. In this chapter, I'm going to share some of my favorites so you can make over your makeup bag. And Lauren and I have also downloaded our best beauty tips and tricks to help you find the magic—and maybe even a bit of that make-believe!—in makeup.

Note: The vast majority of the products that I use are free of all the Dishonest Ingredients I warn you about throughout this chapter and

Honest Beauty Is . . .

* Clean
* Fresh
* Uncomplicated
* Healthy
* Washing your face before bed—most nights
* Sun kissed (with SPF)
* Smiling
* Kid friendly
* Sexy
* Casual
* A little shimmer

Honest Beauty Isn't . . .

* Fake
* Worrying about crow's-feet
* Fretting over every tiny blemish
* Complicated
* Untouchable
* Unkissable
* A lot of work
* Formal
* Serious
* Toxic

have a safety score of 0 to 2 (the best you can get) in the **Environmental Working Group's Skin Deep Cosmetics Database (ewg.org/skindeep).** Remember, Skin Deep is awesome but not perfect —it can't stay on top of every new product, particularly some of the great brands I've discovered on my travels in France or Japan—countries with much stricter safety standards than the USA. But I've consulted environmental health experts like Christopher Gavigan to make sure they meet our safety criteria.

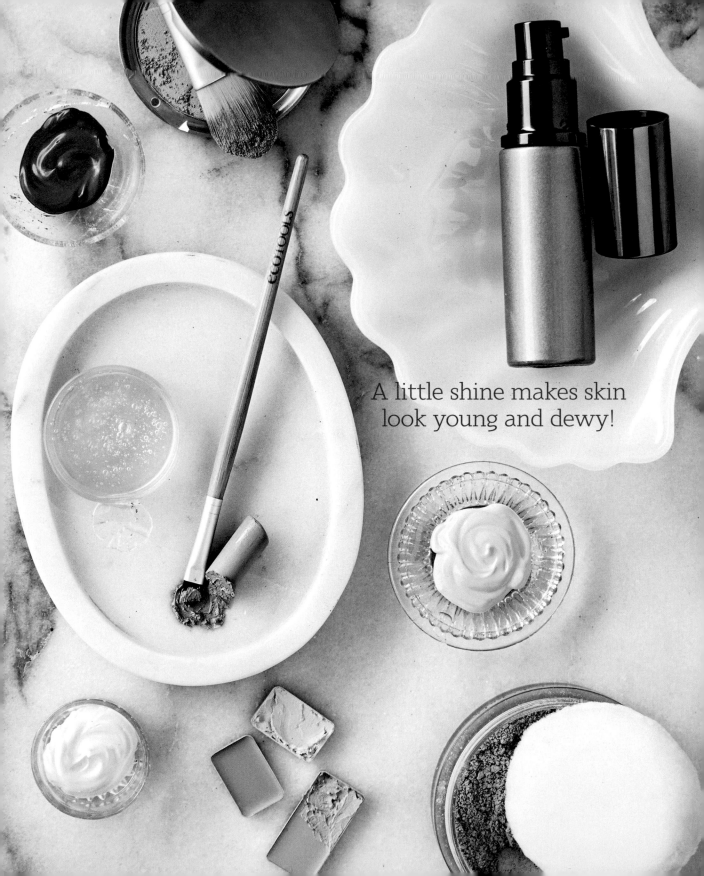

A little shine makes skin
look young and dewy!

Pure & Simple: Base Layer

THIS IS THE makeup that has the most contact with your skin and (in a perfect world, anyway!) stays put all day long. Make it a priority to choose the cleanest products possible to protect your pores and give you a safe, healthy glow. A great base layer minimizes flaws, but it's really about letting your true beauty shine through.

TINTED MOISTURIZER

Most days, I have no desire to do the full primer-foundation-concealer routine, but I still need a little something. Enter tinted moisturizer: It evens things out and makes you all glowy but takes 2 seconds to apply.

I'm particularly fond of tinted moisturizers with SPF because it helps me do even more product multitasking; 100% Pure makes a nice one. And I really love Hourglass Illusion Tinted Moisturizer with SPF; it's a bit pricier, but you cannot beat how well it glides on and never cakes.

Whatever moistur-izer you use, let it sit and absorb for a few minutes before you layer on more cosmetics. This gives your skin a chance to drink it in and get thoroughly hydrated, which makes everything else easier to apply. And always insist that your moisturizer (and all your cosmetics) be synthetic-fragrance free. It's a key way to avoid phthalates (see page 70), since this product sits on your face all day, and you want to minimize chemical absorption into your bloodstream.

PRIMER

Primer is one of those products that I thought was a total waste of time—until a makeup artist made me try it. Then I realized how completely poreless it makes your face—and how much longer the rest of your makeup stays in place. I was a convert! Think of it as a 3-second investment in the rest of your face. (Plus you'll break out less because it prevents everything else from gunking up your pores.)

I tend to skip primer if I'm just using tinted moisturizer, but if you're very oily or have the kind of skin where everything seems to wear off by noon, primer can help make it last. Otherwise, use it after moisturizer but before foundation. You might also want to look for a mattifying primer (Hourglass and Korres make nice ones), but

don't over-matte yourself—I like a little shine because I think it makes skin look young and dewy! Plus it can look weird if your face is super matte and the rest of you is normal.

Most primers are white or clear, so they'll be invisible. I'm also a big fan of Koh Gen Do Maifanshi Makeup Color Base, which comes in shades of yellow, purple, and green and lets you correct color imperfections (like dark circles and red spots) before you layer on your foundation.

CONCEALER

I apply my concealer over tinted moisturizer or foundation—I know that sounds a little counterintuitive, but it gives me a much cleaner application. (When I

HONEST TIP

DIY TINTED MOISTURIZER

Mix a pea-size blob of your suncreen with a pea-size blob of your base to get a homemade tinted moisturizer with SPF.

put concealer on first, I find the moisturizer just wipes it all off!) The trick is to apply concealer with a small brush or a Beautyblender sponge (see page 77) so it mixes in seamlessly with your base—and you can avoid that globby raccoon-eyes effect.

I also stash a concealer in my purse at all times (RMS Beauty "Un" Cover-Up and Hourglass Hidden Corrective Concealer are my favorites) because it's the fastest way to do touch-ups without having to set up for a full foundation redo. I'm always whipping it out in the car or my office— 10 seconds of dabbing and I'm good to go!

FOUNDATION

I'm a liquid foundation girl all the way—with my dry skin, powder can get cakey, or worse, just settle into every little line. I'm completely obsessed with Koh Gen Do's Maifanshi Moisture Foundation. It's from Japan (but you can find it at Sephora) and is so smooth, it almost feels like moisturizer. (It's a little pricey,

but you can always make it last longer by mixing a dab with your tinted moisturizer.)

If you're oily, however, powder might be a better choice—the wrong liquid foundation can make you more prone to breakouts. That's why it's always smart to do a patch test with any new product (but you knew that, of course). Just make sure that *any* powder cosmetics you choose are talc free and 100 percent pure minerals— you don't want any of the cheap fillers some of those greenwashing mineral lines use.

POWDER

Powder is strictly optional for everyday but is useful for setting makeup and preventing shine. My favorite (Koh Gen Do again) is a translucent loose powder that's magical for spot illumination—it's as if a TV lighting crew were following you around. Jane Iredale PurePressed Base SPF 20 is more heavily pigmented and is a great option for an all-over matte finish.

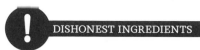

DISHONEST INGREDIENTS

PHTHALATES

FOUND IN: Anything that lists "fragrance" on the label, plus some nail polishes

WHAT IS IT? A plasticizer (which makes your nail polish strong and flexible) or fragrance component (which gives products that "fresh" scent)

WHY IS IT SKETCHY? Twenty years of research suggests that phthalates can mess with our hormones and damage our reproductive health, so it's especially critical for pregnant women, babies, and young children to steer clear.

TEA AND DEA

FOUND IN: Concealer, mascara, sunless tanning lotion, and conditioner

WHAT IS IT? Triethanolamine (TEA) and diethanolamine (DEA) are proteins used to adjust the pH level of a product or as a wetting agent.

WHY IS IT SKETCHY? When TEA is combined with certain preservatives, it can create cancer-causing compounds called nitrosamines.

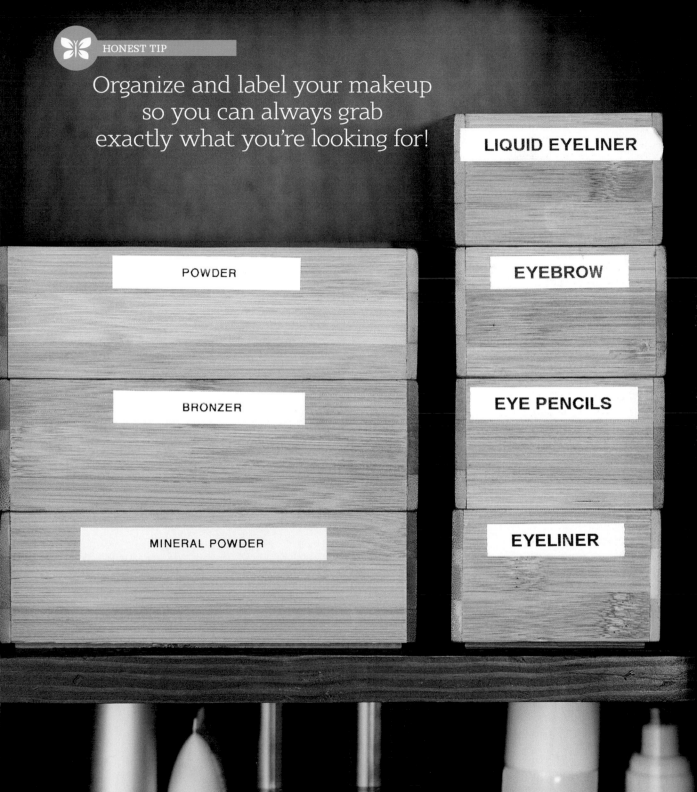

Organize and label your makeup
so you can always grab
exactly what you're looking for!

LIQUID EYELINER

POWDER

EYEBROW

BRONZER

EYE PENCILS

MINERAL POWDER

EYELINER

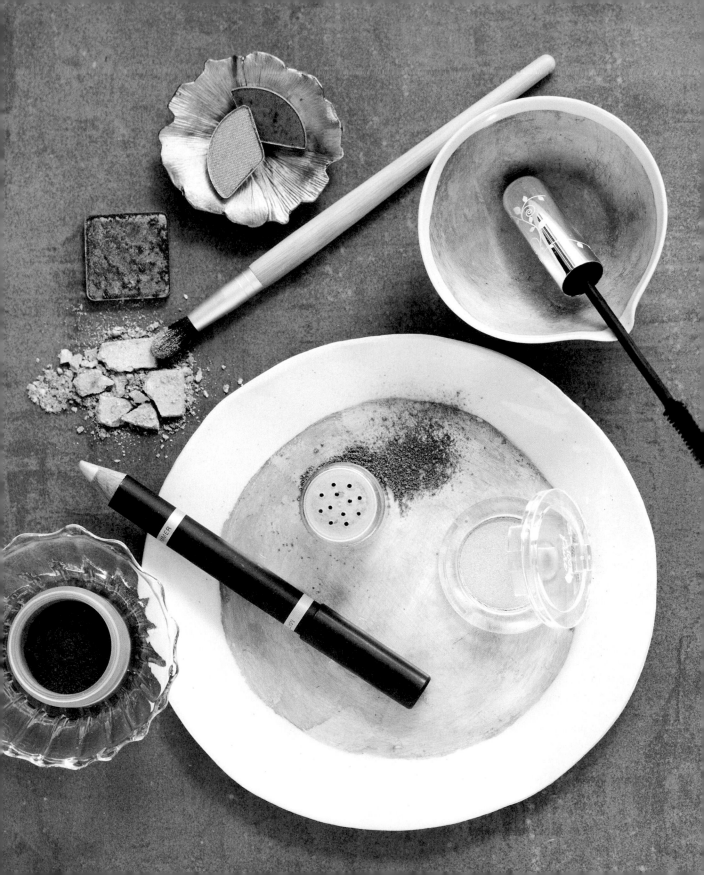

Pure & Simple: Add Color

COLOR IS ONE OF my favorite ways to express myself, whether it's a dramatic eye or a bold red lip. But it can also be a landmine because there aren't always clean alternatives that work as well as synthetic-filled brands. Go as toxin free as you can on the everyday stuff, but don't feel bad if you need to put performance over purity at times.

BLUSH

I opt for cream blushes or cheek stains (100% Pure makes a fabulous one; I also love Tarte's) because I find that powder blushes can look chalky. But it's a personal preference! There are some great powders out there—like Korres' Zea Mays Blush and 100% Pure's—if that's your thing. Whichever type of blush you use, Lauren Andersen advises applying it only where you would naturally flush (the tops of your cheeks) with a big powder brush or Beautyblender, using loose, circular movements for a natural, not-painted-on look.

HIGHLIGHTER

The point of highlighter is to reflect light, which brightens your whole face—so again, this is about creating a natural, healthy glow that lets your authentic beauty shine through . . . not spackling on tons of product. Lauren likes to apply highlighter to the tops of the cheekbones, the bridge of the nose, and just under the brow bones, as well as to the inside corner of each eye. The effect should be very subtle—but it wakes up your whole face!

BRONZER

I'm super into bronzer because it's a much healthier way to look sun kissed and golden than to actually, you know, tan. (It's also way better for you than using most sunless tanners, which can contain sketchy chemicals—see page 83.) Again, Lauren says, think about where you'd naturally go golden if the sun's rays *were* allowed to penetrate your SPF—tops of cheeks, around the hairline (not brows!), and bridge of the nose. Use a big loose powder brush or a Beautyblender to apply the bronzer with big circular motions—this way, you'll avoid that not-so-natural tiger stripe effect. Hourglass has a great crème-to-powder bronzer that looks very authentic. I'm also a fan of Jane Iredale's 24-Karat Gold Dust, for special occasions. And if I'm going to show some leg, I'll mix a little into my body lotion—it creates a subtle shimmer that makes cellulite lumps and bumps a tad less noticeable!

❗ DISHONEST INGREDIENT

MERCURY

FOUND IN: Mascara and some face paints

WHAT IS IT? A preservative that prevents bacterial growth

WHY IS IT SKETCHY? Mercury is a known neurotoxin that can also cause allergic reactions or skin irritation, plus it's easily absorbed through your skin and accumulates in your body. As a result, it's one of the few cosmetic ingredients that the FDA does restrict—mercury can only be used in eye makeup in very small amounts and only "if no other safe and effective preservative can be found." Gosh, that's a big loophole! I think we can do better.

EYE SHADOW

The first rule of Honest Beauty is that there really aren't any rules— you should feel free to play around with any color that excites you! But I'm also all about playing up your assets —and a lot people have great eyes. So choosing shadow colors that truly complement your natural eye color is a pretty effortless way to highlight your natural beauty. Here are Lauren's suggestions:

EYELINER

Eyeliner is what keeps your smoky eye looking sharp, not sloppy, but the key is not to overuse this powerhouse. If your eyes are small or closely set, just line the outer third of your lid, to make the eyes look larger and wider, says Lauren. Tarte makes a nice fat crayon liner called Smolder with a good smudging tool on the other end. I also adore Hourglass liquid liners— they have one called Calligraphy, which is almost like a felt-tip pen and perfect for smoky lines, as well as one called Script Precision, which is great for lower lids.

MASCARA

This is a category where the eco-brands are still working out the kinks. When I need totally smudgeproof, lasts-forever lashes, my favorites are still conventional brands like L'Oréal Voluminous and Diorshow. But 100% Pure and Hourglass have solid organic formulas. Hourglass Film Noir Lash Lacquer is an inky black topcoat with a really dramatic look.

BROW PENCILS

I prefer to use a non-sharpening brow pencil and always go a shade lighter than my actual hair color—it makes the whole operation way more foolproof. The goal here isn't to draw a whole new brow. Just comb your brows and use the pencil to shape and fill in bare spots.

LIPS

For everyday, I'm all about glosses (Koh Gen Do's glossy lip gloss is a favorite, along with Korres Lip Butter Glaze). For a fancy night, I love a glam red pout—and for that, you need to go old school with lipstick. But be careful—red is the lipstick color most likely to contain high levels of lead (see the Dishonest Ingredient box, opposite) according to the Campaign for Safe Cosmetics, so it's especially crucial to shop around for a trustworthy eco-brand here; Hourglass, Tarte, and 100% Pure make great ones, from orange reds to deep reds to purple reds. For more low-key days, if you do nothing else to your face, dab on some tinted lip balm. It's so easy— you were probably going to use lip balm at some point, right? A little color just wakes up your whole face. Try Korres Lip Butters as a base and then top with the Korres Lip Butter Glaze. Use a matching shade, or play around and layer them.

EYE COLOR CHEAT SHEET

If You Have . . .	For a Natural Look, Try	For Drama, Try
BLUE EYES	Gold-toned browns and beiges	Dusty silvers; smoky eyes
BROWN EYES	Bronze, browns (any shade), pewter, and other metallics	Navy or cobalt blue—in a small amount, like an eyeliner (and skip the shadow)
GREEN EYES	Peach, champagne, or another soft, red-toned brown	Light purples, plums (just the eyeliner if you want a pop of color that isn't garish)

LEAD

FOUND IN: Lipsticks and some children's face paints

WHAT IS IT? Lead and other heavy metals such as cadmium and nickel are contaminants (which naturally occur in some pigments). Detectable levels of lead were found in 400 lipsticks tested by the FDA in 2010!

WHY IS IT SKETCHY? There is no safe level of lead exposure: It's a known neurotoxin and can play a role in the development of learning delays, autism, and other neurological problems for babies and children. It also can reach a developing fetus, so if you're pregnant or thinking about it, you want to avoid lead, full stop.

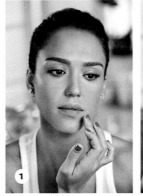

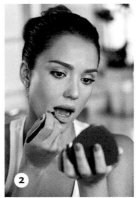

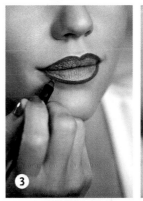

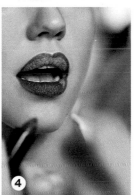

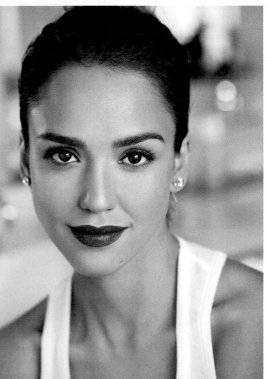

HOW TO MAKE THE PERFECT RED LIP

1. To keep your red lip from feathering out on you, apply foundation all the way around the lips, to the outer edge.

2. Line your lips, starting from the inner crease.

3. Even out any mess by retracing the line.

4. Completely fill in your lips with liner, then top with a matching lipstick. If you want, use a brush for greater accuracy. Lauren also likes to go in and clean up the edges with a Q-tip; she'll even use a small brush and some concealer to make the edges really crisp.

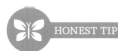

HONEST TIP

MANI-PEDIS FOR KIDS

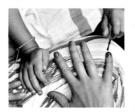

I've come to accept that almost every little girl loves to play beauty parlor. We'll let Honor have her nails painted for a treat, but we always make sure to use a kid-safe water-based polish—I love Hopscotch Kids WaterColors, which is the little sister brand of Scotch Naturals. It contains none of the chemicals found in regular nail polish but still holds up pretty well. I even make sure to bring our own polish and remover if I take Honor with me to the nail salon.

DISHONEST INGREDIENT

TOLUENE

FOUND IN: Nail polish, strengtheners, and cuticle treatments

WHAT IS IT? A clear, colorless solvent that helps suspend little particles of color throughout your nail polish and form a smooth finish

WHY IS IT SKETCHY? As your polish dries, toluene evaporates into the air so you (and your manicurist) breathe it in. This can cause nose, throat, and eye irritation as well as headaches, dizziness, and fatigue. At high levels of exposure, toluene is toxic to your kidneys and liver and may also damage reproductive health, so pregnant women need to avoid it.

NAIL POLISH

Nail polish is super frustrating because it's one area we thought we had sorted—back in 2006, almost all of the big mainstream polish brands promised to reformulate their products and remove the "toxic trio" (formaldehyde, toluene, and dibutyl phthalate or DBP). But in 2011, the California Environmental Protection Agency tested a bunch of nail polishes from local salons and found that 10 out of 12 products claiming to be toxic-trio free actually contained some or all of the chemicals. This is a perfect example of why we need better regulations: Someone needs to be checking that companies are actually doing what they claim.

That being said, of course I'm still wearing nail polish. I love corals and reds, or sometimes (if I'm feeling sort of rocker-glam!) blue. Zoya and Priti NYC are two excellent three-free natural brands. I also love Priti NYC's Soy Nail Polish Remover Wipes because they are far more effective than any other soy polish remover I've tried and so convenient for travel. Dermelect ME Anti-Aging Colored Nail Lacquers also promise to be three free and last forever.

PERFUME

I generally skip perfume—between body wash, lotions, and shampoos, perfume isn't really necessary, and it's one less product to layer on and fuss with. But sometimes I do like to have a special scent, and I'll create my own by adding a couple drops of essential oils—gardenia and jasmine are my favorites—to a body oil. (Play around, but be careful about getting into the patchouli and such, unless that's your move—the goal is to still smell like yourself.) For special nights out, I can't get enough of the Honoré des Prés fragrance line by Olivia Giacobetti; it's completely phthalate—and other sketchy fragrance ingredients—free and smells *ah-mazing*. Her Vamp à NY is my favorite scent.

MUST-HAVE BEAUTY TOOLS

If you aren't using quality brushes, sponges, and other tools to apply your product, you might as well throw your credit card down the drain—because even the best-quality cosmetics will look like hell if you're spackling them on with cotton swabs and thumbs. (Well, sometimes finger painting works . . . if you're going for a bohemian look.) Professional makeup artists invest serious dough in their tools because they know how crucial they are. Lauren and I put together this list of favorites.

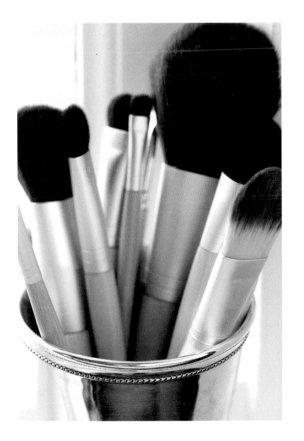

❊ **SHU UEMURA EYELASH CURLER.** This is The Only eyelash curler I will use—it's world famous for a reason. The only bummer is that you have to order it online unless you're going to be in Asia anytime soon; I'd order two and a pack of refill eye pads while you're at it.

❊ **BEAUTYBLENDER.** The best makeup sponge ever—it's shaped like an egg, so you can stipple and twist with the narrow end and blend, blend, blend with the round end. Also I love that the company will recycle your old Beautyblenders for you if you mail them back in once you're done through their "blend-ersender" program.

❊ **ECO TOOLS.** This is a great, comprehensive line of tools that won't break the bank, and their brush sets are second to none. If you are willing to spend a little more, Hourglass brushes are extra-soft, PETA-approved (no animal hair!), and have nice weighted handles that make them easy to work with. Also, I'm fanatical about washing my brushes after every use. It doesn't have to be a big ordeal—just swish them around in some warm water, natural hand soap, and tea tree oil to kill bacteria, then air-dry.

BIG NIGHT BEAUTY

Day to day, I keep it simple (see "My 10-Minute Face," opposite). But for big nights on the red carpet, Lauren and I love to serve it up with some bold looks. Here's how to get three of my favorites.

BRONZED LOOK

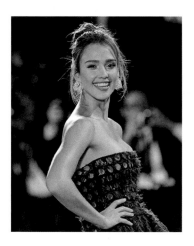

MODIFIED MOD

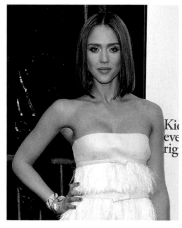

SMOKY EYE

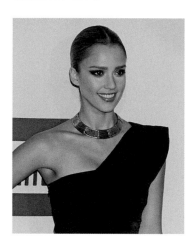

WHAT TO DO:

START: Sweep the eyelid with a golden or bronze-toned eye shadow and line with a black eyeliner. (Use a crayon liner and smudge it a bit as you go.)

NEXT: To soften the eyes, smudge the shadow into the lower lash line, then apply a coat of black mascara.

FINISH: Complete your golden glow by applying bronzer softly to the hairline and contours of the cheek to warm and shape the face. Then dust a soft, shimmery peach blush onto the apples of the cheeks and use a touch of sheer pinky peach gloss on the lips.

WHAT TO DO:

START: Brush a nude shadow on your lids, then contour with a soft brown shadow in the crease.

NEXT: Add a touch of golden glitter on the lid for extra sparkle. (Mac makes a loose glitter that you can press on the eyelid with a small brush.) For a classic wing tip, use a black liquid or cream liner and draw a thin line starting from the inner corner of the eye at the lash line to the outer corner, flicking the line upward.

FINISH: Keep the lips and cheeks a soft peach, letting the eyes be the focus. Apply mascara.

WHAT TO DO:

START: Apply cream metallic black eye shadow from the base of the lid to the crease of the eye. Blend a warm brown into the crease to soften up the edge.

NEXT: Trace a black coal eyeliner along the top lash line and the bottom water line, blending it in with a small brush. To extend the smoky eye outward, place a folded tissue under the eye and use the edge as a guide while blending a black eye shadow at the outer corners of the eye. Curl lashes and apply black mascara.

FINISH: Keep lips and cheeks neutral with a soft peachy blush and a nude lipstick and gloss.

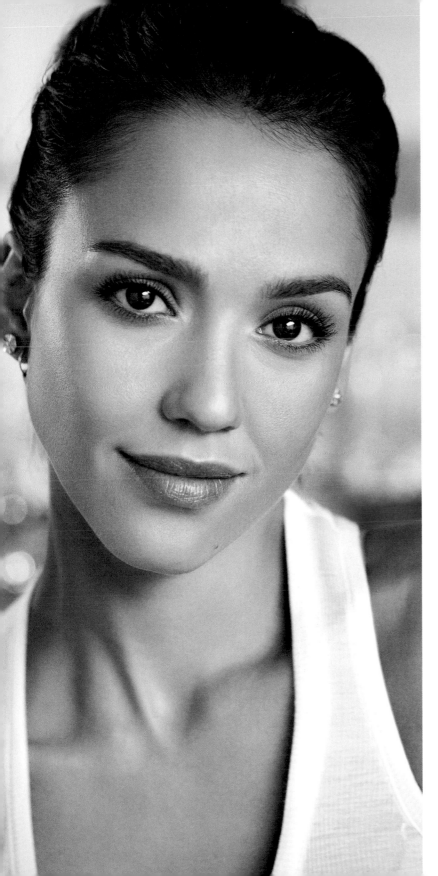

MY 10-MINUTE FACE

So what do I actually do, day in, day out, to get out the door every morning? I keep it simple—because Honest Beauty isn't really about the slew of products you're painting on. It's about being comfortable in your own skin and showing your inner glow.

WHAT TO DO:

1. **Apply tinted moisturizer and sunscreen.** Mix them together in the palm of your hand if you're really time pressed; then go finish your hair or whatever so the moisturizer and sunscreen have a few minutes to absorb into your skin.

2. **Spot conceal** any breakouts, dark circles, red spots. I always go under my eyes and along the sides of my nose and use a little angled brush to blend, blend, blend it smooth.

3. **Curl lashes.** Shu Uemura. Enough said.

4. **Apply mascara.** If needed, use a lash comb to quickly comb out clumps.

5. **Tap cream blush** onto the apples of your cheeks.

6. **Apply a tinted lip balm.** Always dab the center of your lower lip; that's where light hits first.

PS. 1 or 2 minutes more? Use a brow pencil to perfect the brows. Boom—done.

The Honest Salon

IT'S ONE THING to make over your very own bathroom cabinets and makeup bag. But what happens when you take your beauty routine out into the real world—as in the salon? Unless you want to be the weird girl toting in her own sulfate-free shampoo to a blowout, chances are you're going to have to make some occasional compromises if there aren't any great eco-minded salons in your area.

From a health perspective, I think this is mostly okay. I *am* very concerned about the health of hair stylists, nail technicians, and other salon workers who are in these places, breathing the usually toxin-laced air day in, day out . . . especially because they often don't have much control over the health and safety measures taken in their workplace. (If this is an issue that concerns you, you can help by letting the owners of the salons you frequent know that you want to see them prioritizing their workers' health and safety—send them to the National Healthy Nail & Beauty Salon Alliance at nailsalonalliance.org for more info.)

But for consumers who are only popping in to salons every now and again, the exposures are minimal—unless, of course, you're pregnant, breastfeeding, or planning to bring your kids with you (their bodies are still developing and so much more vulnerable!). Nevertheless, it's definitely worthwhile to avoid the most toxic treatments on salon menus:

Avoid

ACRYLIC NAILS

These plasticlike substances that shellac your own nails contain ethyl methacrylate (EMA)—that's the stuff that generates that eau de nail salon scent, and it can cause serious eye, skin, and throat irritation. Plus some salons still use liquid methyl methacrylate monomer (MMA), a related chemical that's now been banned or restricted in at least 30 states because it may cause liver damage and is much harsher and more difficult to get off your nails.

TANNING BEDS

I'm not going to mince words here because I want to scare you: Tanning beds are killing girls, and you should never, ever use them. Skin cancer is not a joke; my mother lost a piece of her lip, arm, and back to melanoma, and I'm grateful it wasn't worse. It's so bizarre to me that tanning salons are even legal in this country—after all, it's not like we don't know tanning can cause cancer. Yet one in three Caucasian women aged 18 to 25 said they had used a tanning bed in the past year, according to a 2012 report by the Centers for Disease Control and Prevention. Frequent indoor tanners are three times more likely to develop melanoma than the rest of us, and skin cancer is now the most common cause of cancer among young women. This has got to stop. Don't waste your money, time, or health on tanning salons. I get wanting a healthy glow, but try the bronzing techniques on page 73, or apply a healthy self-tanner (that meets the safe criteria on page 83).

KERATIN HAIR STRAIGHTENERS

The Brazilian blowout has been making headlines for ages now because its shockingly high formaldehyde content has caused so many hair stylists and some customers to become sick. But did you know that many other

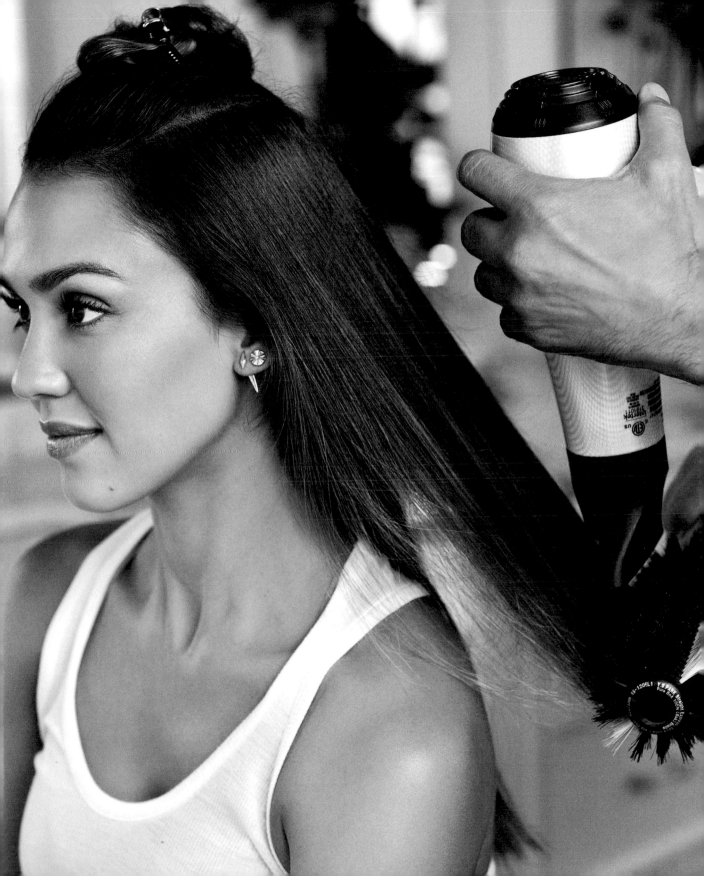

brands of keratin hair-straightening treatments also off-gas formaldehyde once they're heated? Oregon OSHA (Occupational Safety & Health Admininstration) followed up its initial testing with an analysis of 105 hair-straightening samples representing 11 brands and found higher-than-safe formaldehyde levels in all but 3. In 2011, the Environmental Working Group conducted its own lab tests and found 16 brands containing formaldehyde—15 of which claimed to be low or no formaldehyde! Steer clear of any keratin straightening treatments that promise to last longer than eight weeks until we know for sure that all the formaldehyde-containing formulas are off the market. If you want super-straight hair, stick with a flat iron and elbow grease and stay out of the rain—or try a temporary keratin straightener that lasts less than eight weeks, but know that formaldehyde (unfortunately!) is the ingredient that makes the ultra-long-lasting formulas effective. So without it, a keratin straightener may be safer, but it won't do much to straighten or de-frizz your hair.

Proceed with Caution

GEL NAILS

Some salons are now advertising gel nails as a safer alternative to acrylic, but honestly? Those formulas are still plenty full of allergy-causing ingredients, so I'd proceed with lots of caution. I will get gels done if I'm going to be on the road doing events for two weeks straight and won't have time for a regular manicure, but it's definitely a once-in-a-while thing. You don't want to surround yourself with these fumes on a monthly basis. And if you're pregnant, it's probably best to steer clear of nail salons altogether unless they're well ventilated or an "eco" nail salon—it's impossible to avoid the fumes from other customers while you're in there, plus it's so tricky to know whether the regular nail polish is truly of the so-called "toxic trio" (though most places are fine with you bringing your own).

! **DISHONEST INGREDIENT**

TOLUENE

FOUND IN: Hair dyes, brow bleaches, skin lighteners, antiaging creams

WHAT IS IT? Bleaching ingredient used to lighten and brighten top layers of skin and outer hair cuticle

WHY IS IT SKETCHY? Can cause cancer and screw up your immune system and reproductive health. Also associated with developmental problems when little kids are exposed. All-around bad news.

I love highlights, but I ask my stylist to stay away from my roots. Then I can go longer without a touch-up, and the dye can't penetrate my scalp.

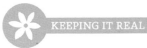

AT THE SALON

SUNLESS TANNING

For years, I was all about the self-tanner as a tanning alternative. Yes, back in the '90s, it used to make us all kinds of orange, but the formulas have gotten much more natural-looking. Yay, right? Until the summer of 2012, when new research surfaced showing that the main skin-tinting ingredient in self-tanners and spray tans—a chemical called dihydroxyacetone, or DHA—could damage your DNA and even cause genetic alterations and cancer. Some health experts think we should avoid these products completely.

So now there's really no such thing as a safe tan? Well, that's just awesome. However, there's still scientific debate over how much DHA can actually penetrate your skin. (Spray tanners, where it's easier to inhale particles, seem like more of a clear no-fly zone.) So DHA rates a 1 to 4 ("fair") safety score in EWG's Skin Deep Cosmetics Database, as long as you aren't ingesting it or rubbing it in your eyes.

Nonetheless, I think caution is warranted: I am still using self-tanner, but sparingly—and I look for brands that use natural DHA, derived from cane or beet sugar, without any added dyes or other harmful stuff. One winner: Chocolate Sun Cocoa Glow Sunless Tanning Cream.

HAIR REMOVAL

For permanent hair removal, I think laser is the way to go if you can swing the hefty price tag and withstand the pain—but most of the time, I stick with waxing and shaving. I like Alba Botanica's shaving cream—or, in a pinch, mixing Honest Conditioner with Honest Shampoo & Body Wash works well!

From an eco-perspective, waxing is not that great because the material is all petrochemicals—the market for hair removal wax developed when oil refineries wanted a way to sell a by-product of their manufacturing process! Seek out natural waxes that are petrochemical free. Sugaring is a more sustainable alternative that you can totally do at home. Parissa Body Sugar is affordable and contains nothing but sugar, water, glycerin, lemon, and chamomile; Shobha Sugaring Kit for Body & Bikini is similarly natural—their strips are made from denim and totally reusable.

HAIR COLOR & HIGHLIGHTS

In a perfect world, I wouldn't color my hair. Numerous studies have connected hair dye with a host of cancers and other adverse health effects; hair stylists have higher rates of bladder cancer, non-Hodgkins lymphoma, fertility issues, and other problems. Salon clients don't have the same level of exposure, but even so, the federal Office on Women's Health in the Department of Health and Human Services advises that "you may reduce your risk of cancer by using less hair dye over time." Common hair dye ingredients can also cause skin rashes and respiratory issues, especially if you're allergy prone or chemically sensitive.

But in my career, going au natural on hair color is not an option. I have to be willing to dye my hair for roles, and you don't usually get a lot of say over what the stylists use. And even when left to my own devices, I do love me some highlights—but I ask my stylist to keep them away from my roots. This means I can go longer without a touch-up (always nice!), and this approach may also offer a layer of protection since the dye can't penetrate my scalp. If you want to use darker colors, always choose semi-permanent dyes, which have been shown to be a little less toxic than the permanent colors.

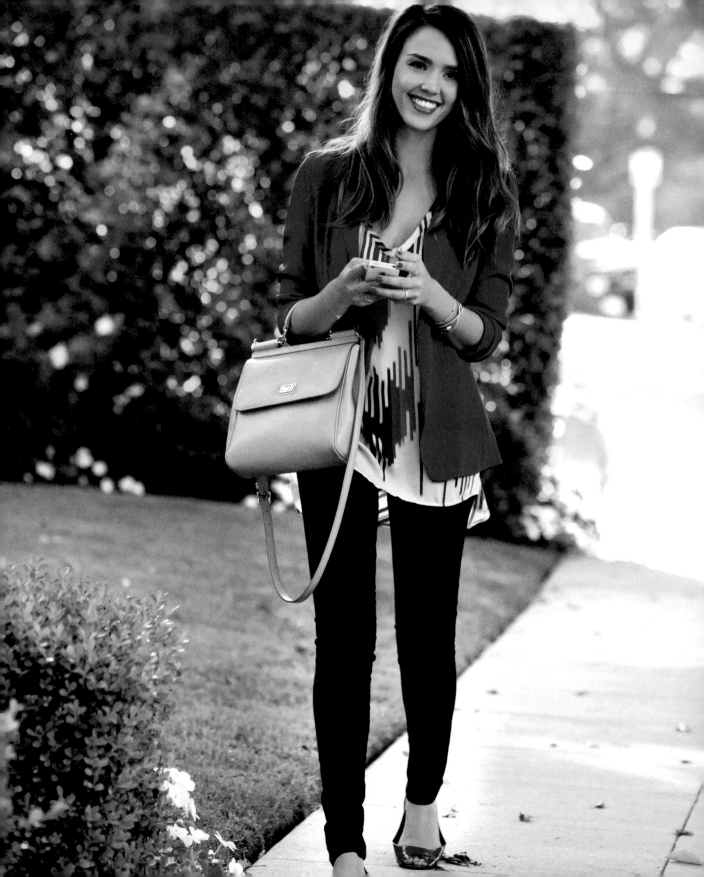

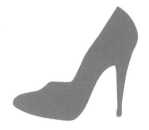

chapter 4

HONEST
style

CURATE YOUR
CLOSET AND
FIND YOUR
SIGNATURE STYLE

IT'S NO SECRET THAT I LOVE FASHION. AND ONE OF THE best things about fashion, beauty, and style of any kind is that it's always changing—I love how my definition of style has evolved since I reached my thirties and even more so since I became a mom. But first, a quick flashback.

You wouldn't think it now, but as a little girl, I was a total tomboy. My major passions were baseball, He-Man and She-Ra, and the ThunderCats. Plus I spent a ton of time watching *Batman* reruns and playing my own make-believe games as those characters. I wanted to be an action hero—*not* one of the girl characters. I was not into princesses or dress-up or needing to be rescued by Prince Charming. Punky Brewster and Madonna were my fashion icons as a kid—it was all about the mismatched scrunchy socks and LA Gear sneakers. I'd wear a pair of heels from my mom's closet out to the living room—and then lose them for my dance routines. Outside of dress-up for a performance with my brother and cousins, I felt like heels were impractical. *You can't even run in them!*

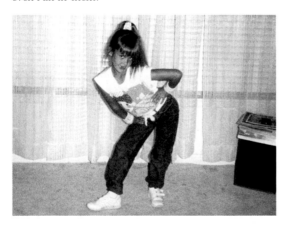

Working my Punky Brewster style!

I got more interested in clothes as I got older. I was funky, not prissy, and preferred tomboyish versions of hippie chic—think if Madonna and Prince had a love child, with a dash of Stevie Nicks and Gwen Stefani. Slip dresses and combat boots, ripped jeans with bedazzled embellishments, Pepe jeans and body suits—you get the idea. During my teenage years and even in my twenties, it felt like everyone expected me to be the tough, sexy action girl because of my character in *Dark Angel*. To me, she was almost a dude—tough, yes, but totally unemotional and barely aware of her sexuality, unless she needed to use it for a hot second to break somebody's neck. Since I was young and still figuring out how *I* felt about my appearance, it was weird to be forced into that box. All that pressure and attention made me super critical and self-conscious of my looks.

Before I had babies, I worried constantly that my body's days would be numbered. But as it turns out, getting older and having kids have only made me much more comfortable in my own skin. A few years ago, I couldn't even use the word "sexy" to describe myself without feeling funny and awkward. Now that I've had two kids, my idea of physical perfection has changed completely—and I finally feel confident, secure, and, yes, sexy.

Now that I've had two kids, my idea of physical perfection has changed completely.

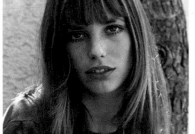
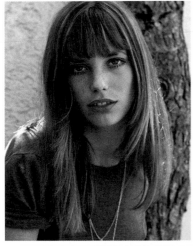
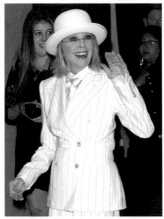

MY STYLE ICONS

JANE BIRKIN: This English actress, singer, and style icon almost singlehandedly created the bohemian-chic look.

DIANE KEATON: She's always had such a clear sense of her own style—she took menswear and gave it a unique spin without losing her femininity or sense of fun.

AUDREY HEPBURN: Her striking gamine style helped make daywear and ready-to-wear chic; whether it was a cropped cigarette pant with flats or a knee-length skirt, she always looked graceful and sophisticated.

GRACE KELLY: So ladylike and polished; her flawless style will always be timeless.

KATE MOSS: I love her minimalist, edgy, sexy, and no-fuss taste; no matter if she's wearing the most insane McQueen gown or a slip dress, she's always effortlessly chic.

ANGELA CHASE: Claire Dane's character on *My So-Called Life* rocked layered flannel and combat boots like nobody else. I tried my hardest to emulate her fashion.

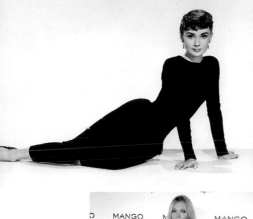
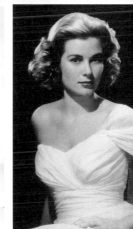
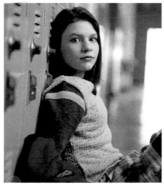
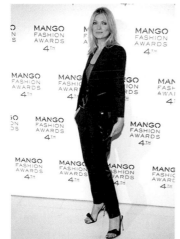

Developing Honest Style

HONEST STYLE ISN'T about pleasing other people with your fashion . . . quite the opposite. It's owning your choices confidently. I love mixing high and low styles, for instance. Of course, I take into account where I'm going and whom I'll be with, but I'm not a slave to trends or expectations. I don't want to look like a store window display or spend 4 hours getting ready to pop out for milk, but I'm also not going to run around in my workout clothes. I want to look pulled together, not schleppy. I wear what makes me happy.

That sounds simple, but it can be tricky. It's easy to get a bit obsessed with what's "hot"—driven by advertising, pop culture, and our own insecurities—and fall into the trap of dressing more for other people's expectations than for ourselves. Think how often you open your closet and say, "I have nothing to wear!" even though this is absolutely false. I promise, your closet is brimming with things that would cover your body beautifully. It's most likely brimming with things that you loved last season, last month, or even last week . . . but now they look dated and you're over it. Maybe they really are worn out—in this age of disposable fashion, clothes are made much more cheaply, and they often fall apart after just a few wears. Or maybe the clothes themselves are fine, but you can't see what you used to love about them because you've stopped

listening to your own authentic sense of style.

Figuring that out is what my definition of Honest Style is all about. Your look shouldn't be the same as your best friend's look, or mine, or the look on page 34 of the J.Crew catalog. Not because those other looks aren't awesome—I get inspired by designers, film heroines, fashion trends, and my friends. This is about taking an idea and putting your own spin on it, in a way that's right for you and your body.

And Honest Style is definitely about making peace with your hips, waistline, bust—or whatever your body hang-ups happen to be. These days, I rarely worry about my flaws because I don't spend a lot of time or energy being negative about my body, period. If something doesn't fit or doesn't work on my body? That's fine. That just means it isn't for me, and I'm on to the next thing that plays to my strengths.

Honest Style is also about being thoughtful about how you shop. Since becoming a mom, I think a little differently about how I consume in every area, and that certainly extends to my closet. It's really exciting to see how the eco-fashion industry is evolving. There are some cool brands and amazing designers (big and small!) who are trying to make their manufacturing processes more sustainable, which I love. Everything we wear has to be farmed (if it's made from a natural fiber like cotton or wool), manufactured, and shipped to stores—so it's great to see companies thinking about how they can lighten up that

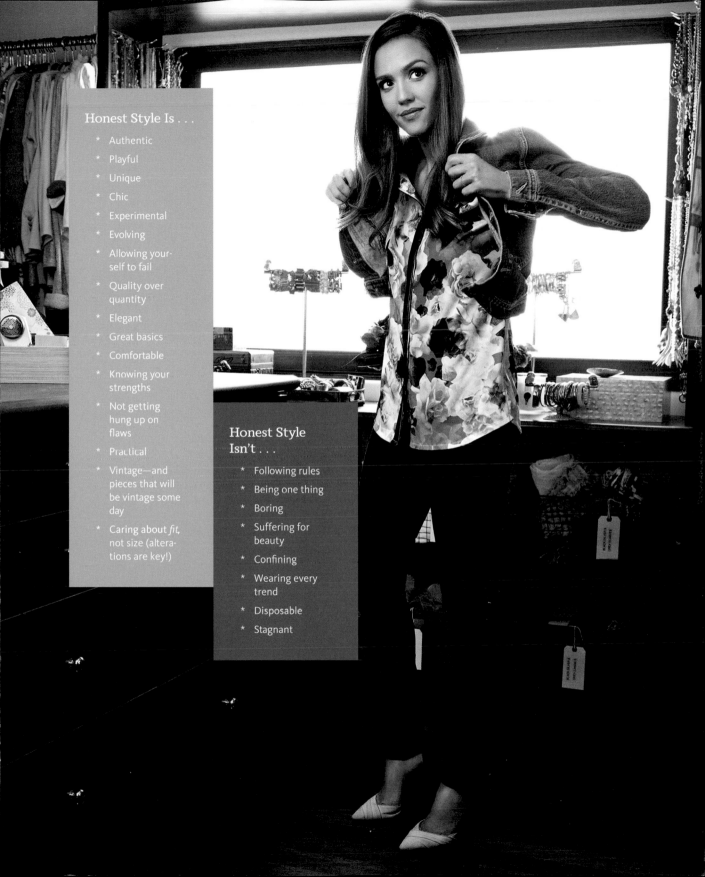

Honest Style Is . . .

* Authentic
* Playful
* Unique
* Chic
* Experimental
* Evolving
* Allowing yourself to fail
* Quality over quantity
* Elegant
* Great basics
* Comfortable
* Knowing your strengths
* Not getting hung up on flaws
* Practical
* Vintage—and pieces that will be vintage some day
* Caring about *fit*, not size (alterations are key!)

Honest Style Isn't . . .

* Following rules
* Being one thing
* Boring
* Suffering for beauty
* Confining
* Wearing every trend
* Disposable
* Stagnant

carbon footprint, whether that means incorporating more organic cotton and safer fabric dyes, or making their business models more socially responsible. But for you and me, it's not necessarily about buying "responsibly." It's also about buying quality—investing in beautiful, well-made pieces that you'll be able to wear for years.

And it's about ending those "I have nothing to wear!" fights with your closet. (Not that these clothing crises *never* happen—when I have to get dressed for a big tech conference or a friend's birthday party, I still get stumped occasionally!) But here is what's important—and this is where my six-year-old tomboy self would so approve: Everything I wear these days is simultaneously about feeling good on the inside and out—yes, even when I'm wearing heels and getting dressed up. If you can't carry yourself well, and you're worried the whole time that something's going to pop out or you can't breathe, then the dress won't look right, no matter how beautiful it is.

So, finding a personal style? Gosh, that can be a bit daunting—there is so much "fashion" to sift through. But the challenge of choosing a signature look that expresses who you really are should be a fun exercise, not a stressful one. It's about figuring out what really inspires you, what you feel fabulous in, and what works for your lifestyle. As you've noticed in previous chapters, I love an expert! So I asked my friends Hillary Kerr and Katherine Power, cofounders of WhoWhatWear.com, for some helpful pointers.

YOUR SHORTCUT TO PERSONAL STYLE

Ready to embrace your best-dressed self? Simply follow our suggestions! —Hillary and Katherine

1. PICK YOUR INSPIRATION

There is one style weapon everyone in the fashion industry uses and that we swear by: the mood board. While we have entire walls of these ever-changing collages, you don't need to dedicate so much space. A bulletin board works, or you can create a Pinterest board and keep it virtual.

* Use anything you like. As for what goes on your board, everything is fair game: runway looks, red carpet shots, street style photos, fashion editorials, movie stills, fabric swatches, album covers, ad campaigns, personal mementos, product shots from your favorite stores—the list is endless.

* Add with abandon. You don't need to understand why you're picking things, just go with your gut instincts. If you like it, pin it.

* Embrace randomness. Your board is all about tapping into your inner desires. It doesn't need to go together or have a theme—in fact, it shouldn't! Don't second-guess yourself; you can always edit it later.

So what does it all mean? Sometimes it's easy to see patterns: If you're pulling lots of fringed suede boots, embellished tunics and caftans, and old photos of Janis Joplin and Anita Pallenberg, you're clearly drawn to a bohemian look. Is your board full of crisp button-up blouses, vintage photos of Lauren Hutton, and lots of chic suits? You like all-American classics. Most people are more of a mishmash, though—and

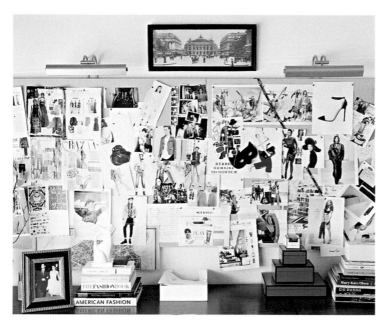

Katherine's inspiration wall at work: a patchwork of magazine tears and mementos.

that's wonderful, too. Don't be afraid to mix together the things you love. For example, you might be drawn to the ladylike look of the 1950s and also adore Kate Moss' dangerously cool style. Though very different on the surface, all it means is that you like to give your girly silhouettes a little edge and should style your full-skirted dresses with some model-off-duty staples, like a cropped leather jacket and super pointy stilettos.

2. FIND YOUR BODY DOUBLE

Not every trend is ideal for every body type—it's sad, but true. That said, if you love a particular look, there's usually a way to adapt it so that it's flattering for your figure. Our suggestion: Make someone else do the work for you by finding your body double. Look for someone—a celeb, fashion blogger, or stylish friend—who shares your basic body type and take note of her most flattering outfits. If you're top heavy and looking for new jeans, see how like-bodied ladies wear them when they're out running errands. (Hint: Go for lower or mid-rise jeans. High-waisted jeans will shorten your torso and make you look squat.) Or maybe you want to buy an of-the-moment dress, but aren't sure if a particular silhouette would work on your petite frame. Simply check out your body double and see what looks she's worn lately.

3. CHOOSE YOUR GO-TO PIECES

Once you've identified your general style and shape, it's time to shop! Our advice is to invest in timeless everyday basics that really fit and flatter, then add personal flair by mixing in a few inexpensive, on-trend pieces. Think about your lifestyle: If you're a busy mom, focus on finding the perfect pair of blue jeans and a trench coat (timeless), then add of-the-moment personality with a print scarf (thrifty thrill). Are you always in the office? You need some gorgeous black pumps and a flawless blazer (timeless), plus a fun bag or clutch in the season's key color (thrifty thrill).

Personal style = fashion inspiration + timeless everday basics + thrifty thrills

Your Guide to the Basics

INVESTING IN HIGH-QUALITY, timeless basics gives you a solid foundation on which to build your Honest Style—think of these as your blank canvas, and now you're free to run wild. (Just remember: Yoga pants are for yoga!) You'll also save money in the long run because with a good core wardrobe, you don't need to constantly top up with cheaply made "disposable fashion" that doesn't last (and isn't very sustainable)—not that I'm against an occasional fun splurge!

A FITTED BLAZER

Blazers are a quick and easy way to look chic. Pair one with an A-line dress, maxi skirt, and tank or T-shirt and jeans. It's really one of the most versatile staples in your closet. Whether it's a cropped boxy blazer or fitted boyfriend blazer, make sure the silhouette complements your look. With one in navy or black, you've always got an insta-outfit, something professional for work, drinks, or what have you. At the high end, I love Céline, Narciso Rodriguez, and Givenchy; for more budget-minded options, check out J.Crew, Topshop, H&M, and the boys' section at Brooks Brothers.

THE LITTLE BLACK DRESS

Every girl needs a good go-to for a night out with friends or a romantic date. Azzedine Alaïa or Dolce & Gabbana if you're going there (Tory Burch and Diane von Furstenberg also have beautiful options); J.Crew, Theory, or Target if you're not.

YOUR PERFECT JEANS

I say *your* perfect jeans, because you're going to have to kiss a lot of toads to find the brand that cuts just right for your body. Right now I'm loving slim boyfriend jeans because you can wear them out at night with heels (so chic!) and they're comfy for day. Avoid crazy stitching and bedazzling on the back pockets; a little stretch is nice because it hugs your curves. Skip the low-cut that shows off your undies—that's one reason high-waisted can look so cute. You can't go wrong with Levi's if you don't want to drop a lot of cash; the Gap is great, too. For premium denim, I love Sevens, J Brand, Earnest Sewn . . . the list goes on.

A DENIM JACKET

Some years it's out, but it always comes back. I like it pretty shrunken and fitted to wear over flowy dresses and skirts (my fave is by Elizabeth and James). You can also never go wrong with a black leather moto jacket—Ralph Lauren and Simone make great ones— timelessly chic!

A SMART COAT

So worth the investment—if you live in a cold climate, your outerwear is all people see half the year! Look for quality stitching, heavy buttons, nice linings— these are signs that your coat will last for decades. This is also a place to go vintage (you might need to have a new lining sewn in— any tailor can do this) because then you know it already *has* lasted for decades. Plus retro coats are just adorable.

BASIC T-SHIRTS OR TANKS

Figure out a neckline and sleeve length that works with your body and cleavage-showing preferences. Then buy tons in white, gray, and black, to layer. I love C&C California, LNA, and Cheap Monday— and Target's long and lean tanks hold their shape surprisingly well for under 10 bucks a pop.

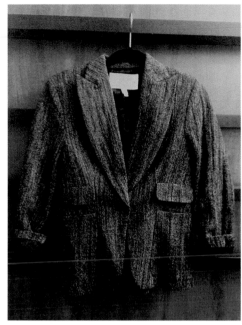

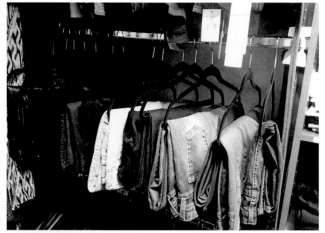

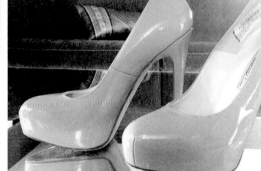

Good basics end
those "I have nothing
to wear!" fights

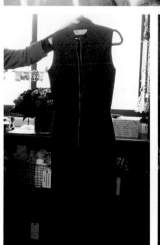

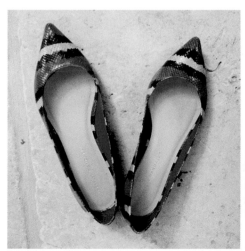

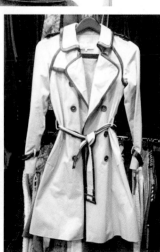

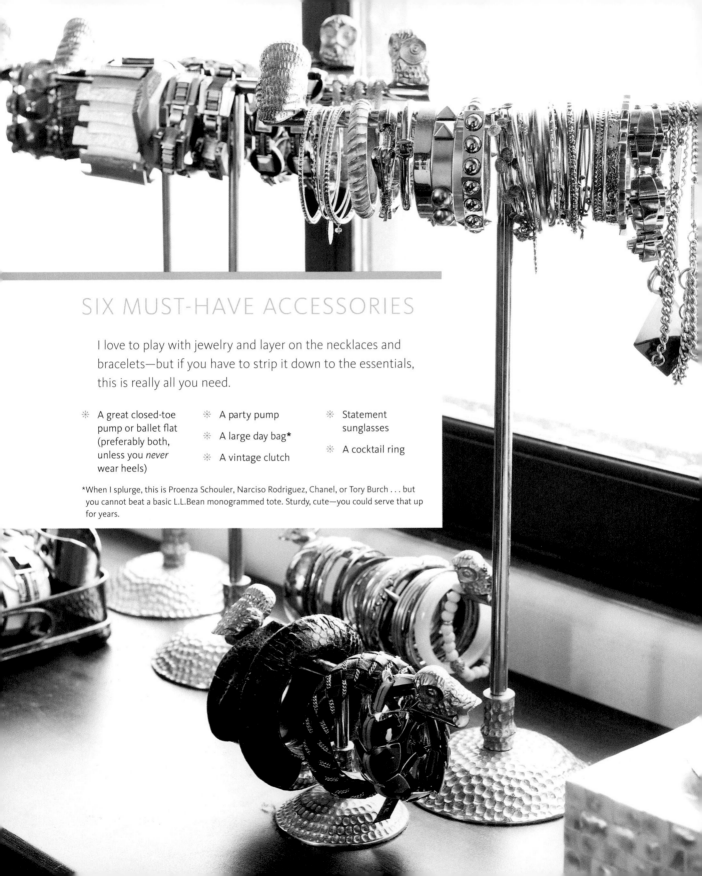

SIX MUST-HAVE ACCESSORIES

I love to play with jewelry and layer on the necklaces and bracelets—but if you have to strip it down to the essentials, this is really all you need.

* A great closed-toe pump or ballet flat (preferably both, unless you *never* wear heels)
* A party pump
* A large day bag*
* A vintage clutch
* Statement sunglasses
* A cocktail ring

*When I splurge, this is Proenza Schouler, Narciso Rodriguez, Chanel, or Tory Burch . . . but you cannot beat a basic L.L.Bean monogrammed tote. Sturdy, cute—you could serve that up for years.

Honest Organization

YOU CAN HAVE all of the Honest Style in the world—but if your closet is a hot mess, there's no helping you. When we moved into our current house, I was determined to finally have my dream closet—and actually, I'm lucky enough to now have two: one for every day, where I keep all my jeans and work clothes, and one for the stuff I wear to events . . . plus my collection of shoes and boots and a separate area for my purses.

But trust me: You do not need a fancy walk-in closet to stay styled. The key organizing principles of my closet would apply to any space, whether you're working with a standard-size closet, a rolling garment rack and a dresser, or an armoire. I don't think organization should be rocket science. Most of this is good old-fashioned common sense—the way your grandma, or mine, would have kept her closets tidy (if she'd had a label maker!).

LABEL!

The label maker is probably our household's most prized possession. Everything in my closet is labeled. This makes putting away laundry fast (and foolproof when it's your husband's turn . . .) and finding what you need even faster. For items that need to be stored in boxes, like purses, I take Polaroids and attach the pics to the outside of the container. No more wondering where you stashed last summer's beaded clutch.

This is also *essential* when it comes to your kids' closets, by the way. Plus if you use pictures (and then upgrade to simple words when the kids are a bit older), you can get your little ones to help put things away themselves—and isn't that the dream?

KEEP LIKE WITH LIKE

Does this ever happen? You want to wear a skirt—but as you're digging for skirt options, you get distracted by those black pants or boyfriend jeans you keep meaning to wear. When I want a skirt, I just head directly to the skirt end of my closet. I don't let myself get sidetracked by poking around in jeans or dresses. This is a huge time-saver when you're trying to lay out outfits in a hurry or if you're overagonizing about what to wear for a certain event. (There is definitely such a thing as too much choice!) Within each category, I hang garments by style and color. So yes, all my skinny jeans are stored together—and all my colored skinny jeans are grouped separately from the regular blue jeans.

DISPLAY ACCESSORIES

Find a shelf, a windowsill, or the back of your closet door—any surface where you can keep your necklaces, bracelets, and earrings *out* where you can see them, instead of stuffed inside boxes tucked into drawers. For one thing, accessories are pretty! You can have fun with this—paint a couple of old (empty) picture frames, hang them on a wall, then arrange your necklaces on nails inside each frame. Or pin earrings on a pretty fabric-covered corkboard. I keep my bracelets grouped together on a simple stand, and I hang

Give clothes room to breathe—if they're too jammed, it's time to edit!

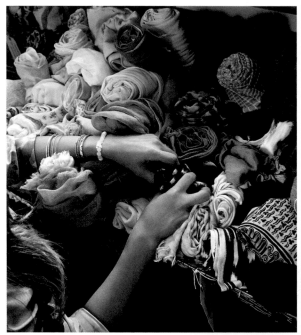

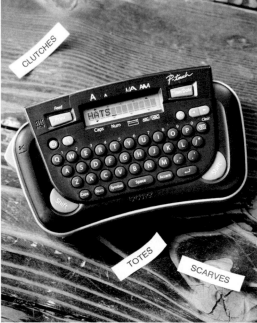

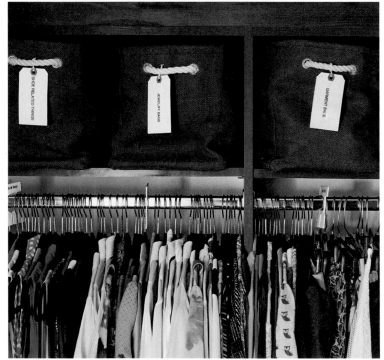

THE HONEST CLOSET

1. Roll your scarves into neat bundles to keep them smooth and wrinkle free. (Never crush or fold such delicate fabrics!)

2. I am a firm believer that you cannot overlabel things. (My family might disagree.)

3. Fabric baskets are great for filling that hard-to-use top shelf in your closet. Use them to sort workout clothes, tights, socks, belts, beach stuff, and other items that you don't use daily but still need handy and are hard to hang or fold.

my necklaces on hooks. When you can see what you've got to work with, accessorizing becomes *styling*, which is really a kind of art. Bonus points if you can position a floor-length mirror nearby—that makes it easier to quickly try combinations with any given outfit and play around.

STEAM, DON'T IRON

Professional stylists swear by their steamers—you'll see them on every photo shoot. They are much gentler on delicate fabrics and work far more quickly than irons (yet are more effective than the old "hang it up while you shower" trick!). I recommend tucking one into your closet. That way, you can pull it out and let it warm up while you're doing your hair or finalizing accessory choices, then give everything a quick steam before you pop it on.

USE THE RIGHT STORAGE TOOLS

If you buy wallet-friendly shoes, shoe trees will help them last longer; if you buy pricey shoes, shoe trees ensure you'll get your money's worth. These tools help footwear hold its shape and keeps leather from sagging.

For anything fragile or very expensive—evening gowns, vintage pieces, nice suits—don't keep them in the plastic bags from the dry cleaners. (In fact, don't let those plastic bags in your house! See "Dry-Cleaning Don'ts," right.) Do keep these items protected from humidity, sun, dust, pets, sticky-fingered kids, and so on. Fabric garment bags—even ones fashioned from old cotton sheets—give your special clothes the protection they deserve.

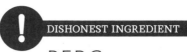

DISHONEST INGREDIENT

PERC

FOUND IN: Most dry cleaning formulas

WHAT IS IT? A colorless, nonflammable solvent used to clean delicate fabrics

WHY IS IT SKETCHY? Perc off-gasses when it's exposed to air, which means we can breathe it in. Short-term exposure can cause dizziness, fatigue, sweating, and headaches. Long-term exposure may cause liver and kidney damage, memory loss, and cancer. Yikes!

DRY-CLEANING DON'TS

I dry-clean as little as possible; sweaters and jackets can absolutely be worn several times before you send them to the cleaners, and even most cocktail dresses can survive at least two wearings. This is better for your clothes because the chemicals in dry cleaning start wearing them down. It's also better for your health.

Dry cleaning involves toxic chemicals like PERC that may be linked to cancer and reproductive damage. When you do dry-clean clothes, ask the cleaners to skip the plastic bags (which just seal in fumes), then hang everything outside to air for an hour or so before you put them away. Better yet, look for "green" or "eco" dry cleaners, which are popping up everywhere, thanks to new demand for a healthier alternative.

How to Rock Vintage

IF YOU WANT to shop and dress more sustainably, vintage is a great place to start. After all, it's the ultimate form of recycling!

You reclaim and reuse clothes that might otherwise have lived out their days in a Goodwill bin or, worse, a landfill. (It would shock my Depression-era grandma to her core, but people really do throw away clothes—almost 100 pounds of them every year.)

But vintage can be a bit intimidating if you haven't gone there before. Here's my advice:

START WITH JEWELRY

This is the best entry point for anyone new to vintage. It doesn't smell, there are few size issues, and it's almost always fabulous. In fact, most new jewelry today is a reinterpretation of older styles—so why not go with the originals? In particular, I tend to buy lots of silver pieces this way—I think they age better than some other types of metals.

THEN MOVE TO PURSES

Bags, and other accessories like scarves and hats, are another not-so-scary way in to vintage. You don't have to use vintage every day, but you can find something great for evenings out or for retro flair on your beach trip.

ALWAYS SHOP WITH A PURPOSE

Flea markets and thrift stores can be overwhelming and chaotic. If you have a goal in mind ("beaded cardigans" or "Pucci scarves"), it's a lot easier to wade through racks and bins and zero in on the good stuff.

SHOP ONLINE

There are no awkward in-person haggling sessions or musty dressing rooms to contend with on eBay or Etsy Vintage. The downside is you can't inspect the goods in person before you buy—so always check a seller's ratings and feedback to make sure he or she seems legit. Bonus: You'll avoid the extra price markup of the retail store.

MAKE FRIENDS WITH YOUR TAILOR

That frees you up to consider purchasing anything a size or two too big—especially if it's a deal. Having the garment altered will add to the total cost, but you'll end up with a one-of-a-kind piece.

 HONEST TIP

SHOE STORAGE TRICK

I always line up my shoes the way you see here, with one heel facing out. They take up less space this way (meaning you can have so many more pairs—yay!). Plus I'm always considering heel height when I plan an outfit, so it's helpful to know at a glance what I'm dealing with. (I keep all my flats together on another wall—if I need to walk a lot, I don't even contemplate the heels!)

When you wear vintage, you never have to worry about showing up in the same dress as someone else.

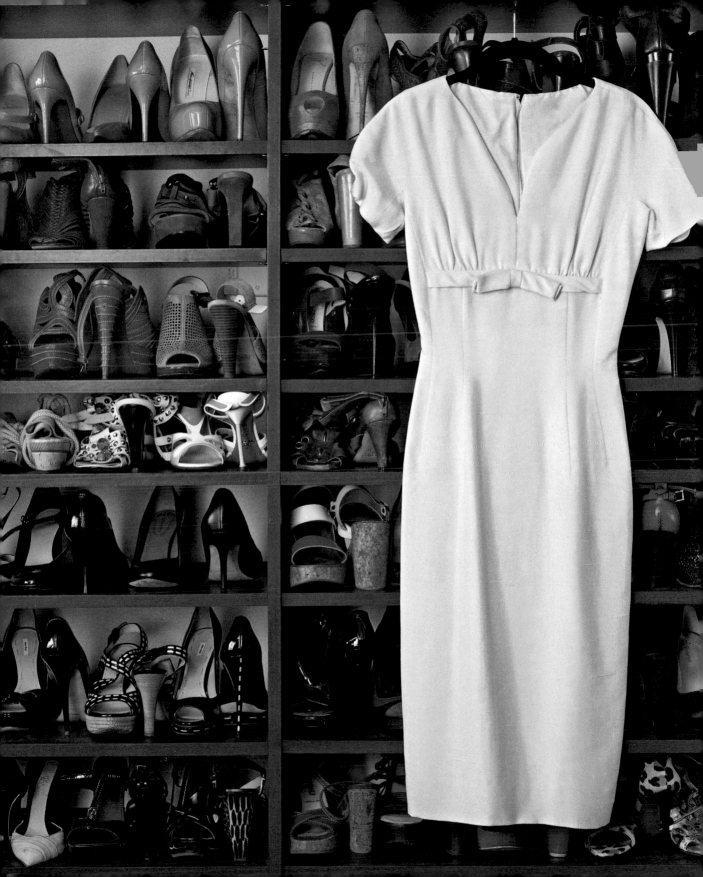

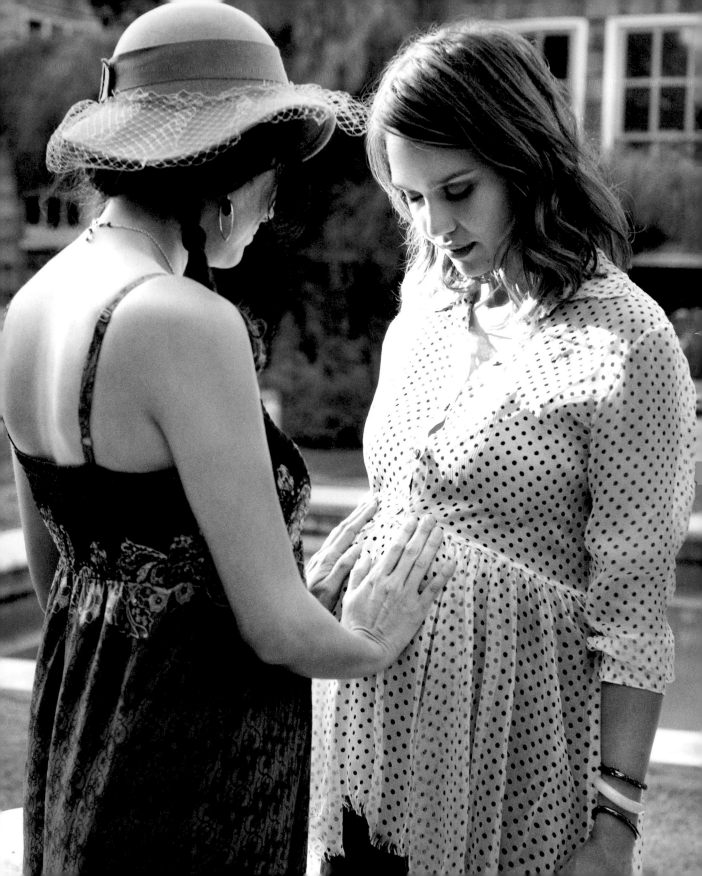

Pregnancy Style

GETTING DRESSED WHEN you're pregnant is a whole new ballgame. Your old clothes stop fitting fast. And no, you can't necessarily wear the same looks (especially if you loved, say, a fitted button-down shirt or sky-high stilettos) because they just won't feel or look good right now. But that's okay. Your body is growing a person! Give it the respect it deserves and dress so that you and that bump are comfortable—you absolutely can still look like your gorgeous self. It's a little daunting at first, but it's also an opportunity to try styles you might not have bothered with before when you couldn't, oh, fill them out.

PLAY WITH PROPORTIONS

I did a lot of fitted jackets over full skirts and dresses; think empire-waist maxidress with a denim jacket or cardigan. (Your pre-baby cardigan will be snugger but luckily it's just a layering piece so you don't need to button it.)

You can also flip the look and pair a flowy peasant top with leggings or skinny jeans.

EMBRACE THE V-NECK

Depending on your pre-pregnancy shape, a voluptous chest might be a new experience for you—it was for me! Go with it and work your new assets, honey! V-necks, camisoles, and scoop necks are your new allies. So are bold statement necklaces.

WHEN IN DOUBT, WEAR A WRAP DRESS

You can adjust it as your belly grows—and cinch it back in afterward.

Such a versatile piece works on almost every body—I have several, in solid colors and cute prints, for each season. My favorites are by Diane von Furstenberg.

WEDGES ARE YOUR NEW BEST FRIENDS

As your due date approaches and your center of gravity shifts, you might find that heels may not feel as great as they used to. I wore a lot of flats, but there are times when you'll want to make your legs look longer. Enter wedges, and boom: sexy, no suffering. Keep in mind that you may need to wear a half size larger during your later months or you'll pay the blister price.

INVEST IN PIECES YOU CAN WEAR AGAIN

Think pull-on skirts, long layering tanks, oversize men's dress shirts, and a bold lipstick collection.

SISTERHOOD OF THE TRAVELING MATERNITY PANTS

Cute maternity clothes cost a fortune, and it stings to spend that much on stuff you'll only be able to wear for a couple of months. After I had Honor, I stuck all of my pregnancy jeans, bras, Spanx, and more in a bin . . . and before I knew it, I was passing it on to a girlfriend who had just become pregnant. That bin got passed along to another mom and then another. At least four people wore my pregnancy clothes, and then they came back around to me for Haven. When you calculate the cost per use, they're now a downright bargain!

New Mommy Style

AS A MOM, it's so easy to fall into that trap of yoga pants and unwashed hair. After all, any outfit you put together is likely to end up covered in puke or poop. Why bother? Because you are a person as well as a mama. And putting on a clean top (even if it stays that way for 5 minutes) or some cute earrings will remind you of that important fact.

INVEST IN GOOD NURSING BRAS

Because nothing kills your mojo like nursing bras that look like . . . nursing bras. My favorites are by Elle Macpherson—they are so beautiful, you'd never know they're for nursing! Avoid underwire, which may interfere with your milk production.

EMBRACE YOUR PREGNANCY JEANS FOR A LITTLE WHILE LONGER

It's really okay! Every body bounces back differently after pregnancy, and you need to be patient with yourself. This is why you invested in those hot maternity jeans in the first place—so you wouldn't hate having to wear them for a while.

SCARVES!

These are one of my signatures. I wear them constantly because they're the easiest way to dress up your basic jeans outfit and make sure you have an extra layer on hand in case it gets cold or your baby throws up on you.

AS SOON AS YOU DO GET BACK INTO JEANS—BREAK OUT THE HEELS

Put on a cute top, blow out your hair, throw on a little makeup, call a babysitter, and go on a date. Because yes, you're a mom now, but you're still *you.*

THINK BOOTS AND BALLET FLATS

Platforms aren't really the right move once you're balancing a baby, and even wedges can be precarious when you're lugging diaper bags or chasing after little ones. You want flat, comfy shoes—but that doesn't have to mean you never get out of your sneakers. I love Roger Vivier, Tory Burch, and Toms flats because they're comfortable and adorable; J.Crew and Kate Spade also make great options. If you do go for a heel, pick something chunky and stacked for support.

KEEPING IT REAL

MY SNAP-BACK SECRET

Sometimes, I still do suffer for beauty. Case in point: After both of my pregnancies, I took a tip from my girlfriend Zoya and wore a girdle. Actually, I opted for two corsets layered over each other (Frederick's of Hollywood are my favorite) for the first 3 months, day and night—I only took them off to bathe. I won't lie—it's the worst! You're hot and sweaty and all of that—but it did bring my stomach back down to normal faster than my friends who didn't wrap their post-baby middles. To be clear: This isn't for everyone. But if you've ever wondered how some people get their bodies back so quickly after pregnancy? Well, here's some insight.

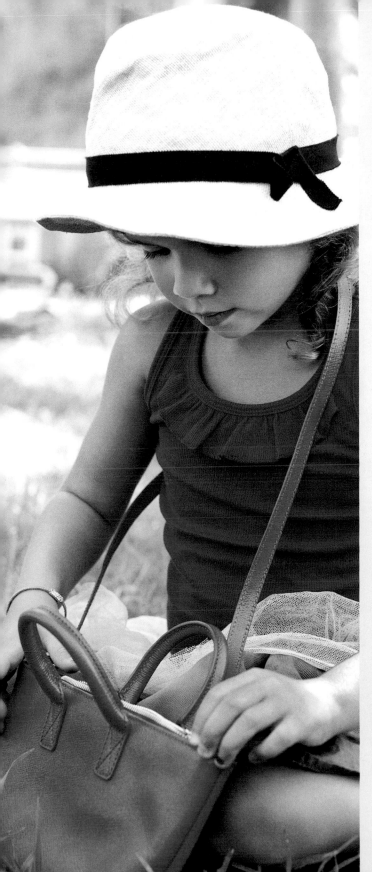

HONEST KIDS STYLE

Basically, with kids, you blink and the pair of shoes or new pants you *just bought* no longer fit. Lately, with Honor, it's been every three months. So as much as I disliked my mom always buying me one size too big when I was a child, now that I'm a mom, I understand what my parents were up against. It can cost a fortune to clothe your little ones. We love to swap clothes with family; there is nothing sweeter than Honor wearing her older cousin Nea's little dress or coat. We hand down Honor's clothes to her younger cousins and eventually they come back to Haven, which is so cool.

There's a health and environmental benefit to dressing your kids in nearly new duds, too. Chemicals used in the manufacturing process (like flame retardants, which are often sprayed on kids' pajamas) will have washed off by the time you get them.

When I do buy new, I try to invest in organic and natural-fiber clothing for the girls. This is getting easier—you can find organic cotton everywhere from Garnet Hill to Walmart now. But my girls absolutely do not wear all organic all the time. It's just too limiting, especially now that they're getting old enough to have opinions. (Let's just say that if there's an organic mermaid costume on the market, I have not been able to find it for Honor.)

At the very least, I suggest picking up a pair of organic cotton pajamas—I adore the ones by Hanna Andersson. Kids spend so much time in their PJs, and this way, you can avoid flame-retardant chemicals. Just make sure the label indicates that the pajamas meet the federal safety requirements for sleepwear (which for most untreated, natural-material jammies means they must be snug fitting).

Chic Everyday Style

As with most busy women, my clothes have to multitask and go from work to play or from day to night. This is where having a developed sense of your own Honest Style really helps. All you need are a few signature pieces you can rely on day in and day out, plus some fun accessories to switch things up. That way, no matter where you go or what you're doing, you'll always look like yourself. And that's appropriate for every occasion!

IF YOU LOVE IT, BUY IT IN MULTIPLES

Some of the most stylish women in the world stick to a basic uniform. It makes getting dressed so much less complicated because you always know at least one outfit will work and look good on you. If I find a T-shirt that fits perfectly (see "Your Guide to the Basics," page 93), I'll buy two, so there's always a clean version in my closet.

LOVE ON COLOR

I do wear a lot of black —but it's easy to end up with a very chic but very neutral and monotone closet. This is where your accessories come in. I'm always doing a pop of color with a scarf, chunky cocktail ring, or bag. And you can layer in multiple colors, too— just keep them in the same tone. So go all neon or all pastel— nothing in between.

PICK AN ACCESSORY FOCAL POINT

If I do big earrings, I leave the big, statement necklace at home. (Though a big ring or bracelet can work.) If I stack layers of skinny rings, I keep everything else more low key.

DRESS FLEXIBLY FOR DAY-TO-EVENING

If you're going to be running around all day and need to make a seamless transition to a dinner party or cocktails, try these ideas:

* **Stash a clutch inside your day bag.** Trust me, it will fit! And don't be afraid to go for an oversized clutch; you can cram a surprising amount of stuff into one.

* **Upgrade your outerwear.** There's nothing about a work blazer that says "party," so switch out your power jacket for something appropriate for your after-hours event. A little leather motorcycle jacket, embellished bolero, or even a sleek tux jacket can transform your work outfit into a cocktail-ready ensemble.

* **Add a bold lipstick.** Any color can work— fire engine red, hot pink, or a vibrant berry; just make sure it complements your skin tone. The look is chicest when worn with a bare face and uncomplicated eyes (mascara, that's it!). If you hate lipstick, play up your eyes instead. A fat eye pencil, the kind that looks like a crayon, is basically foolproof and will make you look like you tried (even if you didn't).

PLAN YOUR OUTFIT THE NIGHT BEFORE.

I always pick out my clothes for the next day before I go to bed. It's such a time-saver in the morning when you can get dressed and go on autopilot!

Stock your car or desk with a mini—makeup bag plus a change of shoes and accessories. Then you can upgrade any outfit from "work" to "play."

MY HONEST SIGNATURES

Eventually, you'll know exactly what you like and how you like to wear it—so you can find easy ways to update your look. Here are a few of my signature pieces that I rarely leave home without.

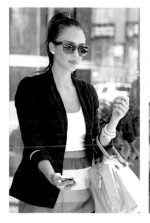 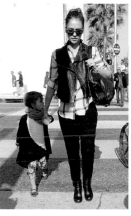 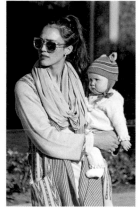 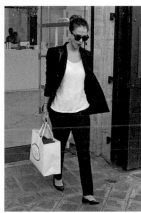

❋ COLOR. I love a chic black look for evening, but for day, I'm all about my pop of color. Red, pink, turquoise, purple . . . they all make me happy.

❋ LAYERS. A great way to make pieces look different in combination and to work surprising contrasts; you can mix different colors, fabrics (I love to pair sweet, floaty florals with deconstructed denim or leather), or shapes (say, a shrunken cardigan over a flowy dress or a tunic over leggings). You probably want to limit your layers to three to avoid too much bulk!

❋ SCARVES. Basically another way to layer—a smart scarf can make any old T-shirt and jeans look more polished. And they're genius for hiding jam smears, juice stains, and other kid grime.

❋ BALLET FLATS. Because during the day I'm running around from meetings to lunch to pick up Honor at school, I'm all about comfy flats—you can be on the move but the look is more polished than flip-flops or sneakers.

❋ A GREAT DAY BAG. To carry my whole life in—be it my tablet and work files or diapers and wipes. Plus my makeup kit and probably a spare scarf, jewelry upgrade, or change of shoes.

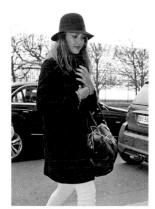

❋ HATS. They're a stylish form of sun protection. A floppy felt hat adds an Ali MacGraw, boho-chic vibe, while a fedora lends a touch of flair.

❋ STATEMENT SUNGLASSES. To finish the look, I have lots of sunglasses. I love to mix it up with chunky frames, metal frames, or color, depending on my outfit.

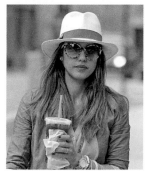

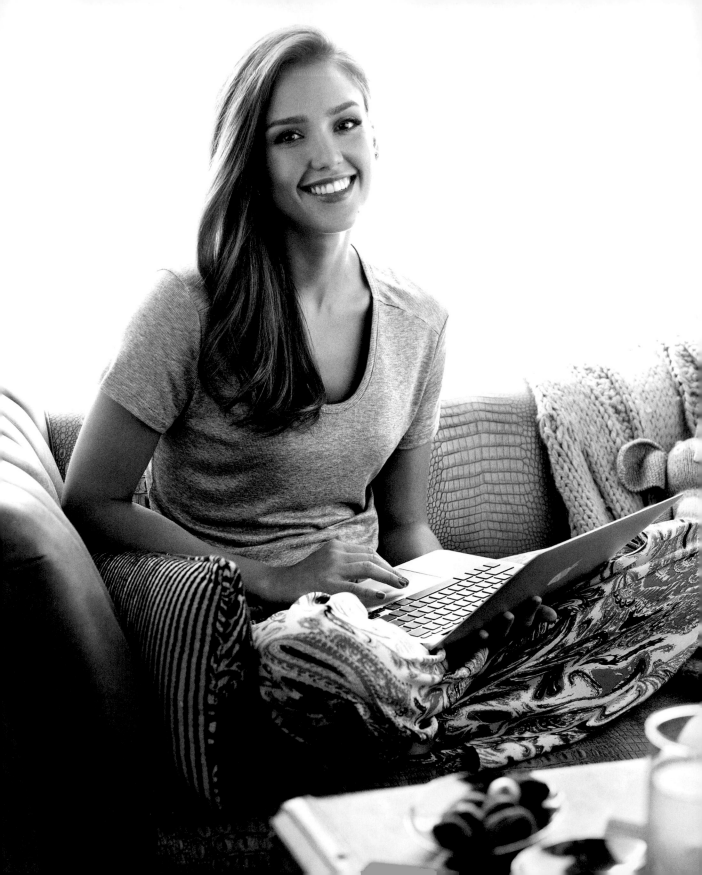

chapter 5

HONEST
home

CREATE A SPACE
THAT'S COZY, CLEAN,
AND TOTALLY YOU

ONE DAY, SOON AFTER I HAD HONOR, MY GIRLFRIEND Ramona Braganza—who is a personal trainer I met when I was 17 while working on a TV show—came over for a workout. As usual, we were chatting (I need to be distracted when I'm exercising!), and she told me about another client of hers, who'd also just had a baby.

"You should see her house now—it's amazing! It's all organic, natural, and eco-friendly," she said.

I looked around. We had just finished a big pre-Honor renovation on our house, too: PVC-free vinyl chairs that wipe clean, couches stuffed with nontoxic filler and covered with flame-retardant-free fabric, organic area rugs? Check. Nontoxic wallpapers? Check. No-VOC paint? Check again. (Don't worry, I'll tell you what all that stuff means in a minute!) "Mona, *my house* is organic, natural, and eco-friendly!" I said.

She looked a little confused. "Really? Because in her house . . . everything is *beige* or *white*."

Oh, right.

So I'd really love to know: Who made this design rule that if it's going to be eco, it's got to be beige, brown, muted, or full of earth tones? If that's truly your style, great. Layer on your neutrals, paint all your floors white, arrange your books in architectural stacks, and be your bad minimalist self. But our house is a fun, busy, kid-friendly place. We have yellow-and-gold wallpaper in the kitchen, deep blues and browns in our den—where we cozy up to watch movies and play board games—and pink and purple *everything* in Honor's room.

I love to play with colors and patterns in home design just as much as I do with fashion. After spending countless hours living in hotels, I find I gravitate toward that kind of cleanliness and organization, where everything has a place. But I also crave personality and coziness, because hotel spaces can be so impersonal and sterile—it's always been important to me to create my own sense of space where I can return home. And

everywhere I travel, I fall in love with a new aesthetic—the Midcentury Modern ranch houses in Southern California, a modern beachy condo I lived in when I was in Australia, the old-world classic Provençal style my mother-in-law inhabits in the south of France, or the unbelievable hand-carved teak furniture you see in Indonesia. The place that most inspired me when I was first figuring out my home style was the bar at Round Hill, a resort in Montego Bay, Jamaica. It was designed by Ralph Lauren and has such a sense of history—so many famous writers, artists, and musicians have lived there—but it doesn't feel like a cloistered museum. Instead, it's light and airy, with lots of open space and this great juxtaposition of heavy, dark wood and clean, white linens with bold pops of color like turquoise or royal blue.

In every space I decorate, I'm always playing with that relationship—how do you keep the space clean, light, and uncluttered yet also layer in plenty of warmth and personality? In our current house, I struck the balance by using lots of textured fabrics and wallpapers and by finding interesting-shaped lighting while keeping the overall color scheme on the lighter side of the palette.

And as much as I want color and style, I also need everything that I bring into our home to be completely safe and healthy—and this cannot be a compromise. Our home is our sanctuary at the end of busy workdays and must be a calm, welcoming place. But even more important, it's where our daughters spend most of their time. Babies' and little kids' bodies are growing and developing *so* rapidly—any exposure to chemicals that can harm development can do maximum damage at this time. And babies breathe in twice as much as adults (per pound of body weight), so if the air they're breathing is polluted with harmful toxins, they're getting a double dose. You might think of air pollution as an outdoor problem—I sure used to, growing up in the "Inland Empire" just outside of LA with its awful smog situation—but it turns out that tons of household items release fumes or off-gas chemicals that pollute the indoor air as well. Not to mention, little kids often have an even more direct route of exposure since they'll put everything they can reach into their mouths. In the next chapter, we'll talk more specifically about the best nontoxic teething toys and other gear for babies and young children. For now, consider this chapter your whole-house guide to developing your home's style *and* ensuring that you're decorating and maintaining it in the safest and healthiest ways possible.

We transformed a bunch of flea market and Craigslist finds into a library. Here, I found a vintage suitcase that's fastened to a table.

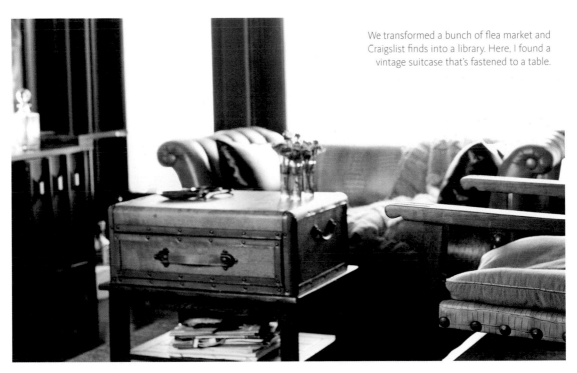

"Have nothing in your home that you do not know to be useful or believe to be beautiful."
—William Morris

Hip, Healthy Home Design

"**Have nothing in your home** that you do not know to be useful or believe to be beautiful." That's a design rule from the famous British designer (and pioneer of the Arts and Crafts Movement) William Morris, which I try to keep in mind whenever I'm considering something new for our home . . . or editing what we already have because clutter is starting to pile up!

Just like Honest Style, Honest Home style is intensely personal—you'll never walk into my house and wonder if you've stepped into a home décor catalog. Nothing against any one store—I've pulled my home's look from all sorts of sources, from mass market (I love Target's Missoni plates!) to flea market to handmade to designer vintage. I'll definitely get ideas from catalog pages and tons of other places, but then it's all about how I can put my own spin on it and make it unique.

When you have a really strong sense of your own aesthetic, you make fewer design mistakes—which is more sustainable in the long term. You don't find yourself getting sick of a room after six months or a year and wanting to redecorate it completely. At the same time, you understand that your home is a living, breathing space and it's always evolving—there's no "done"—so tweaks are always fair game because that's how we keep a space fresh and functional for our family's evolving needs.

Whenever I travel, shop, eat in a new restaurant, or even just walk down a city block I haven't explored before, I'm always keeping an eye out for inspiration—some of the things I love most in my house have been accidental finds, like the vintage postcards I stumbled on at a New York City flea market or colorful fabrics at a thrift store in France. Here are more ways to find inspiration, develop your eye for interior decorating, and hone your own style.

Everything you see in this picture I bought used. The woodsy chandelier was forest green but I spray-painted it silver. The chairs were upholstered with an ugly silk fabric but I recovered them in an outdoor-safe, PVC-free vinyl. Each one was under $30!

KNOW YOUR REFERENCES

All the furniture you see in stores today was inspired by something old—so why not go for the real thing instead? The key is to know what the looks you like today are referencing from the past. This helps me zero in on the right shapes and styles when I'm in a cluttered antiques store or flea market.

IF YOU LIKE:	HUNT FOR:
Modern/Minimalist	Midcentury Modern
Shabby Chic	English Tudor
Glam	Hollywood Regency, Art Deco

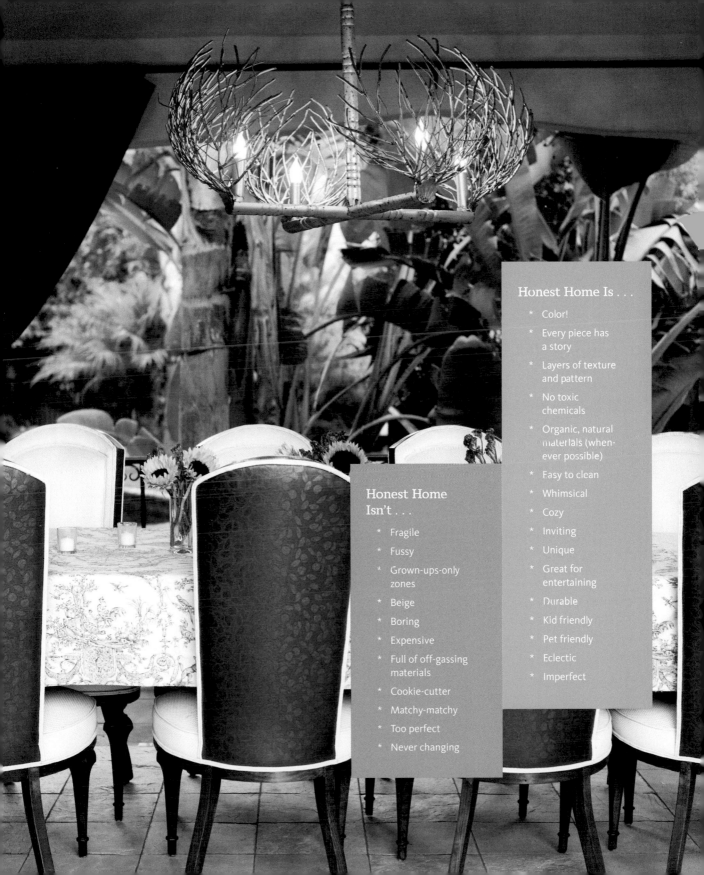

Honest Home Isn't . . .

* Fragile
* Fussy
* Grown-ups-only zones
* Beige
* Boring
* Expensive
* Full of off-gassing materials
* Cookie-cutter
* Matchy-matchy
* Too perfect
* Never changing

Honest Home Is . . .

* Color!
* Every piece has a story
* Layers of texture and pattern
* No toxic chemicals
* Organic, natural materials (whenever possible)
* Easy to clean
* Whimsical
* Cozy
* Inviting
* Unique
* Great for entertaining
* Durable
* Kid friendly
* Pet friendly
* Eclectic
* Imperfect

ANATOMY OF AN INSPIRATION BOOK

Before I decorate a room, I always compile an inspiration book. In fact, even once a room is "done" (except it's never really done!), I'll refer to the book whenever I want to make a tweak or a more major update to remember what my initial idea was and ensure I'm staying on track. This is because whether I'm working with an interior designer or not—at the end of the day, my house is all me. And I can fall in love with everything if I'm not careful . . . so I've found inspiration books are the best tools to help me stay within my original theme and not go off the deep end, trying to cram too many ideas into a room at once.

I like to build my inspiration books the old-fashioned way: on paper. I do mine as collages—they're almost like scrapbooks! It becomes a fun creative project where I can involve Honor—I love that when we made the book for Haven's room, Honor added her own artwork to the cover. It was a cool way to start talking to her about the new baby and becoming a big sister. But I also find tons of inspiration online at Pinterest and other sites that let you create virtual inspiration boards—this is so helpful when you're trying to remember where on earth you saw that specific type of recycled glass bathroom tile or whatever.

Here's a peek at one of my inspiration books, with tips on how to create your own.

✳ TEARS FROM MAGAZINES. I'm a magazine junkie. I read everything from the kitchen renovation guides you find in the supermarket to *Lonny* (an online shelter magazine; lonnymag.com) and *Milk* (an amazing French children's design mag; milkmagazine. net). Don't limit yourself to design mags only—I'm often tearing out catalog pages, cool advertisements, fashion spreads shot in gorgeous locations, and more. Sometimes, I pull out a specific idea I want to try—like pictures of tree decals behind a crib, which is what we did in Haven's room. But I also keep an eye out for less literal inspiration photos, like a bouquet of flowers or a sunset that inspires a color scheme.

✳ FABRIC SNIPPETS. These might be real fabric or pictures of it—either way, use them to represent potential color schemes or ideas of how you want to use fabric (favorite curtain styles, flag bunting, framed as art, etc.), plus, of course, the actual linens you'll want to source for the room.

✳ GRAPHIC ELEMENTS. Stencil lettering and glitter are obviously optional! But they make the inspiration book more fun . . . and they do end up subtly informing my design projects. In Haven's room, we added a string of lights around the perimeter of her ceiling for a little touch of nighttime glitter that also helps soothe her to sleep.

✳ NOTES. I don't write a ton on my inspiration books, but a little note here and there (to remind yourself why you love an image or to keep track of a specific thought on how you want to use it) can be helpful when revisiting a page later on.

✳ PAINT CHIPS. Free at any hardware store or home improvement center, chips are the best way to play around with color combos. Stockpile a bunch in a little box or if you use them a lot, you might consider putting them all on a key ring or even investing in a Pantone Color Chart—I organize mine by room and color scheme in baggies! Chips are also great for craft projects, gift tags, place cards . . .

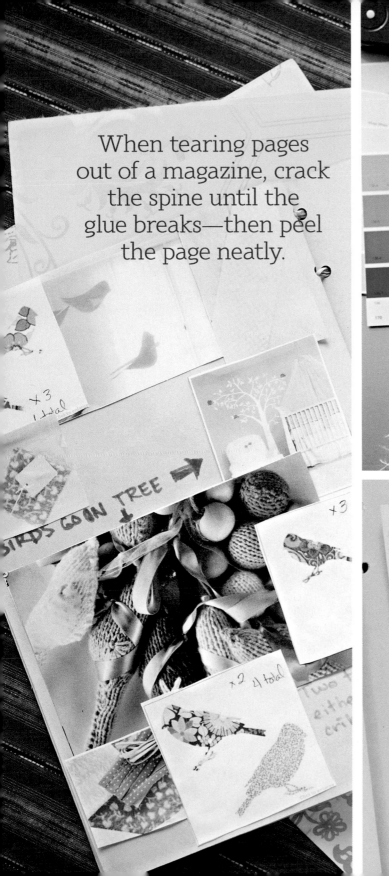

When tearing pages out of a magazine, crack the spine until the glue breaks—then peel the page neatly.

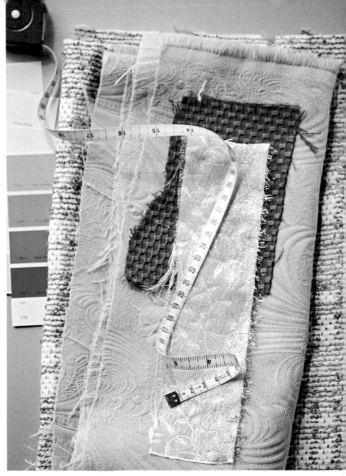

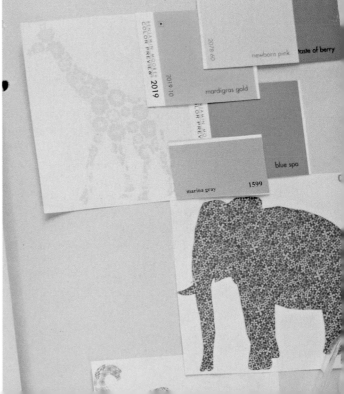

Pure & Simple: Stylish, Sustainable Home

WHETHER YOU'RE in the market for new sheets or undergoing a major renovation project, here's what to look for when you're making a home décor purchase—plus some of my favorite brands. See "The Honest Details" (page 207) for resources.

FLOORS

Safer carpets. Skip wall-to-wall carpet—it's too toxic because it releases (or "off-gasses"—you're going to hear me use this word a lot!) chemicals from the glue and synthetic fibers. FLOR modular carpet tiles are made with renewable and recyclable materials and are endlessly customizable—and if you spill something on your wall-to-wall tile carpet, you can simply swap out one tile to have it cleaned or replaced, no problem! For area rugs, I look for natural fibers made from pesticide-free wool, cotton, jute, hemp, coir, cornhusk, coconut fiber, or woven silk. You can easily remove them to clean and air outside. Vintage area rugs are fantastic—old wool rugs (especially oriental) were most likely made without synthetic fibers and coatings and they're gorgeous. Your house instantly looks lived-in and stylish. For new, I like Capel Rugs, which offers a huge selection of rugs, even hand-braided, that are made in the USA so they don't guzzle energy being shipped from halfway across the world.

Sustainable floors. If you're having your existing hardwood floors refinished, consider skipping the usual (super-toxic!) polyurethane coating in favor of a PVC-free finish like tung oil or the polywhey floor finishes from Vermont Natural Coatings.

If you're installing new floors, look for sustainably harvested hardwood (it should be certified by the Forest Stewardship Council), or consider cork, which is a highly renewable resource. We used this in Honor's room—I prefer the floating floors, which click together and don't require toxic glues or adhesives. I also love salvaged wood floors, which repurpose old wood (often from barns or vintage flooring), though they can get very expensive; the Vintage Wood Floor Company is a great resource.

WALLS

No-VOC paint. You know that new-paint smell? That's the scent of harmful chemicals! Always look for a no-odor paint—then read the label to make sure the manufacturer has really taken out the nasty stuff (instead of just masking it with yet more chemicals). My absolute favorite is Mythic Paint, which is completely zero-VOC (which means it doesn't contain any "volatile organic compounds"— see page 133—and is also free of many other toxins), is ultralow in odor, and comes in tons of gorgeous colors. But pretty much every brand has a no-VOC

DISHONEST INGREDIENT

FORMALDEHYDE

FOUND IN: Kitchen cabinets, carpeting, mattresses

WHAT IS IT AGAIN? A preservative

WHY IS IT SKETCHY? Chronic, long-term exposure has been linked to cancer, plus it can trigger more immediate allergic reactions, rashes, asthma, nosebleeds, and other respiratory issues.

line now, so make sure you opt for that, no matter what.

Toxin-free wallpaper. Many wallpapers are made from vinyl and require toxic adhesives—even after these glues dry, they continue to off-gas for years (it takes about two years for vinyl wallpaper's fumes to completely dissipate). Instead, try to find nonvinyl paper, organic cotton, or recycled content wallpaper and use a nontoxic paste or adhesive. Natural fiber covers (arrowroot, bamboo, cattail, jute, paper weaves, reed, rush, sea grass, or sisal) are also nice, although not great in moist rooms. I like Graham & Brown and Phillip Jeffries; both carry nontoxic papers made of recycled or natural materials.

TILE & COUNTERTOP

With tile, head to the nearest discount tile warehouse and ask to see all of their recycled glass or other environmentally friendly lines—pretty much every dealer has some now. For counters, consider kitchen salvage depots, which can have great deals (and save somebody else's old granite or marble counter from going to a landfill). Or look for recycled glass or concrete for more sustainable options. We used IceStone, which is made from 100 percent recycled glass mixed with concrete and comes in tons of beautiful colors.

CABINETRY

Most mainstream brands of cabinets are made with pressed wood or particleboard that's stuck together with glue containing formaldehyde and other preservatives that off-gas chemicals you won't want in your kitchen. Cabinetry is a great opportunity to go used—look for architectural or kitchen salvage depots in your area that specialize in pulling out kitchens when other people are renovating and selling the cabinetry (often for much less than you'd pay

WALLPAPER ACCENT

If you can't afford to wallpaper an entire room, consider using paper as an accent on the inside of built-in bookcases or on one wall, like I did here in my kitchen cabinets. You can even frame beautiful wallpaper inside molding as a giant piece of art!

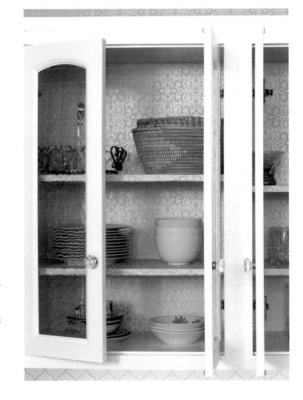

new). Or look for a local cabinetmaker who will work with all wood and nontoxic glues; we opted for an Amish-run company that did wonderful work, though a bit slowly, since they don't use electricity or glue! On the budget but stylish end, IKEA has made a big effort to get the toxic stuff out of its cabinetry.

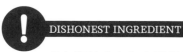

DISHONEST INGREDIENT

PHTHALATES

FOUND IN: Flooring, windows, plastics

WHAT IS IT AGAIN? The same plasticizer in nail polish also makes your shower curtain strong and flexible; it typically turns up in PVC (polyvinyl chloride) plastics.

WHY IS IT SKETCHY? It's a known endocrine disruptor, so avoid exposure in pregnant women, babies, and young children.

BEDDING

Natural mattresses. You spend about 20 percent of your life in bed—which means it's worth investing in a mattress that doesn't make you sick. Conventional mattresses are full of synthetic foam that's been coated with flame retardants and other toxic particles . . . so we can't be sure they won't fall into the "doesn't make you sick" category.

If you're stuck with your current mattress, at the very least, put a strong, organic, allergen-blocking cover on it to help mitigate the off-gassing. If you're in the market for a new mattress, make it organic cotton, wool, or another natural material like natural latex, which can be slightly less expensive and deters dust mites and bacteria (avoid this last option if you have a latex allergy, of course!). If you can't afford to entirely upgrade your mattress, consider topping your old one with an organic wool mattress pad. Wool is naturally flame resistant and comfy, and will provide a layer of protection between you and the chemicals below.

Then add an allergen-protecting cover—this will keep dust mites from saturating your mattress (key for allergy sufferers) and may also help block any chemicals that are off-gassing.

Organic bedding. Look for duvet, comforter, and sheet sets made from unbleached, untreated organic cotton or other eco-friendly natural fibers if you can—again, you spend so much time in bed, why not have the purest materials next to your skin? I like Simply Organic and Naturepedic; West Elm's organic cotton line is a good affordable option. Always wash new bedding before you put it on the bed to rinse away manufacturing residues from the no-wrinkle coatings that many sheets are treated with these days.

Protected pillows. Always encase pillows in protective covers with strong zippers; this helps them last longer and eases allergy symptoms. Regular pillows are filled with polyester and treated with chemical finishes, so I like natural fills like wool, kapok, buckwheat (which deters dust mites), or organic cotton; Gaiam, Garnet Hill, and Pristine Planet are good resources.

BATHROOM

Toxin-free towels. Pesticide-free organic cotton or bamboo are best, with no trace of triclosan (that nasty antibacterial chemical, which often gets coated onto towels that bill themselves as "antimicrobial"). Turkish-style linen towels are also lovely, natural, and get softer as you wash them. I love Gaiam, Garnet Hill, and Pristine Planet—we also stock up at Bed Bath & Beyond. If you buy regular towels, wash them first in hot water to remove any unwanted residues.

Shower curtains. Whatever you do, skip the vinyl—the kind of curtain that stinks up your bathroom as soon as you hang it up!—in curtains *and* in liners. Organic cotton, linen, canvas, and hemp are all good choices because they don't off-gas and you can throw them in the wash once a week to keep bacteria buildup at bay. Rock Candy Life makes adorable ones.

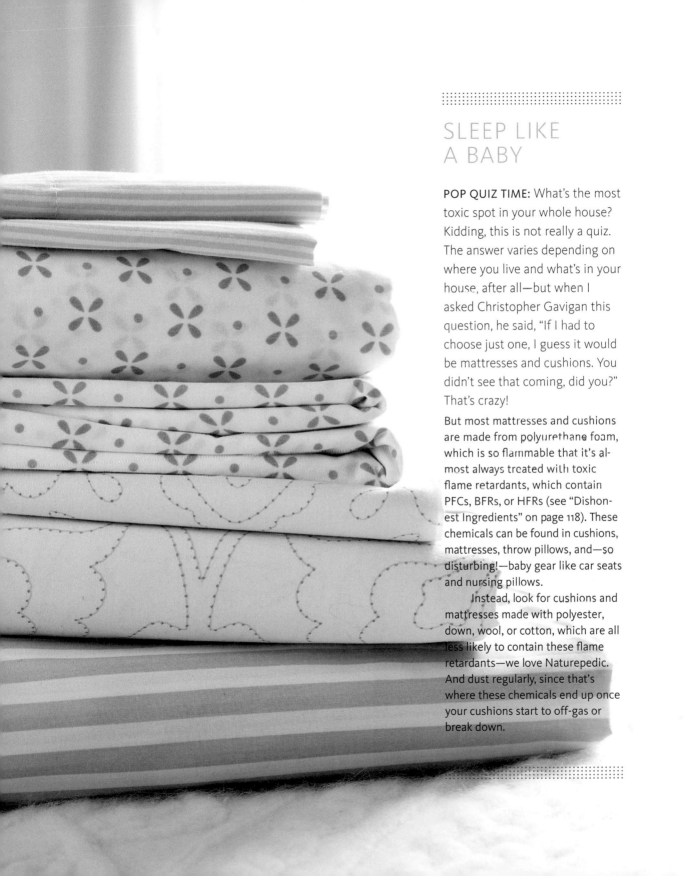

SLEEP LIKE
A BABY

POP QUIZ TIME: What's the most toxic spot in your whole house? Kidding, this is not really a quiz. The answer varies depending on where you live and what's in your house, after all—but when I asked Christopher Gavigan this question, he said, "If I had to choose just one, I guess it would be mattresses and cushions. You didn't see that coming, did you?" That's crazy!

But most mattresses and cushions are made from polyurethane foam, which is so flammable that it's almost always treated with toxic flame retardants, which contain PFCs, BFRs, or HFRs (see "Dishonest Ingredients" on page 118). These chemicals can be found in cushions, mattresses, throw pillows, and—so disturbing!—baby gear like car seats and nursing pillows.

Instead, look for cushions and mattresses made with polyester, down, wool, or cotton, which are all less likely to contain these flame retardants—we love Naturepedic. And dust regularly, since that's where these chemicals end up once your cushions start to off-gas or break down.

FURNITURE

Buying used. Craigslist! I troll it endlessly when there's a particular item I'm after. You get the automatic environmental win of buying something used—plus you'll often find more unusual, one-of-a-kind pieces at way better prices, which you can then refinish and reupholster in the eco-friendly materials of your choice. Note: Always take a guy you trust with you when you go to check out a piece from an ad. Better safe than sorry! Usually, I wait in the car and send Cash or a guy friend inside and have them text me pictures so we can be sure it's the right piece.

One of my favorite sites I've bought a ton from is This Is Not Ikea (thisisnotikea.com), a well-curated vintage site. I also love Etsy.com, the online resource of artisan-made products, including tons of unique household stuff.

Buying new. I try to shop indie boutiques where I can support local craftspeople as much as possible.

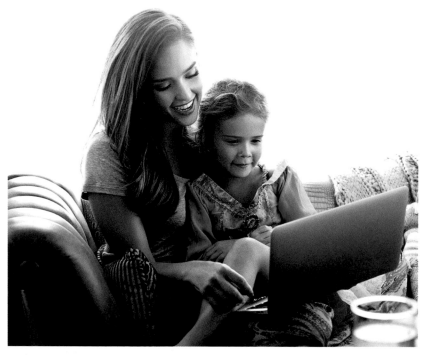

They're often more likely to be working with upcycled and repurposed materials, and you're guaranteed to get a one-of-a-kind piece. That being said, I have seen lots of mainstream places—West Elm, Restoration Hardware, the Sundance Catalog, Anthropologie, Urban Outfitters, and so on—incorporating more vintage and repurposed elements into their furniture. I think it's great to support those efforts whenever we can.

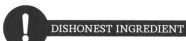

DISHONEST INGREDIENT

FLAME RETARDANTS

* Includes perfluorinated compounds (PFCs), brominated flame retardants (BFRs), and halogenated flame retardants (HFRs)

FOUND IN: Stain-resistant fabric, foam cushions, mattresses, carpeting, and paints

WHAT IS IT? A group of chemicals that make things stain, water, and flame resistant

WHY IS IT SKETCHY? PFCs, BFRs, and HFRs are endocrine disruptors: They interfere with healthy hormonal development and can lead to reproductive and developmental disorders. They're also associated with certain cancers.

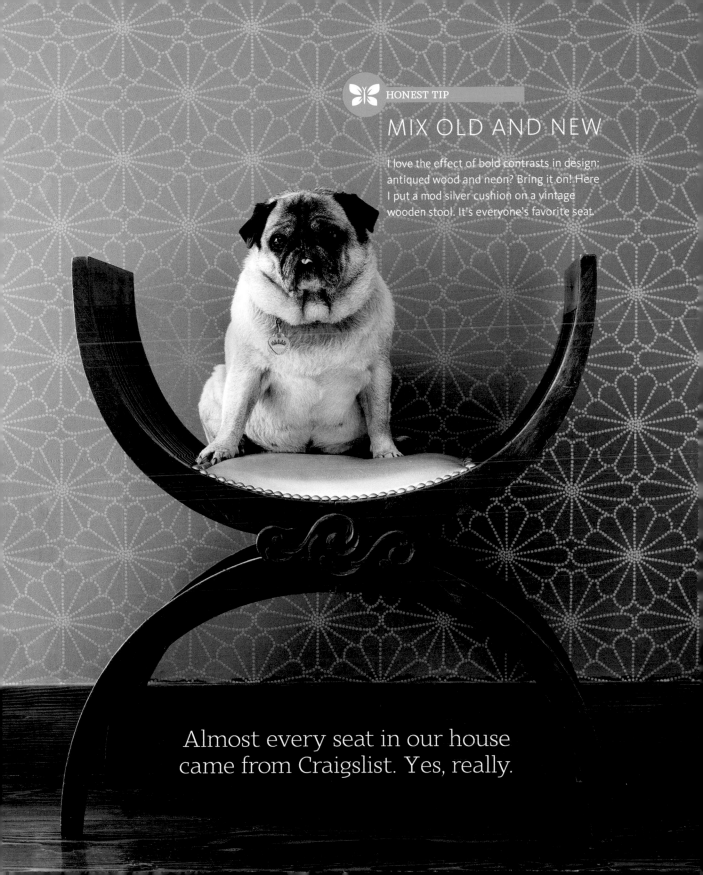

HONEST TIP

MIX OLD AND NEW

I love the effect of bold contrasts in design: antiqued wood and neon? Bring it on! Here I put a mod silver cushion on a vintage wooden stool. It's everyone's favorite seat.

Almost every seat in our house came from Craigslist. Yes, really.

Vintage Décor

VINTAGE IS A huge part of Honest Home style. Not only do antique or secondhand pieces instantly lower your home's carbon footprint because you're reusing instead of buying brand-new—it also ensures that every room will look unique and especially "you." As I mentioned, I always check Craigslist, eBay, thisisnotikea.com, and my local thrift stores whenever I'm on the hunt for a specific furniture item—almost every piece of furniture in our house has an entire life history that started well before it met us!

Buying secondhand also tends to be more affordable—or, at least, on par with what you'd pay at the big box stores and other lower-priced furniture outlets, where, frankly, the quality isn't as great. When I was younger and decorating my first apartment, I made too many mistakes buying cheap pieces quickly, just to fill a room—only to have those furnishings fall apart, sag in the middle, or look like crap after a couple of months. Not to mention that all the while this cheap stuff was probably off-gassing toxic chemicals in the air I breathed. Formaldehyde and other VOC chemicals dissipate significantly after the first five years of a piece of furniture's life, so vintage finds are often a safer bet than buying new.

But you do have to be careful to check for quality with older pieces and watch for a few safety hazards like rusty nails, splintering wood, and lead paint. I always have upholstered pieces

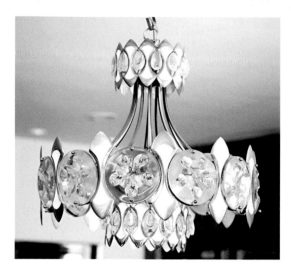

I found this chandelier in a local vintage store. I had it "dipped" to take it from icky brass to silver.

thoroughly checked for bedbugs; restuffed with natural foam rubber, organic cotton, or wool fill; and recovered in organic cotton, wool blends, or silk (untreated and low-impact dyes only) or non-toxic vinyl. Wood gets repainted and sealed with no-VOC paints and stains. Depending on your time, budget, and talents, you can do some or all of this yourself—for example, I'll handle the basic refinishing and painting but usually send upholstery to the pros because it's so much more complex.

HONEST TIP

BUFF UP VINTAGE WOOD FURNITURE

When you get your vintage wood furniture home, it's going to need some TLC. Skip the toxic furniture polish and instead combine 2 cups olive oil and the juice from one lemon in a glass or ceramic container. Apply to the furniture with a soft polishing cloth, rub briskly to shine, and allow to dry. (Always test first on a small, inconspicuous area.)

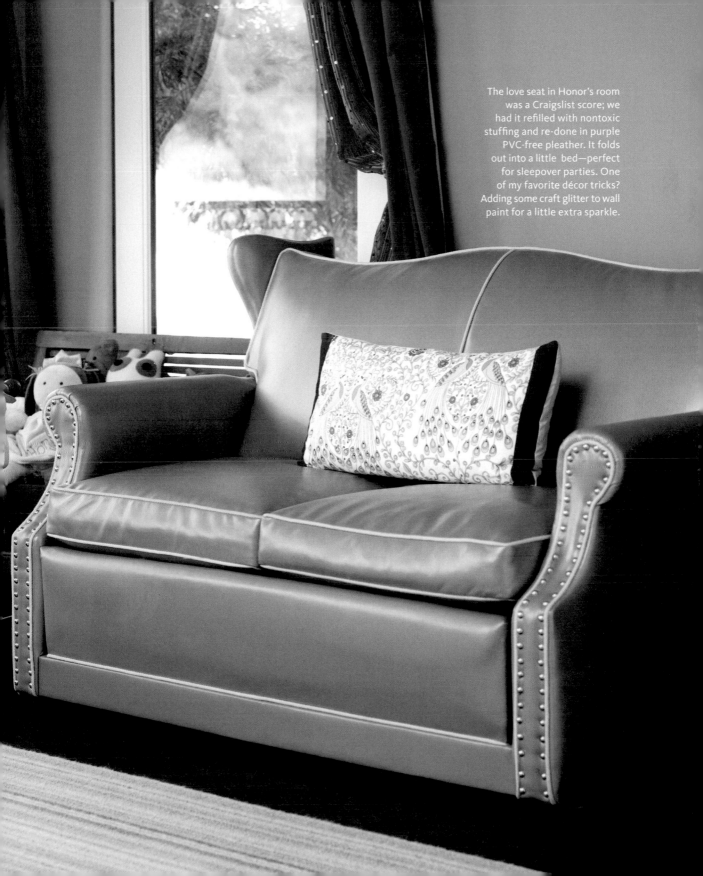

The love seat in Honor's room was a Craigslist score; we had it refilled with nontoxic stuffing and re-done in purple PVC-free pleather. It folds out into a little bed—perfect for sleepover parties. One of my favorite décor tricks? Adding some craft glitter to wall paint for a little extra sparkle.

HOW TO SCORE SOME QUALITY VINTAGE

Avoid . . .	Look for . . .
* Fiberboard—it tends to fall apart and can emit formaldehyde and other toxins	* Solid wood construction
* Plastic or sticker veneers (these can't be refinished and look cheap)	* High-quality wood veneers (common in more-expensive antiques, especially if the piece features inlay or multiple kinds of wood in the design)
* Staples, nails, or visible glue	* Joint construction (dovetail or mortise and tendon) or at least dowels and screws
* Anything that twists or squeaks when you lift one corner	* Weight evenly distributed on all four corners—no drunken tilting!
* Visible rust	* A furniture manufacturer's name printed somewhere—this means you can go home and Google your new find to see when it was made and how much it's worth!
* Knots (unless you love the character they add), cracked, or soft, easily scratched surfaces	* Smooth, hardwood surfaces
* Wood-on-wood sliding drawers (they stick)	* Metal glide rails on drawers
* Springs more than a few inches apart—or that chair or couch is going to sag	* Hand-tied coil springs, grouped closely together to provide even resistance

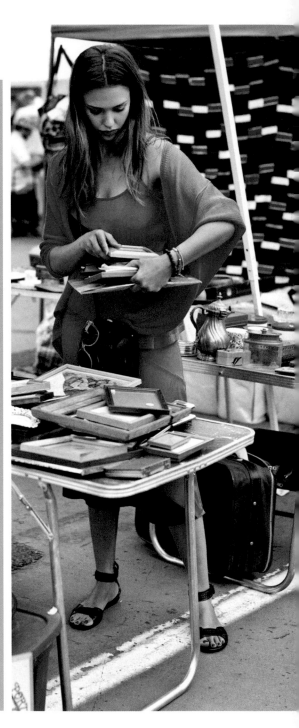

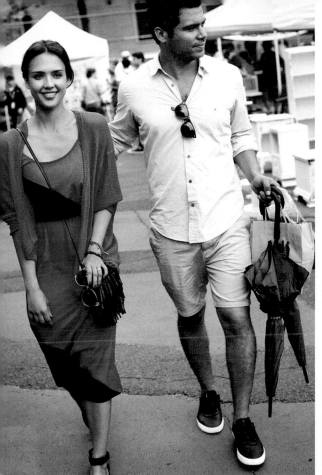

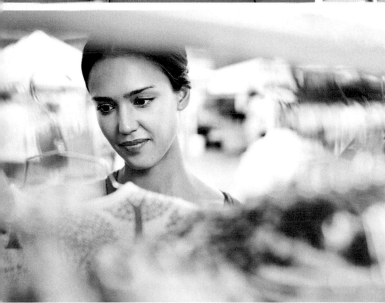

Our family has so much fun at flea markets—I love finding treasures like inexpensive frames I can paint (far left) or one-of-a-kind jewelry. Honor gets excited about the most random, fun things (like that traffic light!), and Cash is a great sport about toting bags.

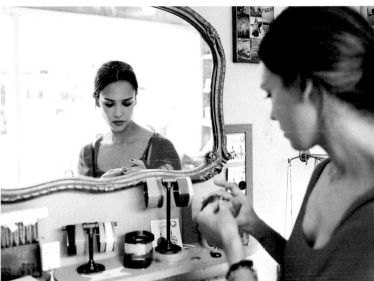

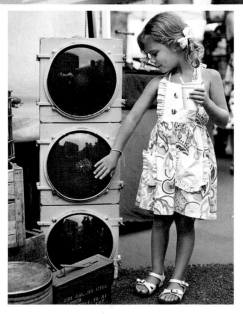

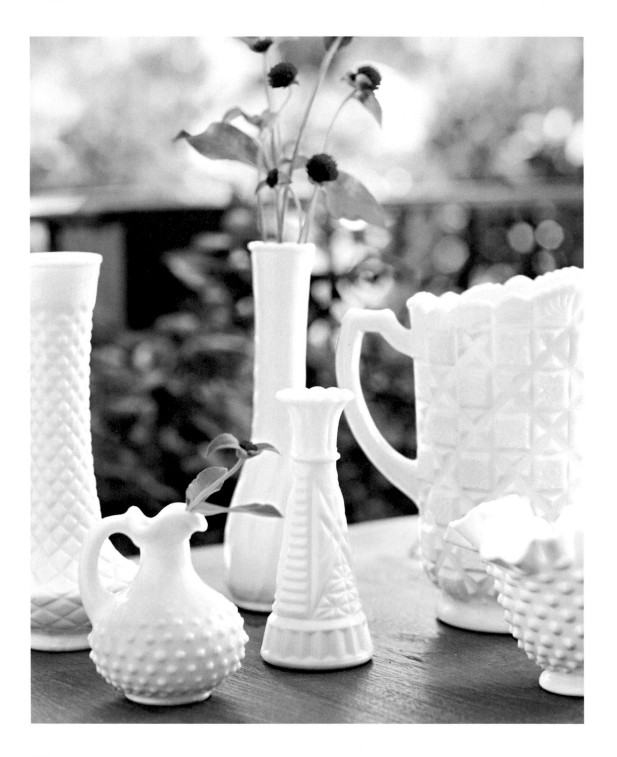

My Vintage Moments

WHENEVER I HIT UP a flea market, antiques store, thrift store, or tag sale—or just log some quality browsing time on eBay or thisisnotikea.com—there are a couple of things I'm keeping an eye out for. Call them my vintage moments—some are true heirlooms (certain milk glass serving pieces can be quite valuable); some have zero value beyond putting a smile on my face. But they fit our aesthetic and life, and I love adding to my collections.

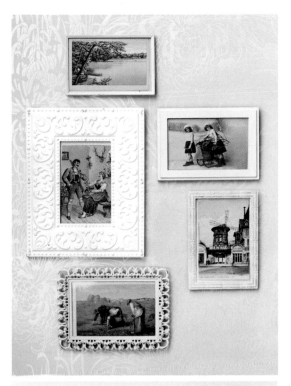

MILK GLASS

I get tons of this as gifts, too. I display all of my vases, serving pieces, and cake stands along the tops of our kitchen cabinets—the creamy white glass really pops against the yellow-and-gold wallpaper.

POSTCARDS

I have a little work-in-progress collection of vintage postcards framed on one wall of my kitchen (top right). There's a great farmers' market in New York City where I found the first batch—eventually, I'd love to cover the whole wall.

LINENS

When I first picked up a bunch of vintage animal-print sheets from a bin outside this thrift store in the south of France, I didn't have any idea what I'd do with them—I just loved the happy colors! Then, when it came time to decorate Haven's nursery, inspiration struck: I collected gently used frames, painted them in complementary colors, and cut animals out of the sheets to frame as art for her walls (see page 193 for the how-to).

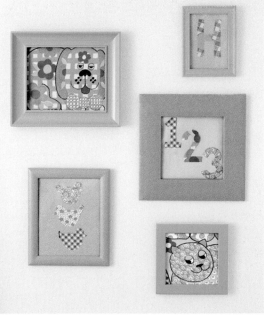

The Honest Remodel

As I've been describing, so many of the pieces of furniture, mattresses, shower curtains, candles, and other goods we bring into our home affect our quality of life (read: our health) in invisible ways, by off-gassing or releasing microscopic particles into the air that we breathe. The impact of home materials multiplies during a renovation, because of the high concentration of dust or construction by-products—as well as the risk of opening up a Pandora's box of toxic exposures, from mold to lead paint. This section might read like a bit of a downer, but it's important to scrutinize if you're considering a renovation so you can be sure to take the safest precautions.

CHECK FOR EXISTING LEAD PAINT HAZARDS

If your home was built before 1978, it probably has some of this. Contractors are required by law to be certified in lead-safe work practices, but if you go the DIY-route, you'll need to check with your state's Environmental Protection Agency for guidance on how to handle any lead paint you find. Visit epa.gov/lead/pubs/renovate rightbrochure.pdf for more info. This also applies to any salvaged or upcycled materials you might be incorporating into your renovation—people are so hot on furniture made from old shipping pallets, but they tend to forget that wood can contain all sorts of nastiness!

CHECK FOR ASBESTOS

Again, older homes? Asbestos could be a major bummer, especially if you've got any of those delightful "popcorn" ceilings, vinyl flooring, or old insulation. You'll need to hire a certified asbestos abatement contractor to test for and remove or seal in any asbestos in your house.

CHECK FOR MOLD AND MOISTURE ISSUES

Remodeling can expose hidden mold, water damage, or leaks. If the affected area is larger than 10 square feet, the EPA recommends hiring a professional mold-abatement contractor (homeowners' insurance may help defray the cost!) who knows how to do this right (contain spores, minimize exposure). Definitely factor in any potential moisture issues when you're choosing building materials. For instance, carpet in the bathroom? Not so much.

LOOK FOR THIRD-PARTY ECO-CERTIFICATIONS

Unfortunately, no single certification covers all health and environmental issues. Look for products certified by Greenguard (required in California), the Forest Stewardship Council (FSC), and other organizations that are independent of any industry. Visit healthybuilding.net for more info.

TAKE SAFETY PRECAUTIONS SERIOUSLY

Just because your building materials say they're "safe for pets

Never sand old paint yourself without first making sure that it doesn't contain lead!

and kids" or "no-VOC" doesn't mean they're totally free from hazardous chemicals. Always use adequate ventilation, contain dust, and wear masks, protective goggles, or respirators if directed.

CHOOSE DURABLE, LOW-MAINTENANCE MATERIALS

A) Having to repaint, retreat, or waterproof something every few months or year is a huge pain. B) It's yet another opportunity to dump more chemicals on your house on a regular basis. Buy the higher-quality stuff that's made to last for years without the constant upkeep.

LET IT BREATHE

Whether you've just painted a room or purchased a new sofa, it's a good idea to open up the windows and run a fan to air it out for a day or two before you use it, especially if there's a strong chemical smell right off the bat. You won't vent out all the toxins, but doing so can reduce your exposure.

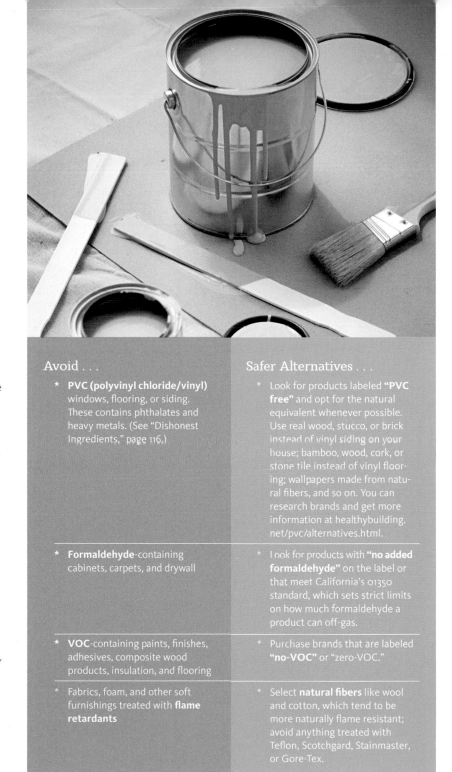

Avoid . . .

* **PVC (polyvinyl chloride/vinyl)** windows, flooring, or siding. These contains phthalates and heavy metals. (See "Dishonest Ingredients," page 116.)

* **Formaldehyde**-containing cabinets, carpets, and drywall

* **VOC**-containing paints, finishes, adhesives, composite wood products, insulation, and flooring

* Fabrics, foam, and other soft furnishings treated with **flame retardants**

Safer Alternatives . . .

* Look for products labeled **"PVC free"** and opt for the natural equivalent whenever possible. Use real wood, stucco, or brick instead of vinyl siding on your house; bamboo, wood, cork, or stone tile instead of vinyl flooring; wallpapers made from natural fibers, and so on. You can research brands and get more information at healthybuilding. net/pvc/alternatives.html.

* Look for products with **"no added formaldehyde"** on the label or that meet California's 01350 standard, which sets strict limits on how much formaldehyde a product can off-gas.

* Purchase brands that are labeled **"no-VOC"** or "zero-VOC."

* Select **natural fibers** like wool and cotton, which tend to be more naturally flame resistant; avoid anything treated with Teflon, Scotchgard, Stainmaster, or Gore-Tex.

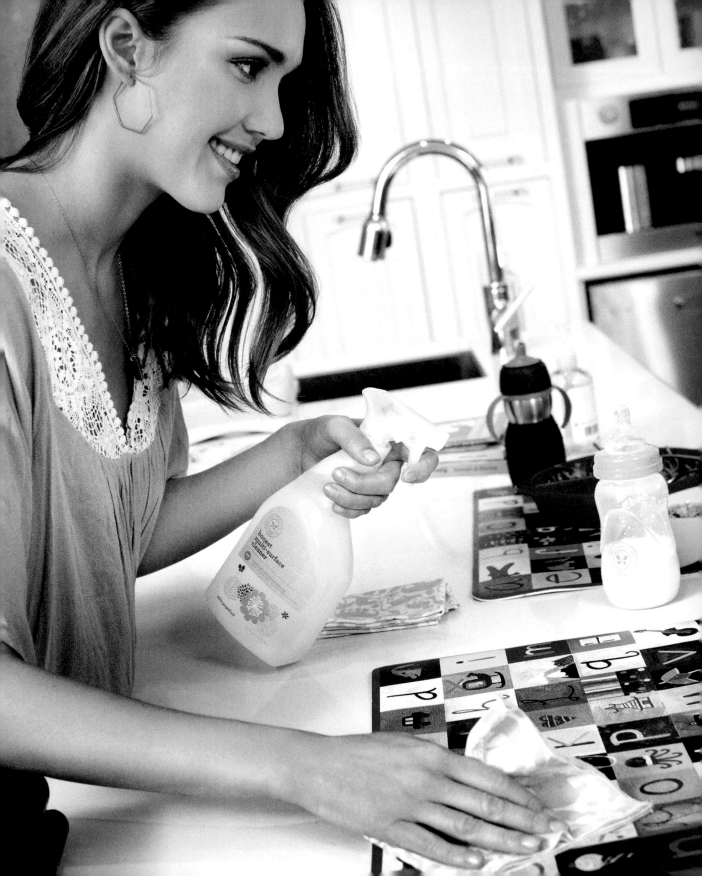

Pure & Simple:
Honest Clean

WHEN I WAS GROWING UP, my mom or grand-mother always scoured every surface of our homes. Their idea of "clean" was a floor you could serve dinner on—meaning bleached to within an inch of its life. But now we know that conventional cleaning products are actually making your house dirtier—because they contain hundreds of toxic chemicals that you don't want to inhale or absorb through your skin. Frankly, even back then, I had to suspect something was up—when you can't be in the same room as a freshly "cleaned" sink or bathtub because the chemicals make your eyes water and your nose run (not to mention the label's marked poison) . . . how is that *clean*?

A Healthy Dose of Dirt

SO NOW THAT you know how to style up your house—and know what you definitely *don't* want in your house—let's talk about how to take care of your lovely home. Keeping your house Honest Clean doesn't have to mean floors you can eat off of and everything perfectly pin-straight at all times—we don't make every bed every day at my house, and you'll certainly find the occasional pile-up of clutter (although too much clutter makes me crazy!). The Honest Home is lived in. It's tidy, yes, and clean in a safe and healthy way—but also laid-back, friendly, and sometimes overflowing with (organized) chaos.

In fact, you don't want a completely sterile, germ-free house. Christopher Gavigan is a big proponent of raising kids with "a dose of dirt" to help prevent allergies—because our overcleaning, sterilization, and sanitization can get in the way of building healthy, mature immune systems. More and more science is suggesting that there's some hard truth in the "hygiene hypothesis," that our culture of antibacterial soap and obsessive allergy monitoring has only led our kids' immune systems away from fighting infection to developing more allergic tendencies. And all of this germ killing may end up leaving us *more* vulnerable to infection, as those antibacterial products get over-used and kill off the healthy bacteria we really need. Besides, the active ingredients in antibacterial products have been linked to everything from thyroid damage to the explosion of superbugs (bacteria that have become resistant to antibiotics).

So when you clean, don't worry about whether you're getting everything 100 percent science-lab sterile. That's not the goal. Instead, focus on using healthy products to clear up obvious dirt (the kind that leads to ants in the kitchen!) and dust (that can be filled with those toxic chemicals). This means using nonpetroleum-based cleaning products, like the ones we've designed at Honest, or even simple homemade cleaning solutions you can mix up yourself.

No-Brainer Cleaning Strategies

FOR AN EVERYDAY CLEAN, there are a few low-effort and high-impact things you can do to make sure your home environment stays low on toxins and irritants.

Open the windows. VOC (volatile organic compound) levels are higher indoors than out, so opening your windows for even just a few minutes every day—even in the winter!—can significantly improve your indoor air quality.

Take off your shoes. I love shoes, of course, but their bottoms are nasty. Lead dust, animal feces, gasoline, fertilizers, pesticides, and other chemicals all pack into your soles. When you enter your house, leave your shoes at the door and keep this grossness there, too, instead of tracking it all over. (At the very least, keep your bedrooms and kids' rooms shoe free!) You might even consider leaving a basket of slippers or brightly colored socks at the door for guests to use, if that's your thing (in my house, we go barefoot).

Kick your chemical habit. Switching to nontoxic cleaning products is just about the single most important thing you can do to purge your home air quality of VOCs (see page 133) and other toxic chemicals. Embrace label reading and avoid products with all the stuff listed in the Dishonest Ingredients charts—the biggies in this category are chlorine and ammonia, though cleaning products contain hundreds of other "inert" ingredients that you won't find on labels.

Dust. Most of the stuff in your house, plus the materials used to make the building itself, is slowly degrading and breaking down into microscopic particles that wind up in your dust. So wipe up surfaces regularly with a damp cloth and wipe hard floors with a damp mop (you typically only need water for these tasks). Swipe your screens (some of the most contaminated dust is found on TV and computer screens) and vacuum regularly with a machine outfitted with a HEPA (high efficiency particulate air) filter, which tightly traps the dust rather than flinging particles back into the room.

I like to be creative when it comes to wall décor. In our foyer, for example, we assembled a collection of old family photos from all of our relatives, which I scanned and printed out in black and white for a cohesive look. Then we framed them all in inexpensive black frames. It feels homey and it's great for sharing memories with our family and friends.

Wiping shoes on a mat and removing them at the door can cut lead dust tracked into the home by 60 percent, according to the EPA.

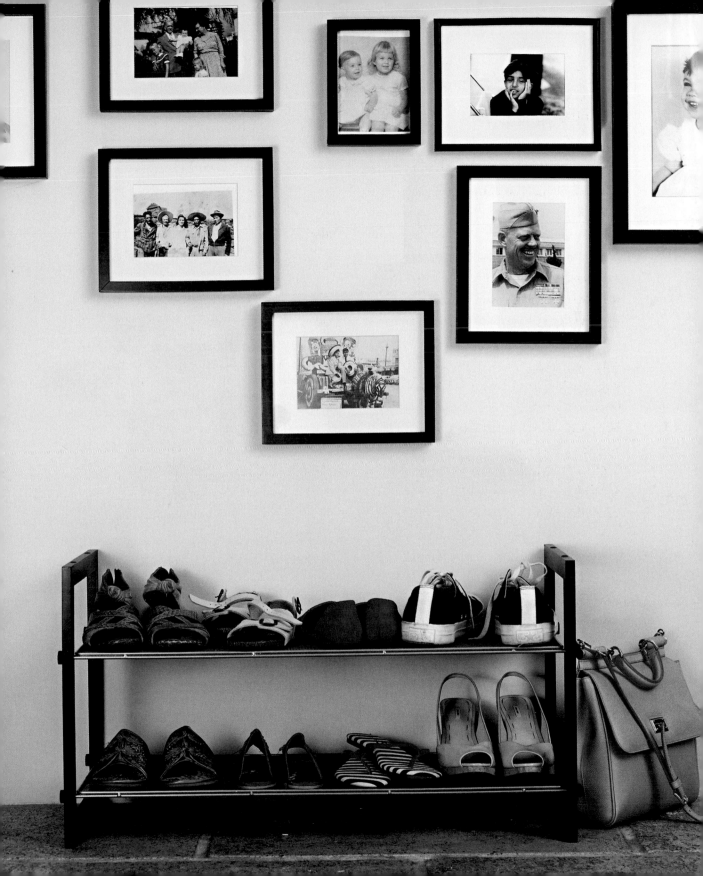

The Honest Cleaning Guide

HERE'S A SURFACE-BY-SURFACE guide to cleaning up every room in your house healthfully. Virtually every synthetic chemical-filled product you use can now be replaced with a nontoxic alternative. It may take you a while to get used to not having that aggressive pine forest or lemon smell that has signaled "clean" for oh, your whole life, but trust me—an odorless (or naturally scented) house is *so* much better for your and your family's health.

Floors

HARDWOOD

Sweep or dry-mop often (daily in your kitchen) to get up the big stuff. Then damp-mop at least once a week to stay on top of dust; plain old water works amazingly well. When things get scummy, I like to add a bit of our Honest Floor Cleaner; whatever you use, make sure it's natural and biodegradable.

CARPET

Vacuum using a machine outfitted with a HEPA filter, which traps small particles and keeps them from spewing back into the room. If you sprinkle baking soda on the carpet and let it stand for 15 to 30 minutes beforehand, you'll naturally deodorize the carpet at the same time.

Area rugs can also be hung outside on cold, breezy days for several hours—this will freshen them up, release toxins, and, if temperatures dip below freezing, also kill dust mites.

For deeper cleaning, professionals tend to use really toxic cleaners on carpet. Instead, rent a steam cleaner from a local home improvement store or supermarket.

Pretreat spots with lemon juice and $\frac{1}{8}$ cup of liquid soap to 2 gallons of hot water (skip the conventional rug cleaners—they're full of harsh chemicals—although I do like Earth Friendly Products Carpet Shampoo and, of course, Honest Stain Remover). Make sure the carpet is thoroughly dry before children are allowed back in, and if your carpet is in a damp room, run a dehumidifier regularly to discourage mold growth (inhaling mold spores can trigger allergies and asthma—or worse, make you seriously sick).

Windows

Clean with a lint-free rag (microfiber cloths are great for this, and reusable!) and a nontoxic window cleaner. This is also one of the easiest products to make yourself: Just mix distilled white vinegar with water in a 1:2 ratio. (Yes, your house will smell acidic—try adding a drop or two of your favorite essential oil, like lavender or eucalyptus, to combat the vinegar scent.) You can find lots of great DIY cleaning recipes at Rodale.com.

When switching to nontoxic cleaning products, it may take you a while to get used to not having that pine forest or lemon smell that has signaled "clean" for, oh, your whole life. But trust me—odorless (or naturally scented) is much healthier!

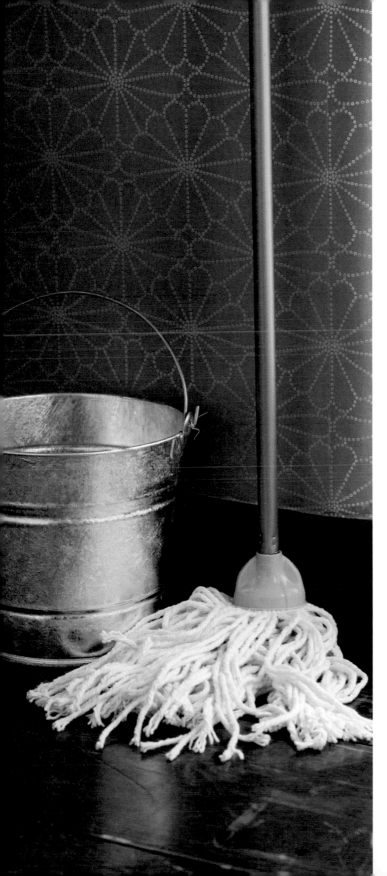

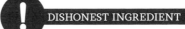

VOLATILE ORGANIC COMPOUNDS (VOCs)

FOUND IN: Cleaning supplies, air fresheners, pesticides, building materials, paints, furnishings—anything with a strong scent!

WHAT IS IT? An umbrella term for a huge group of chemicals that release fumes and gases

WHY IS IT SKETCHY? Some VOCs can cause serious health issues ranging from respiratory illness to cancer, while others are pretty benign. Unfortunately, the EPA doesn't know that much yet about what health effects occur from typical household VOC levels—although they do know that indoor levels are typically much higher than outdoor.

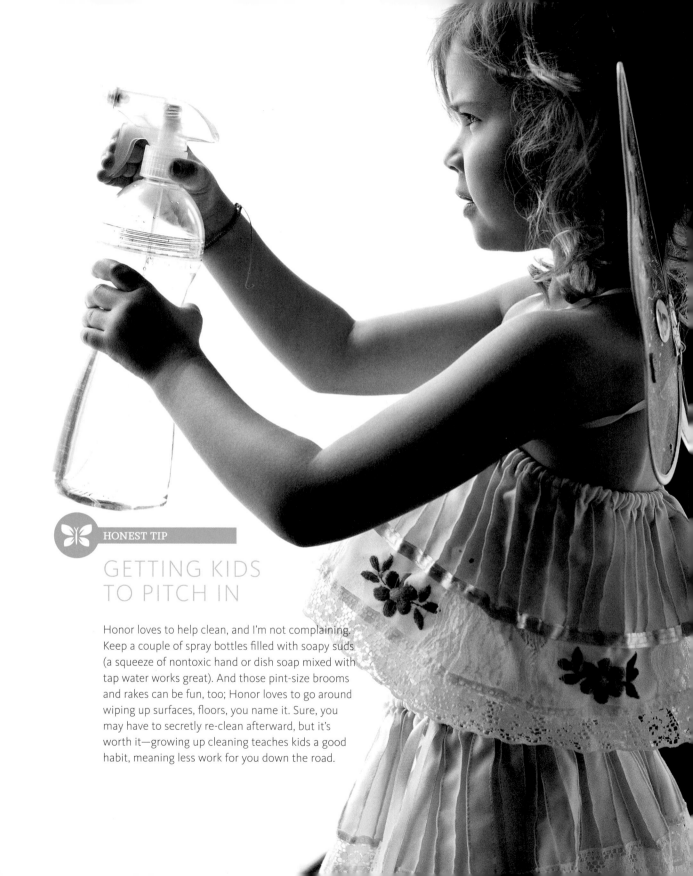

GETTING KIDS TO PITCH IN

Honor loves to help clean, and I'm not complaining. Keep a couple of spray bottles filled with soapy suds (a squeeze of nontoxic hand or dish soap mixed with tap water works great). And those pint-size brooms and rakes can be fun, too; Honor loves to go around wiping up surfaces, floors, you name it. Sure, you may have to secretly re-clean afterward, but it's worth it—growing up cleaning teaches kids a good habit, meaning less work for you down the road.

Kitchen

COUNTERS

Wipe down daily with a damp rag (water only or a splash of white vinegar to keep bacteria at bay); I also love a little counter broom and dustpan for sweeping up crumbs and bigger messes. Clean once a week with a natural spray (I use Honest Multi-Surface Cleaner).

SINK

Wipe it out every time you use it—this helps prevent clogs and build-up. But if you do get a gunky drain situation, pour a mixture of equal parts baking soda, white vinegar, and boiling water (carefully!) down your drain and let it sit for half an hour—the baking soda and vinegar fizz up and eat through clogs.

APPLIANCES

Make sure your cleaner is an eco-friendly brand because stainless-steel cleaners can get pretty toxic. Or just wipe using a cloth doused with white vinegar.

Bathroom

TOILET

Scrub once a week with baking soda and vinegar, nonchlorine bleach, or a natural toilet cleaner (I played with essential oils to help get the scent of our Honest Toilet Cleaner just right!). Pour a little nonchlorine bleach in the base of your toilet brush holder, too; it will keep it from getting super gross, and the brush will last longer. Never use those drop-in chemical toilet deodorizer tablets; most contain a known carcinogen.

SHOWER AND TILE

I rarely remember to spray down the shower after I'm done—I'm too busy rushing to the next thing! Mainly, stick with your Honest Bathroom Cleaner or other natural product and wipe down the shower once a week to stay on top of grime.

The secret to an always-clean shower, sans mildew and other grossness? Sealing your grout. This chemical concoction isn't all that natural—but when you consider that it enables you to lay off the scouring powder, grout whiteners, and other harsh cleansers for six months to a year at a time, I think it's a fair trade. You can buy a bottle of grout sealant at any home improvement center or tile store. Simply follow the directions on the bottle to sponge it on, let it absorb into the grout, and then wipe it off the surrounding tile (or else it will leave a waxy film). If done correctly, you won't be able to see any difference—but you will see a completely clean and mildew-free shower for months to come.

MAKE YOUR OWN CLEANERS

I've always experimented with DIY cleaner recipes—you can never go wrong with the basic ingredients your grandmother probably used: baking soda, lemon, and vinegar. Here are some recipes that totally get the job done from Rodale.com's Nickel Pincher:

- ❋ **All purpose cleaner:** 9 parts water, 1 part vinegar
- ❋ **Window cleaner:** ¼ cup vinegar, ½ teaspoon natural liquid soap, 2 cups water
- ❋ **Tile cleaner:** ½ cup baking soda, liquid soap (enough so it looks like frosting when poured into the baking soda), 5 to 10 drops of your favorite essential oil
- ❋ **Oven cleaner:** 2 cups hot water, 1 tablespoon natural dish liquid, 1 teaspoon borax

Mix all ingredients together in a spray bottle and shake gently.

A Breath of Fresh Air

HERE'S A NASTY FACT: According to the EPA, indoor air can be two to five times more polluted than outdoor air—and we spend 90 percent of our lives indoors! Choosing natural, healthy materials for building supplies and furniture and swapping in safer cleaning products will go a long way. But there are still some key air quality issues that you need to brush up on to make sure your home is as healthy as possible.

Dust

AS ALLERGY GIRL, dust is serious business to me. Whenever I find myself waking up with a stuffy nose, itchy, watery eyes, or trouble breathing, I know it means the dust situation in my house isn't under control—and our bedrooms are ground zero because over two million microscopic dust mites live in the average bed. (I bet you wish you could un-know that fun fact.) Dust gathers on blinds, carpets, and around collectibles filling shelves and nooks, so regular dusting is important but not a complete solution.

Protect your bedding from dust mites by encasing your mattress and pillows in protective covers and washing all linens weekly in hot water. (Some cases also limit the off-gassing from your mattress.) Kill dust mites in stuffed animals and other bulky items by putting them in the freezer for 3 to 5 hours per week.

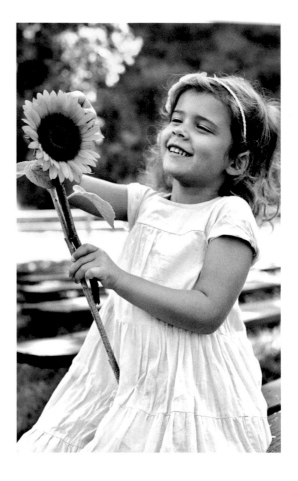

Remove your shoes. As previously mentioned, this keeps all kinds of mess (dust included) out of your house. The exception to that rule: households like mine with an indoor/outdoor pet. Our dogs bring all that same stuff in on their paws and coat, so taking off our shoes downstairs where they hang out becomes sort of moot. It's better to maintain a more rigorous cleaning schedule. Keeping a track-off mat at the front door will also help.

Consider installing forced-air filters with a minimum efficiency reporting value (MERV) of 8 or higher on all air vents if you have central air. Seriously—our HEPA filters changed my life! Cash and I always woke up with stuffy noses—we thought that was just normal—until the filters started pulling dust and other particles out of the air as they circulated the heat and air-conditioning. No central air? A freestanding HEPA filter air purifier in your bedroom or other main living spaces can do the same job—you can pick up one at most home appliance stores.

Mold

MOLDS REQUIRE ONLY MOISTURE and oxygen to grow, so they crop up easily in bathroom corners, dank basements, fridges, or under kitchen sinks. A mold infestation can trigger asthma and allergies, or, in more concentrated doses, dizziness and flu-like symptoms. It's impossible to clear your air of *all* mold spores, but as long as you keep moisture under control, you can prevent the spores from landing on surfaces—which is how they grow. Remember, any mold growth that covers an area larger than 10 square feet, or has spread inside the ducts of your central air system, should be handled by a professional, according to the Environmental Protection Agency.

You can tackle smaller jobs yourself by scrubbing the mold off of hard surfaces with a mixture of detergent and hot water, then fixing the source of the water damage, whether that means tightening leaky plumbing or sealing up cracks in walls and roofs.

DISHONEST INGREDIENT

MOLD

FOUND IN: Bathroom corners, dank basements or under kitchen sinks and fridges

WHAT IS IT? Tiny spores that require only moisture and oxygen to grow—and grow

WHY IS IT SKETCHY? A mold infestation can trigger asthma and allergies, or, in more concentrated doses, dizziness and flulike symptoms.

Unfortunately, it's impossible to salvage a moldy rug or other porous material. It's not worth the health ramifications, so throw out infested carpets or ceiling tiles. Visit **epa.gov/mold** for more info on handling mold in your home.

Check your home's humidity level. Thirty to 50 percent is optimal; any higher and mold, bacteria, and dust mites can flourish. A good digital thermometer or hygrometer can give you an accurate reading on a cool, low-humidity day. And don't forget to check your attic and basement—standing water or humidity over 50 percent in these areas can contribute to mold growth throughout your house. Run a dehumidifier as needed to fix the problem.

Use exhaust fans in bathrooms and kitchens. The best fans vent to the outside and include a HEPA filter to eliminate that nasty mold-causing moisture buildup.

Scents & Smoke

REMEMBER HOW FRAGRANCE is bad news in beauty products? That goes double for anything you want to light on fire—like scented candles or incense—or spray all over your house to make it smell good, like air fresheners and potpourri. Fragrance contains phthalates and God-knows-what-else, and you don't want that fuming up your home—plus some candle wicks actually contain lead.

Wood-burning fireplaces can also compromise indoor air quality. Although, in theory, a fire's heat pulls dirty air out of a chimney, increasing home air circulation, not all chimneys do this effectively and many can aggravate breathing.

Make sure your stove has a range hood with a good fan that vents outside—and use the fan (or, at least, crack a window) every time you cook! Be sure to clean the fan's filter regularly.

Grill outdoors whenever you can—it's a great way to minimize the pollution your stove creates indoors. Plus grilled food is delicious!

Keep your chimney clean with a yearly sweeping to remove buildup, which can block smoke exhaust.

Light fragrance-free candles. Unscented products off-gas less than their scented counterparts. But if you love a light scent, go with a high-quality soy-based candle, which is a better bet than paraffin wax. My fave candle brand is Joya.

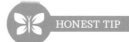

HONEST TIP

NATURAL AIR FRESHENERS

If you have to break up with your plug-in air fresheners and fancy candles, what's a girl to do? Try these natural air-freshening strategies.

Vodka contains ethyl alcohol, which is a main ingredient in most commercial air fresheners—minus all the added chemicals like petrochemicals and synthetic fragrances. Vodka leaves no odor as it dries, so you can spray it straight into your air to absorb odors or add a few drops of a favorite essential oil for a (safe) yummy scent (just don't, um, spray it right at a flame!). And don't worry, inhaling vodka can't get you buzzed.

Baking soda absorbs odors and couldn't be cheaper; sprinkle in your empty trash cans or leave one container open in the fridge.

Essential oils can smell awesome, and many are actually antibacterial, but they are overwhelming unless you dilute them (and definitely don't leave them out to tempt curious kids—they're incredibly potent). Add 10 drops of your favorite essential oil to 7 tablespoons of water in a spray bottle, and spritz. I love the scents of lavender, cinnamon, jasmine, and eucalyptus around the house.

Coffee grounds smell awesome when they're fresh—plus they're amazingly odor-absorbent. Try tying them up in a coffee filter sachet or setting out a small bowl wherever you need a smell removed.

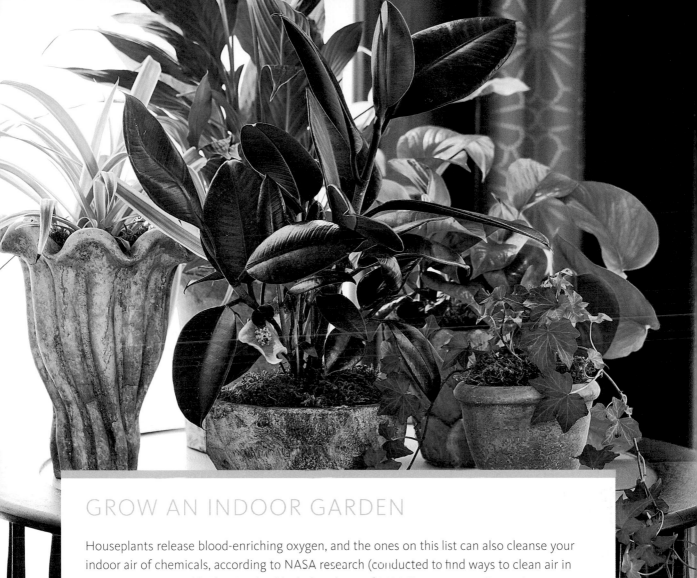

GROW AN INDOOR GARDEN

Houseplants release blood-enriching oxygen, and the ones on this list can also cleanse your indoor air of chemicals, according to NASA research (conducted to find ways to clean air in space stations—cool!). They're also black-thumb-proof. NASA's suggestion: For a 1,800-square-foot house, place 15 to 18 of these plants in 6- to 8-inch-diameter containers. (Take care where you place them if you have young children or pets—some are poisonous if ingested.)

* Bamboo palm or reed palm
* Chinese evergreen
* Cornstalk dracaena
* Elephant ear philodendron
* English ivy
* Gerbera daisy or Barberton daisy

* Golden pothos (devil's ivy)
* Heartleaf philodendron
* Janet Craig dracaena
* Peace lily
* Pot mum or florist's chrysanthemum
* Red-edged dracaena

* Rubber plant
* Selloum philodendron
* Snake plant or mother-in-law's tongue
* Spider plant
* Warneck dracaena
* Weeping fig

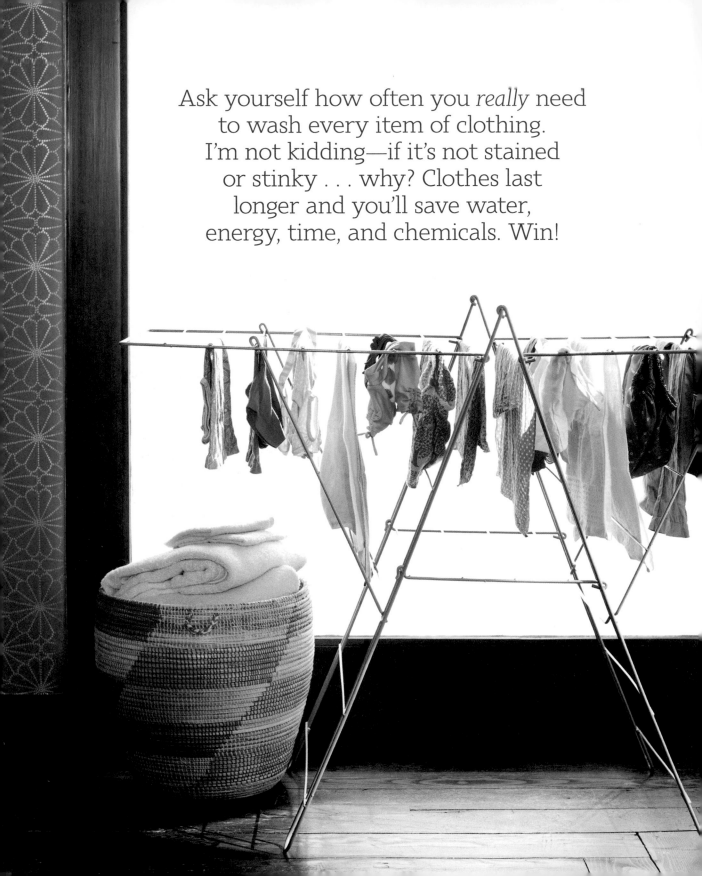

Ask yourself how often you *really* need to wash every item of clothing. I'm not kidding—if it's not stained or stinky . . . why? Clothes last longer and you'll save water, energy, time, and chemicals. Win!

Fresh Laundry —Honestly

You **ALREADY HEARD** the fancy baby detergent story, so you know how a load of laundry more or less changed my life. The fact is, how we wash our clothes has a huge impact on our families' health because the clothes we wear (not to mention our sheets and towels) are the next-closest things to our skin after soaps and lotions. If they're regularly getting dosed with toxic chemicals via detergents, softeners, and stain removers . . . well, you know where this is going. It's also no good for the planet because we wash all that junk down the drain—and it ends up polluting our waterways.

Washing & Drying

DETERGENT

I use our Honest Laundry Detergent, but whichever brand you choose, make sure it contains no petroleum products, phosphates, chlorine, optical brighteners, or synthetic fragrances and dyes.

STAIN REMOVERS

Chlorine bleach reacts with water, forming a group of nasty, cancer-causing by-products called dioxins. Alternatively, look for non-chlorine-based products (like Honest OxyBoost).

These are mostly hydrogen peroxide–based and far less toxic, although you should still keep them away from kids and pets. You can also bleach linens naturally by line-drying them outside on sunny days or adding a cup of white vinegar to every load. (Honest Stain Remover is great, too, for pretreating stains.)

FABRIC SOFTENERS

Chemical fabric softener is mainly fragrance and other toxic stuff. Instead, toss $1/2$ to $3/4$ cup baking soda in the wash and clothes will come out soft and smelling fresh.

! **DISHONEST INGREDIENT**

OPTICAL BRIGHTENERS

FOUND IN: Laundry detergents

WHAT IS IT? Dyes that absorb UV light to make your whites whiter and your clothes brighter by removing yellow tones

WHY IS IT SKETCHY? Optical brighteners bind to the skin and may cause rashes and allergic reactions; they may also be hormone disruptors and we just don't know whether they're safe to use over long periods of time (like the number of years you'll do laundry). One bummer: They're toxic to fish.

DRYER SHEETS

Most store-bought dryer sheets are petroleum based and full of fragrance and grossness, so give them a skip. (I go nuts when I see that cleaning tip about using dryer sheets to dust-proof your baseboards—sure it works, but you're spreading phthalates all over your house!) If you like that extra scent, try a natural brand like Honest Dryer Cloths or a homemade concoction—spritz a washcloth or clean rag with a few drops of your favorite essential oil.

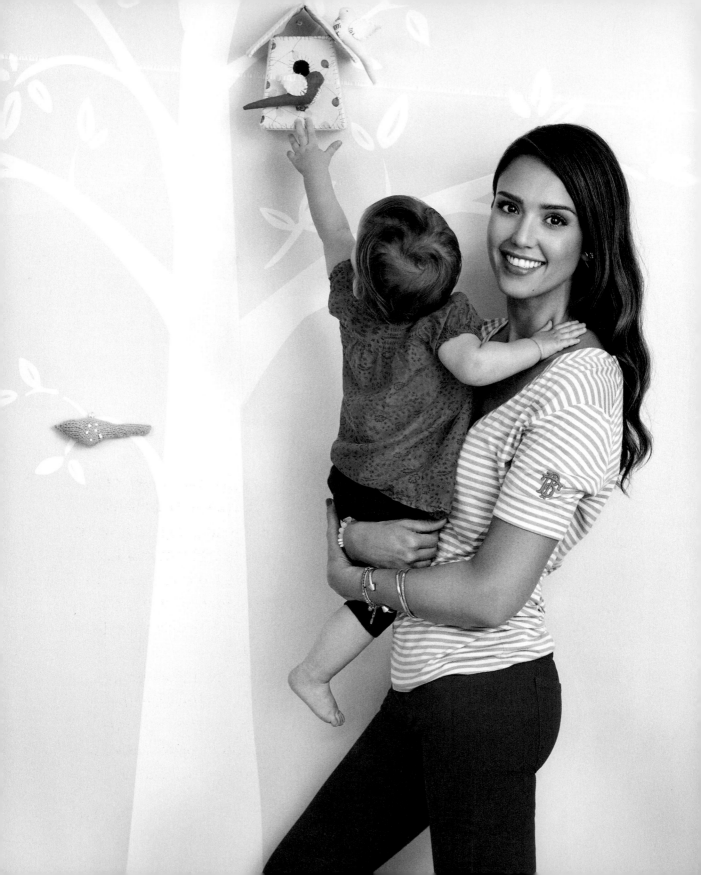

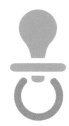

chapter 6

HONEST
baby

PREPARE FOR
PARENTHOOD
WITHOUT LOSING
YOURSELF

BEFORE HONOR ARRIVED, I WAS TOTALLY FOCUSED ON MY career. I was 26 when I got pregnant, and I wasn't sure how I was going to manage juggling both work and family. But when it happened, something just clicked for Cash and me—we realized what a beautiful moment it was and how lucky we were to be able to start a family. The day Honor was born, I discovered the true meaning of love.

As she's started to walk, talk, and have opinions, my love has only deepened. When Haven came along three years later, our family was complete. Today, our home is filled with more pink, dress-up, and giggles than we could ever have imagined.

MY CAREER is still a priority—I think it's so important to show your kids by example how hard work can lead to dreams fulfilled. My relationship with my husband is also super important—having children has made Cash and me a lot closer. Once you've gone through all those late-night feedings and diaper explosions together, you're bonded like nothing else; we share everything now. And I literally could not have survived the past four years without my mom or mom friends—no one else understands how you feel when you've been up all night with a newborn and crazy new hormones. But there's no question: Becoming a mom made me the person I was always meant to be.

If you're reading this chapter because you're pregnant, or you're in that thinking-about-it place, get excited! Having a baby is the hardest, most terrifying, exhausting, overwhelming thing I've ever done—but it's also the sweetest, most beautiful, most profound love I've ever experienced.

What does frustrate me is how much pressure parents—especially moms!—are under today. Almost as soon as you announce that you're expecting, it feels like the entire world wants to know every detail: *Will you have a home birth or deliver in a hospital? Use an epidural or tough it out? Will you breastfeed or use formula? Sleep train or cosleep? Diaper with cloth or disposables? Pacifiers or self-soothing? Wear the baby or use a swing? Attachment parent? French parent? Tiger mom?*

Here's what everyone is really asking: *What kind of mom do you want to be?*

And here's my response: Everyone can back off.

There are no right or wrong answers. It's important to take all the advice, sift through it, and see what resonates—but at the end of the day, you have to go with your gut. You don't have to follow any one parenting philosophy or set of rules to a T. It's perfectly fine to shop around! Be the kind of mom you want to be, and don't worry about how you're measuring up to anyone else's expectations.

Of course, I didn't get to this confident place as a mom overnight. During my first pregnancy, as you know from the fancy baby detergent story, I was pretty much in panic mode. I did tons of research on every aspect of parenting, especially on how to put together a safe and healthy nursery—and there were definitely times when I went overboard and worried way too much about stuff you just can't control. Cash and I had some tense moments, like when we received some baby shower gifts made from potentially toxic plastic and I didn't want to bring them in the house. He thought I had lost my mind. (Okay, I sort of had, but seriously: If you receive something made from a questionable plastic that you really need or love—it *is* a good idea to keep it out on the back porch for a few days until that stinky plastic smell wears off. Let those chemicals off-gas outside, not in your baby's new nursery!)

But even while that whole preparation process was so daunting, it was also unbelievably empowering. Knowing that we had created a safe and welcoming environment in our house for the new baby made me a lot less terrified to bring her home from the hospital and start figuring out how to be a mom. Nothing will prepare you for parenthood (maybe-baby folks, if you're waiting to feel "ready" or for "the right time," there's no such thing!). But doing my homework on, say, the safest crib mattresses made me realize that I had the skills to tackle all these new challenges: I ask questions—and I'm persistent. That was useful when I was trying to figure out which brand of baby sunscreen to buy, and it's important when one of the girls has a weird cough or rash and I need to bug the doctor to figure out what's going on. I do it all from a place of love for my children. Which is why a parent knows better than any book or "expert" what their kid really needs.

This chapter will show you how I put together my daughters' rooms and prepared for their arrival, babyhood, and first few years. I've incorporated plenty of healthy parenting tips from the experts I rely on—my beautiful and loving mom and wonderful pediatricians like Alan Greene, MD; Jay Gordon, MD; and children's toxicology expert Philip J. Landrigan, MD, the director of the Children's Environmental Health Center at New York's Mount Sinai School of Medicine. I also could not have done it without one of my besties, Kelly Sawyer (momma of two), who is the president of the nonprofit Baby2Baby. Kelly and I met when we were pregnant—me with Honor, she with her second daughter, Sawyer. Our husbands were work friends and dragged us along to this

HONEST PARENTING: MY DEFINITION

Figuring out what kind of parent you want to be is an intensely personal decision—and frankly, nobody's business but yours! But here's my parenting philosophy, in a nutshell.

Honest Parenting Is . . .

* Love
* Believing kids flourish within boundaries
* Lots of snuggles
* Laughter
* Telling stories
* Pretend play
* Being positive
* A veggie at lunch and dinner
* A schedule that works for parents and kiddos

Honest Parenting Isn't . . .

* Always saying yes
* No routine
* Tolerating sass
* Being *overly* rigid
* Letting media raise your kids

dinner . . . both cranky and hormonal that night, we bonded instantly—even though Kelly was still so thin she didn't look pregnant and I was *very* pregnant and feeling so fat! And since she already had a two-year-old daughter at home, she became my mom guru as we hit the new-mom circuit of mommy and me classes, playgroups, and the occasional but oh-so-necessary Girls Night Out (GNO).

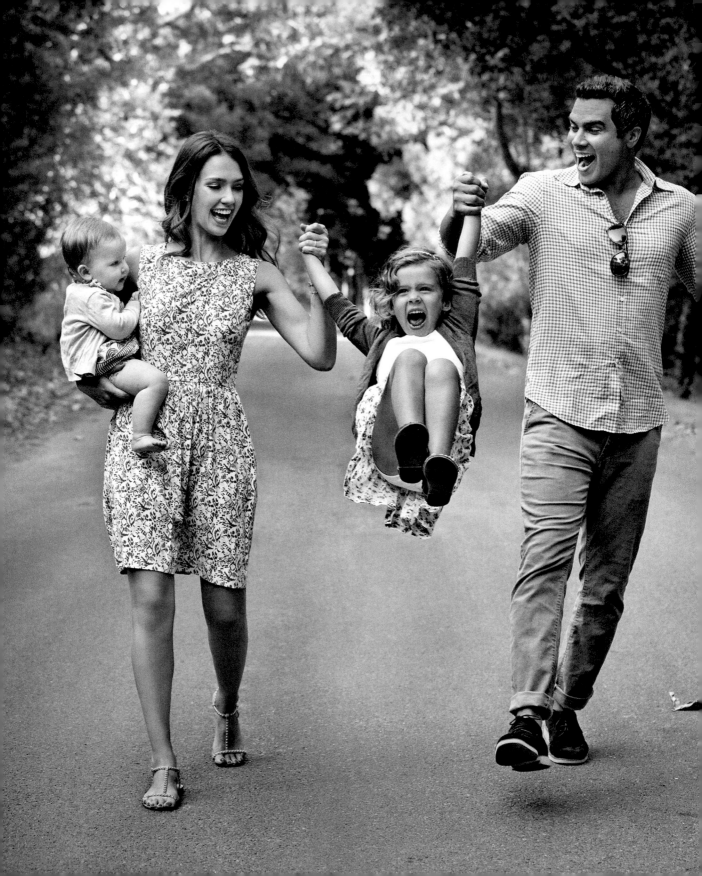

With the help of these experts, I'm also going to weigh in on a few of those Big Parenting Questions we all have. I'm sharing what worked for me, but that doesn't mean you need to do the same—every family's needs are different and special. However, I've been able to gather information and make thoughtful choices by hearing how other parents did it.

Honestly Expecting: Getting through Your Pregnancy

BEING PREGNANT is this crazy roller coaster of paradoxes—for 10 months, you never quite know if you'll wake up feeling like the fattest person alive or all glowing fertility goddess; if you'll be nauseous, achy, and exhausted or weirdly energetic in hyper-nesting mode. Pretty much all you know for sure is that you have to pee. Again.

All that being said, pregnancy was the most incredible experience ever—and the payoffs? Obviously, they are the best. So I'll take the stretch marks. I'll take the sagging boobs and the cellulite that's never going away. But I was also awfully grateful to my mom friends who clued me in to a few things the first time around—and the second time around, there were so many things that felt easier because I'd had a little practice. So here's a checklist of things that helped me keep my sanity and enjoy every little milestone along the way.

CURE CRAVINGS

With Honor, I craved citrus like crazy—I could eat two grapefruits in one sitting and was forever snacking on oranges, tangerines, and clementines. With Haven, I had a fierce, insatiable craving for watermelon—I even had dreams about it! The best way to deal with cravings? Go eat whatever it is your body says it needs, especially if it's fresh and healthy. (Assuming it isn't anything dangerous or highly processed, of course; if you're craving super-processed foods, talk to your OB-GYN or midwife about your diet because you might be lacking nutrients.) Don't question the logic. Your body knows what it's doing.

BUT DO EAT MINDFULLY

With Honor, I took the whole "eating for two" thing a little too literally and let Cash go wild, making half a pack of (nitrate-free) bacon for breakfast every morning and eating tons of dessert every night. It's a vicious cycle where the more junk you eat, the more you crave. Not only did this result in *waaay* more baby weight than I wanted, but I felt a lot more sluggish and uncomfortable in my own skin. I paid closer attention to portion sizes and eating what my body was truly hungry for during my pregnancy with Haven. I always kept a healthy snack on hand, so I wouldn't wind up starving and eating crap because it was right in front of me.

DON'T FORGET TO EXERCISE

You won't want to, but sticking with even a super-basic exercise program will make you stronger going into the delivery and make it much easier to bounce back afterward. I worked out until seven months when I was pregnant with Honor, but then I stopped dead and it was game over. I gained more than 60 pounds during that pregnancy. This was not easy—it took a full year of major concerted

CREATE A BIRTH PLAN

I could not have gotten through either of my deliveries without my birth plan, which my doula, Alisha Tamburri (clearmindhypno therapy.com), helped us write. We took Alisha's HypnoBirthing course, where you learn how to have a very quiet, relaxed, natural birth. Of course, there are many right ways to birth a baby, but whatever route you choose—hospital, birthing center, home birth—do take the time to write out your birth plan, including details about when and how to consider inducement, whom you want present at the birth, what labor technique you want to use, your medication preferences, etc. Share it with your doctor or midwife early in the process, Alisha says. Birth is always full of surprises, but at least you will have discussed your preferences.

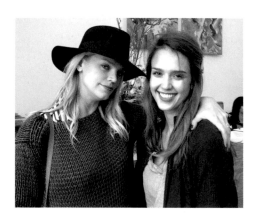

effort to lose the weight. With Haven, I did pre-natal yoga and took 30-minute walks throughout my third trimester. Plus I had a 3-year-old running around. Staying more active was a huge benefit. I gained much less and had more energy. I also felt comfortable a lot more quickly. Not everyone struggles to lose baby weight or ride out mood swings—I'm just letting you in on my experience and how I coped.

FIND THE RIGHT SUPPORT

My chiropractor and yoga teacher were my saviors during my second pregnancy because I had a lot of lower back pain and very tight hips. It's also important to figure out whom you want on your team for the birth. For Honor, I was induced because my fluids were low and we chose a hospital delivery with a "walking epidural" (so I could feel the contractions and walk to the bathroom if necessary). For Haven, we also had a hospital delivery (this time, I went into labor naturally). Through both pregnancies, Cash and I took hypnobirthing classes, where you learn to relax through guided meditation. This was a great tool before birth, and I still apply some of the techniques we learned when I feel overwhelmed and need to unwind.

My good friend Kelly has gotten me through the highs and lows of pregnancy and motherhood.

Finding a friend to exercise with pre- and post-baby is a lifesaver. Kelly and I suffered through a lot of workouts together; I pushed us to stay focused and she kept us laughing the whole time.

Dealing with Pregnancy Paranoia

I **KNOW IT WELL,** since I spent most of my first pregnancy in a mild-to-extreme panic about what environmental toxins could do to my baby. And it's not just the eco-health stuff (although we'll get to that, don't you worry!). Getting ready to have a baby is such a life-altering, overpowering experience and so thoroughly beyond your control. You may or may not have a lot of fears, but here are a few of mine—and how I dealt.

Being a Mom Means Losing Myself

I'VE **ALWAYS BEEN** a fiercely independent person. It was crazy to think that in a couple of months, I'd have to transition from being totally independent to being totally *depended on*. And even weirder, that I'd need to depend on other people—Cash, our baby's grandparents, our siblings, my mom friends and extended family—for support, because there would be lots of times when I wouldn't know what the heck I was doing. Asking for help doesn't come easily to me, so that was hard. But I gradually realized the age-old saying "It takes a village to raise a child" is true—and the closer we got to the delivery, the more I found that to be such a relief. I didn't have to do it all by myself. I could still be me—becoming a parent is about this balance of holding on to the things that are important to you (your sense of self) and knowing when to let go of the ideas that are no longer

crucial to your identity (like the complete fallacy that you have to do it all and be perfect!).

Becoming a parent changed me, for the better—I have a whole new scope of interests and passions that I was only dimly aware of before! I'm proud to be that lame-sauce parent who will bore everyone with pictures of her kids on her cell phone. What can I say—my family is the best thing in the whole world to me, and nothing gives me more joy or greater pleasure than hearing my kiddos say their first words, or see them taking their first steps, or showing off their individuality in gestures, facial expressions, and opinions about the world around them.

My Romantic Relationship Will Change

OKAY, ACTUALLY, IT DID. But that isn't necessarily a bad thing! Going from "we" to "three" (and then four) absolutely strengthened our bond. You have to work together, make tough decisions together, see each other at your most vulnerable and sleep deprived (looking not cute doesn't even begin to describe it, nor will it matter!). Yet you still want to wake up next to the other person every morning and snuggle most

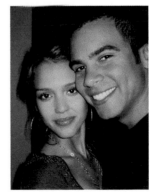

Cash and me in our dating days—we look so well rested!

nights. I was terrified we'd lose the romance—and it's true, romance doesn't mean the kind of grand gestures that it used to when we were first dating. But when Cash gets up to deal with a midnight fever or takes the girls to the park for an afternoon to give me some "me" time, that's crazy romantic.

It Will Never Feel Like "My" Body Again

BEING PREGNANT can be magical and wonderful . . . but it's also like being kidnapped by aliens. I always felt like I'd zipped on this other body, which was now solely focused on making a baby, not on being *my* body as I'd always known it. It was hard to feel so disconnected from myself. It didn't necessarily get easier once my kids were born either, because if you're breastfeeding, you still feel like your body has been taken over to feed this infant. Even if you're not breastfeeding, being woken up constantly and unexpectedly can get super disorienting. So I worried a lot that I'd never feel like myself again.

But you do get there. Trust me. Both times, there was suddenly this one day, many months later, when it felt like everything zipped back into place and I was me again. I wish I could figure out exactly what did it (or how to get there faster)—but I think it's one of those things where you just need to be patient and kind to yourself. Remember that it really is still your body—doing something incredible and wonderful beyond anything you ever imagined!

I'll Go Insane Avoiding the Toxic Traps

SO NOW, the biggest fear of all for me: How to keep a baby safe from all the environmental hazards crowding out the healthy in our world. I mean, everything else—your independence, your relationship—feels pretty abstract and inconsequential compared to this. It's very easy to become toxin obsessed and try to trap your pregnant self in a (biodegradable, nonplastic) bubble for 10 months. But you can't live this way. You have to go on breathing the air, leaving the house, and so on—and even if you took every precaution, you'd still inevitably fail to avoid every single infinitesimal risk *and* drive yourself (and your family) crazy in the process.

My advice is to pay attention to the "Dishonest Ingredients" scattered throughout this book—but remember that you're only human and you can't control the universe. Chances are very good that your baby will be just fine. So let go of what you can't control and just focus on the handful of things that are within your power—what you're eating, drinking, and bringing into your home. If you're relatively careful on these fronts, you can rest easy knowing you've given your baby every shot at a healthy and happy existence.

Pure & Simple: The Honest Nursery

WHEN WE HAD HONOR, we had everything prepped and ready to go months before she arrived—and not just for the initial newborn stage either—even though, of course, as soon as she showed up, I realized there was no way we could ever have been prepared for the new adventure that was about to start.

With Haven's arrival, we had to undergo a major home renovation to make room for another

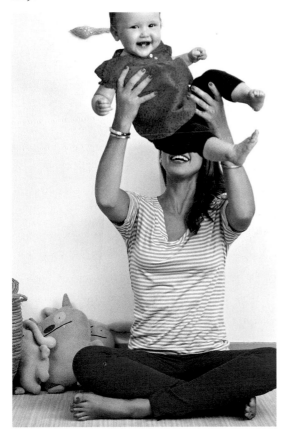

baby, but that meant we had to temporarily move out of the house while the work was being done, since—even with all of my efforts to choose eco-friendly, nontoxic materials—it's not safe for pregnant women or little kids to be around a building site. That meant I didn't have a nursery to decorate or any space to stockpile gear. And you know? It was totally okay. Honor had spent her first five months in a cosleeper in our room anyway, so it wasn't like this new baby would need a perfectly prepared nursery the second we got home from the hospital. Instead, we focused on getting the bulk of the renovation done early and safely, and then we took our time with the fun details for Haven. I was a lot more laid-back and go with the flow—and I bought way less stuff, both because we could use Honor's hand-me-downs and because I'd realized the first time around how much you just do not need all of that excess.

The truth is, new babies don't need much in the beginning. Diapers, a few onesies, swaddle blankets, burp cloths, somewhere safe to sleep, and you're pretty much set. Picking out a color scheme for your nursery, finding the perfect ergonomic rocking chair, stacking up pretty piles of receiving blankets and plush toys? That's your call. If you find the process helpful and comforting—and more important, fun!—the way I did, then by all means, go bananas. But please don't stress if your nursery doesn't look perfectly styled like the ones you see in parenting magazines and design blogs. Your baby

(continued on page 154)

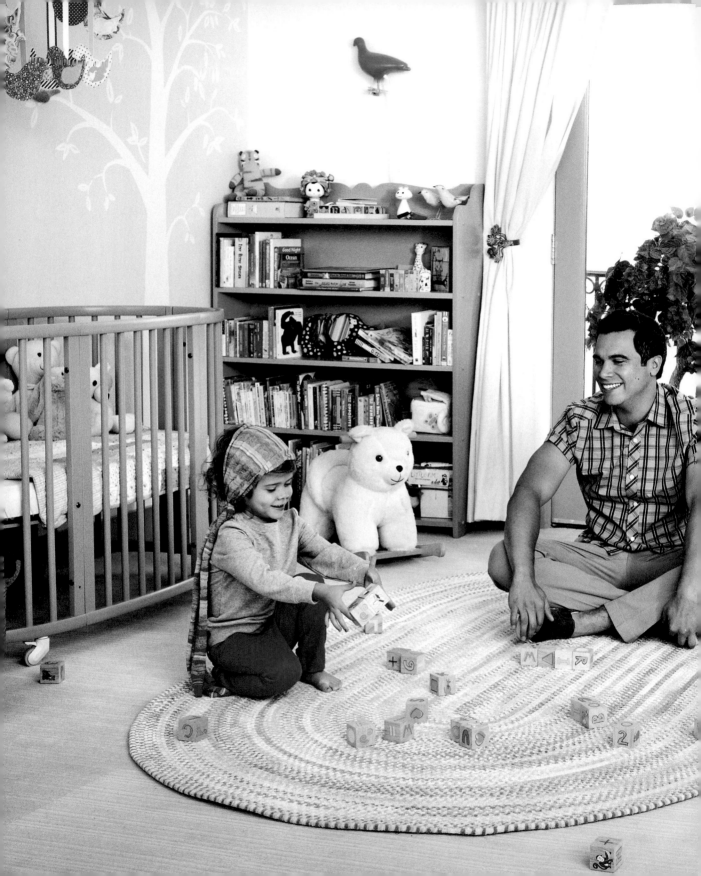

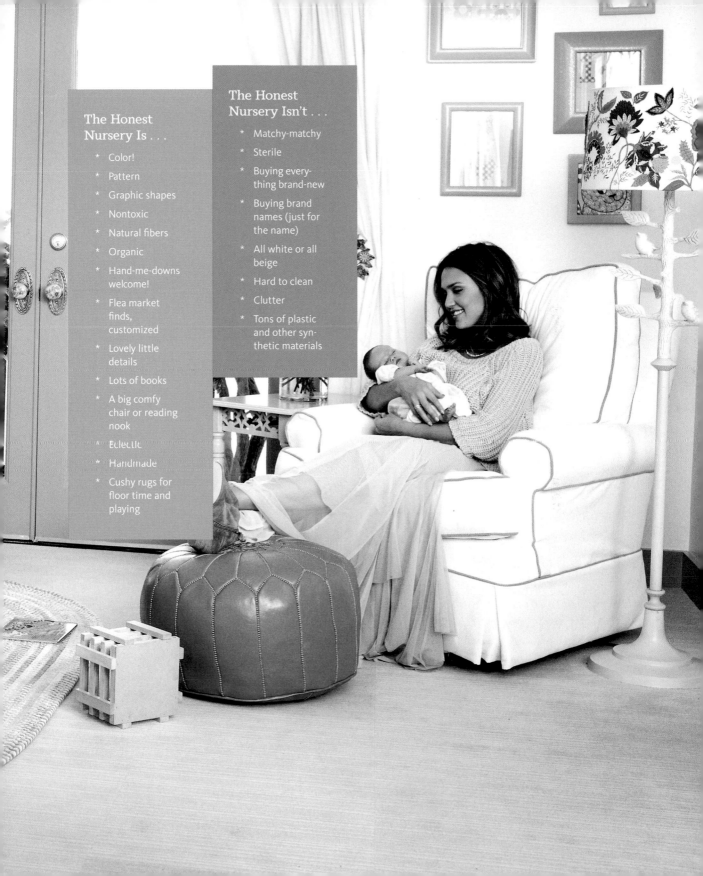

The Honest Nursery Is . . .

* Color!
* Pattern
* Graphic shapes
* Nontoxic
* Natural fibers
* Organic
* Hand-me-downs welcome!
* Flea market finds, customized
* Lovely little details
* Lots of books
* A big comfy chair or reading nook
* Eclectic
* Handmade
* Cushy rugs for floor time and playing

The Honest Nursery Isn't . . .

* Matchy-matchy
* Sterile
* Buying everything brand-new
* Buying brand names (just for the name)
* All white or all beige
* Hard to clean
* Clutter
* Tons of plastic and other synthetic materials

doesn't read parenting magazines or design blogs. Remember that just like with the rest of your home, your Honest Nursery shouldn't replicate a store display—it should be a reflection of your family's needs and style. For my girls, that has meant using an eclectic mix of furniture found at flea markets and online at Craigslist and Etsy, and purchases of my favorite baby brands that put a major emphasis on using nontoxic materials.

Starting from Scratch: Remodel Safely

IF YOU HAVE big plans for your nursery, don't wait until your third trimester to start renovating. Pregnant women and their fetuses are especially vulnerable to contaminants in plaster, paint, lead dust, particleboard (what most inexpensive furniture is made from), treated wood, and carpet fumes. In particular, let someone else do the demo and painting and absolutely avoid scraping and sanding surfaces yourself—that dust is likely chock-full of toxic chemicals, metals, and other bad news. Your safest strategy for a major reno is to consider staying with grandparents or friends while the work is being done. Better yet, aim to

HOW TO CHECK FOR LEAD PAINT

Before you (or better yet, someone else!) pick up a paintbrush, it's crucial to be sure your nursery's walls and trim do not contain any lead paint because lead poisoning can harm a child's developing brain—and babies can be exposed in utero. And never, ever sand down old paint during pregnancy. DIY lead-testing kits are available at your local hardware store, but by far the best thing to do is to have a lead-certified contractor give your home a proper assessment—and then handle the remediation, if necessary. The National Lead Information Center provides a list of EPA-certified labs in your area (800-424-LEAD).

get everything finished at least two months before your due date. That allows plenty of time for dust to be vacuumed and mopped up and new furniture and paint fumes to finish off-gassing. Once you move back in, run HEPA air purifiers in every room where work was done for a week or two afterward. We still have one in Haven's room.

Watch out for lead paint on windowsills; paint peels fastest there, and kids love to spend time looking out of windows. Check your sills for lead if your home was built before 1978.

THE HONEST NURSERY—SAFER SWAPS

Whether you're doing a studs-out renovation or just repurposing the old guest room, consider these healthier alternatives to traditional nursery materials.

Instead of . . .	Consider . . .
Wall-to-wall carpet, which can emit harmful chemicals from the fibers, dyes, adhesives, and flame retardants—especially when newly installed	* **Hardwood floors** topped with organic or natural-fiber rugs. * **FLOR carpet tiles,** which are made from nontoxic, recycled materials (and can be endlessly customized!).
A new coat of conventional paint	* **Working with the current paint** (as long as you've checked it doesn't contain lead). Maybe it's not a "traditional" baby color, but that could inspire a hip and one-of-a-kind nursery theme! And it means fewer chemicals to off-gas right before the baby arrives. * **Running fans, opening windows, and using no-VOC paint** (and having a nonpregnant person do the painting—you should steer clear of the room for at least a week afterward).
Buying a brand new crib, changing table, and rocker—all made from particleboard or other composite woods, which can off-gas formaldehyde and other toxins	* **If you buy new, choosing untreated solid wood furniture,** which can be left bare or refinished with nontoxic, no-VOC paints and sealants. * **Scouring tag sales, flea markets, thrift stores, and your family's attics for used pieces.** Older composite wood pieces are likely to have finished off-gassing (older solid wood pieces are even better!). Just test all finishes for lead.
Buying a brand-new conventional crib mattress covered in baby-unfriendly vinyl, stuffed with polyurethane foam, and treated with flame retardants —all bad news for babies *PS. Whatever type of mattress you choose, make sure it's firm to protect against sudden infant death syndrome (SIDS).*	* **Buying a natural fiber (usually organic cotton) crib mattress.** It's a splurge (often $300 or more), but I think this is one worth making, considering how many hours per day your baby will spend there. If it's not in the budget, put it on your registry—family and friends can all chip in! * **Covering a conventional crib mattress with an organic allergy protective cover**—it will help block out dust mites and off-gassing chemicals.

Pure & Simple: Baby Essentials

THERE'S AN ABSOLUTELY endless list of baby gear available out there, so you will need to spend some time figuring out what will be useful for you and what's just superfluous. I recommend grilling any and all parents you know to figure out what they couldn't live without and what they never bothered to take out of its box—and keep in mind that it's going to vary so much, kid to kid. Here are my must-haves (in addition to everything covered in the "Safer Swaps" chart on page 155).

CRIB SET

Two or three sheets (so you can always have a clean one while you're doing laundry), preferably organic cotton with no synthetic finishes or flame retardants. (I don't see a need for bumpers, but they should also be flame retardant free if you plan to use them.)

SWADDLING BLANKETS

Babies do like to be bundled pretty tightly for the first few months. (Some pediatricians call this the "fourth trimester.") Again, organic cotton if you can; I love the pretty, lightweight organic and bamboo muslin blankets by Aden + Anais.

WATER-RESISTANT MATTRESS COVER

Because babies' diapers will leak.

SLEEP SACKS

I'm obsessed with these—they're so much less stressful than trying to cover your baby with a blanket and worrying she'll get it smushed on her face (Honor was an expert at freaking me out that way!), and your baby still stays warm and cozy at night. Halo's are PFC-free.

REST OF THE LAYETTE

Keep it simple—(organic) cotton onesies, leggings, pajamas, socks, and some booties. Dwell Baby has an adorable organic layette line.

TOWELS

Organic cotton or other nontoxic options. The ones with hoods are particularly helpful. You can't have too many washcloths.

BABY BATH

I prefer the kind that you can use right in your regular tub. And don't forget cups for rinsing, plus a little wooden stool so you can sit next to the tub and save your knees!

 DISHONEST INGREDIENT

FLAME RETARDANTS

* Includes perfluorinated compounds (PFCs), brominated flame retardants (BFRs), and halogenated flame retardants (HFRs)

FOUND IN: Crib mattresses and kids' pajamas (as well as carpeting, paint, and stain-resistant fabric)

WHAT IS IT AGAIN? Makes things water, stain, and flame resistant

WHY IS IT SKETCHY? PFCs, BFRs, and HFRs are endocrine disruptors, which means they mess with healthy hormonal development and can lead to reproductive and developmental disorders—that's why it's super important to minimize exposure in babies, kids, and pregnant women.

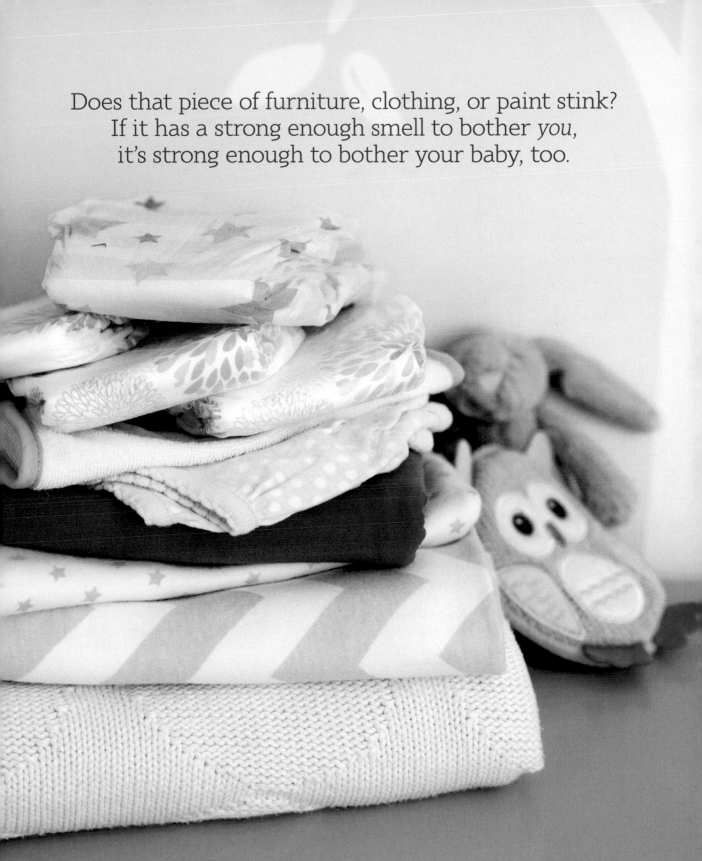

Does that piece of furniture, clothing, or paint stink?
If it has a strong enough smell to bother *you*,
it's strong enough to bother your baby, too.

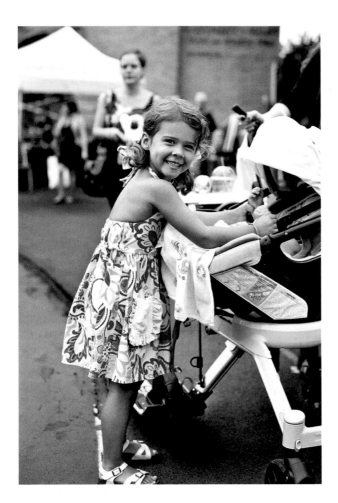

HIGH CHAIR OR BUMPER SEAT

Keep in mind that some foam-padded high chairs may contain polyurethane foam, which off-gasses nastiness. We use an Argington high chair made with sustainable wood and nontoxic finishes; you can find lots of beautiful, du-rable wooden high chairs with natural cushions in stores now. I love ours because it can also be lowered and pulled up to the table as a toddler grows. I also like bumper seats that can snap into a dining room chair—just check that kids are strapped in securely.

CAR SEATS

You can't leave the hospital without one. Fortunately, the Consumer Product Safety Commission regulates car seats pretty tightly for gen-eral safety. But lots of the plastic models leach gross chemicals like chlorine and lead. Visit HealthyCar.org for a list of the best and worst seats. No matter which model you buy, air it out for a few days on your back porch or other covered outdoor space before you stick it in the car. We used YouTube videos to fig-ure out how to install ours—lifesaver!

SWINGS AND SAUCERS

I do swear by these because they are awe-some baby entertainers whenever you need to do something requiring two hands, like taking a shower. But most options on the market use a lot of molded plastic, which can re-lease fumes . . . and offer a lot of plastic parts for your baby to chew on. So maybe consider a

gently used model or the most nontoxic option within your budget? You'll bring fewer fumes into your house that way, and you can pay it forward when you're done by reselling or donating it.

SLINGS AND CARRIERS

You have to experi-ment here to figure out what works for you and your baby; most slings hurt my shoul-ders too badly to use, so I stuck with the tried-and-true Ergo-baby Organic Carrier most of the time. (I have to say having your little one snuggled on you is the best feel-ing ever.) If you do want to try a sling or carrier, start using it right away so your baby will get used to falling asleep in there. Then you're home free—you can go gro-cery shopping or what-ever because you know kiddo is just chilling.

STROLLERS

There are tons of op-tions in the marketplace—the best tip I got was to watch online videos of real parent reviews. Consider your needs, like whether you will primarily stroll in your neighborhood, use a car whenever you take your stroller, or jog with your baby a lot. If you are in an urban environment and rely on public transportation, you might want one that is lightweight and easily collapsible. Strollers can get expensive, so this is definitely a category to try to go gently used if you can—either via Freecycle or Craigslist or from a mom friend whose kids are outgrowing theirs!

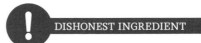

DISHONEST INGREDIENT

BISPHENOL A (BPA)

FOUND IN: Some pacifiers and baby toys (or any plastic labeled #7); recently banned by the government in baby bottles and sippy cups

WHAT IS IT? A plasticizer that makes polycarbonate plastic clear and hard

WHY IS IT SKETCHY? BPA is an endocrine disruptor. It's associated with infertility, obesity, metabolic disorders, thyroid problems, and low birth weight.

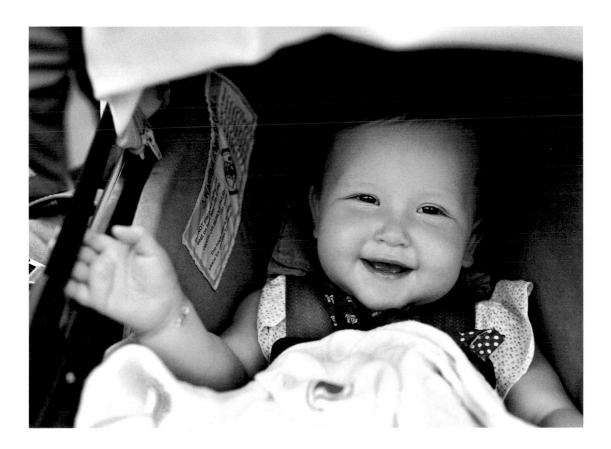

Bringing Home Baby

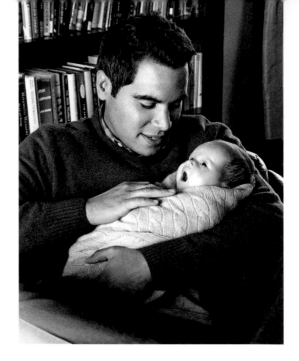

LET ME TELL YOU RIGHT NOW: The first few weeks of having your new baby home are the most surreal of your life. It's mind-boggling to have this person in the world at all—and you're totally responsible for keeping her alive, plus you are recovering from the birth while feeling super hormonal and sleep deprived. I never understood, until we went through it with Honor, that it was actually possible to feel frustrated, delighted, over-whelmed, exhausted, and crazy in love with one tiny person all at the same time—it's this constant state of butterflies-in-your-stomach joy that I could never have grasped before.

After the first three weeks or so, you turn a corner and start figuring out how to function like a person again. But it never gets totally seam-less, especially if you go back to work. Trying to work, be a mom and wife, and do it all perfectly with a smile is tough as heck. In fact, it's impos-sible. As much as I try to prepare and have every-thing planned, there are still—yes, almost five years in, this is still happening!—moments where I didn't pack enough outfits, toys, snacks, or paci-fiers, to avoid a meltdown. And the baby vomits, poops, pees (or some combination), and I only have one diaper left and no extra outfit for her, forget about me. No matter how prepared we are as moms, I've found that we're always going to make mistakes. And most crushingly, for

whatever reason, I always feel like I should be doing more. I think we all need to cut ourselves some slack.

As much as you can, let yourself off that perfection hook. Is your baby happy and healthy? *That's* all that matters—not whether you have the most perfectly packed diaper bag or whether you've managed to color-coordinate her outfit to yours (okay, I do this sometimes by accident!). And again, don't get hung up on whether every-body else thinks you're making the most socially responsible or smartest parenting decision. Go with your gut, do what works for your family, and don't sweat the small stuff.

Here's how I navigated some of those Big Baby Decisions during the first few months with both of my girls—plus some tips and tricks I fig-ured out along the way to make life with a new baby a little easier!

Honest Discussion: Is Breast Best?

THERE MAY BE no other decision you can make as a parent that will open you up to more guilt, judgment, and criticism than whether you choose to breastfeed or use formula. I don't know why, exactly, we've made this *such* a loaded issue—yes, there's lots of research showing the health benefits of breastfeeding over formula, and the official recommendation is that moms should try to breastfeed for at least the first 6 months. But what people seem to forget is that breastfeeding—as natural and wonderful as it is!—can be terribly challenging for many women. Some just plain can't do it, either because their milk doesn't come in or they have a pre-existing medical condition that doesn't allow it. Others press on but struggle with all sorts of complications. And others really want to, but have to go back to work and don't have the means to pump, due to cost, lack of privacy, or some other barrier.

At the same time, society is hypercritical of moms who breastfeed for a super-long time (longer than one year, say), even though this is quite common in other cultures. And people get squeamish about breastfeeding in public at any stage—which sure doesn't help when you're trying to do this really difficult, high-pressure thing because everyone is telling you *it's best for your baby or else*.

So can we please agree that this is one issue where everyone should just back off and let moms figure this out as best they can? Enough with the judgment already! Let's unite in supporting parents' decisions, whatever they are. With both of my daughters, I breastfed as long as I could, but not as long as I wanted. I had to get back to work, and I wasn't able to keep it going. But I am proud to say I did the best for my daughters—and I'm proud of all of my mom friends for doing the best they can on this issue. Whatever you do, trust that you're doing the best you can for your baby.

Honest Discussion: The Diaper Decision

YOU'RE GOING TO change 5,000 to 8,000 diapers before you get your kid on the potty. That, my friends, is a lot of poop. It means whether you go cloth or disposable is actually a fairly important and impactful decision—and this is not an easy call, because you not only have to weigh the environmental health concerns but you also need a diaper that *works*. I mean, if there's one product category where function really matters, this is it.

The bottom line on **conventional disposable diapers** is that they're made out of paper, plastic, and absorptive gels, all mostly nonbiodegradable, so these diapers live in landfills for decades—and we add 3.6 million tons more every year, according to the EPA. Even worse news where your baby is concerned: Conventional disposable diapers contain chemicals that were banned way back in the 1980s for use in women's tampons—yet somehow, we think they're okay to put near babies? This means the average diaper can emit

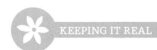

WHY I HAD TO CREATE MY OWN

I put a ton of research into diapers in my pre-Honor days and decided that we would try some of the eco-friendly, disposable options on the market. I wish we could have done cloth, but with the amount of time Cash and I work and travel, it wasn't realistic.

Once I started with those eco-disposables (which looked like brown paper bags—so not cute!), I wished we could have done cloth even more—Honor was constantly having diaper blowouts. Finally, one exhausted night, I put two diapers on her before bed. When I went in to get her the next morning, the diapers had exploded and there was tons of this white plastic popcorn stuff everywhere. It was all over Honor's crib and all over Honor—in her hair, eyes, and mouth. I called 911 in a panic because I thought, If this stuff is supposed to be absorbent, what if it swells up in her stomach?

When I called the diaper company to find out what this white popcorn crap was, they wouldn't tell me! I'm sorry, but that is unacceptable to me—both as a mom and as an environmentalist. That's why Christopher and I decided that The Honest Company would start with diapers—and do it better. Our diapers are nontoxic, made from plant-based ingredients, as biodegradable as possible, and are the most absorbent and disposable on the market (in fact, they have outperformed both conventional and eco-brands by 25 to 45 percent). Oh, and they come in fashionably cute patterns and get delivered every month for a relatively affordable fee. We're definitely considering adding a cloth or hybrid diaper as our company grows.

toxic gases like toluene (see page 76). We don't have a lot of research on how this impacts a baby's health—but I'm not excited about it. And at least one mainstream diaper brand got into some hot water because their "new and improved" diapers were giving babies chemical rashes. No, thanks.

Cloth diapers are a much less toxic and less wasteful option, especially now that they are designed to be laundered in your home washer and dryer (instead of sending them out to a diaper service, where you lose eco-points for transportation and industrial-strength cleaners). They also come in cuter colors—you can treat them like little pants! If washing poopy diapers is not your thing, there are hybrid diapers, where you get cute reusable pants, and you just switch out an eco-safe disposable or flushable diaper liner when your kid needs changing. Cloth and hybrids are both a sizable upfront investment, but they are endlessly reusable, and you usually end up saving money in the long run over disposables. The biggest problem with both cloth and hybrids remains convenience: Most daycare centers won't deal with them, and if you're traveling, I can't begin to work out the logistics.

Enter your fourth option: **nontoxic, eco-friendly disposable diapers.** This is what ended up working best for my family—so much so that I launched my own brand! Beware of "green washing"—like the phrase "chlorine free." No diaper on the market is allowed to use chlorine anymore, so it isn't really something to boast about.

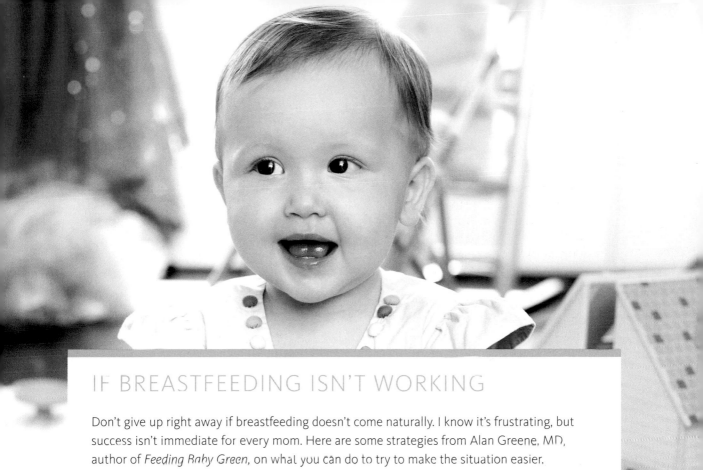

IF BREASTFEEDING ISN'T WORKING

Don't give up right away if breastfeeding doesn't come naturally. I know it's frustrating, but success isn't immediate for every mom. Here are some strategies from Alan Greene, MD, author of *Feeding Baby Green,* on what you can do to try to make the situation easier.

✳ **GET AS MUCH SLEEP AS POSSIBLE.** Let the dishes stack up—or ask a family member or close friend to come help out for a few days. Take naps.

✳ **DRINK AT LEAST EIGHT GLASSES OF WATER PER DAY.** This will help increase your milk supply.

✳ **DON'T FEED YOUR BABY MORE OFTEN THAN EVERY 90 MINUTES TO 2 HOURS.** She may want to eat more often, but if you wait a bit longer, she may eat more and stay full longer, and your milk will have time to replenish.

✳ **DON'T EVEN THINK ABOUT DIETING FOR THE FIRST SIX WEEKS** no matter how worried you are about your baby weight. You need adequate nutrition right now. (Keep taking your prenatal vitamins!)

✳ **GET SUPPORT.** Your pediatrician, lactation consultant, and OB-GYN can all offer useful insights. (*Jessica's note:* But I found that some of the best advice came from other moms I met at mommy and me classes and through mommy blogs!)

Getting Them to SLEEP!

"LACK OF SLEEP" is probably every nonparent's biggest fear. Certainly, your sleep schedule requires the biggest adjustment during the first few months of parenthood. Those first few weeks? It is what it is. Your baby needs to eat every few hours (maybe even every 90 minutes), and if you're breastfeeding, that's going to be your new around-the-clock alarm clock. With Honor, I was just about at my breaking point (especially because I couldn't drink coffee while nursing), when my girlfriend Kelly Sawyer said the magic word: "Schedule!" She had successfully transitioned both of her kids to a consistent 7:00 p.m. to 7:00 a.m. sleep schedule. It totally changed her life—and then mine.

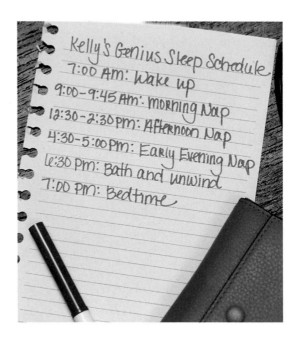

Caveat: This is a (kinder, gentler) form of sleep training, and that's *not* for everyone. Definitely discuss this strategy with your partner and your pediatrician—many experts have written about this subject and there is a wide variety of opinion. I'm simply sharing what worked for us—in the hopes that it can help you and your little ones get a better night's sleep.

That being said, here's what Kelly's Genius Sleep Schedule looks like (see photo, above)—you can start it with a child as young as a few months old, then phase out the daytime naps when your baby stops needing to sleep as much. "It may take your baby a week or so to get used to the new routine, so be patient," Kelly warns. "The key is to wake them up at the end of each naptime right on schedule—as hard as that seems! If they sleep too

much during the day, they *won't* sleep at night. It's that simple." Kelly says she implemented the schedule at four months with her first daughter, and "as soon as humanly possible" with number two. With Honor, we were able to get her on this schedule by about three months. By four weeks old, she was big enough to sleep for 6 hours at a stretch, and at that point, we started letting her be awake and fussing a bit before we'd go in to get her—gradually, we were able to stretch this from 6 to 8 to 10 to 12 hours. Amazing!

With Haven, it took a little longer—maybe four or five months before she had the full 12 hours down. But we got there, and I added my own twist to Kelly's schedule: a midnight feeding (right before I went to bed) that would help her sleep through until 7:00 or 8:00 a.m. (The key was to make sure it was at least 4 hours since her last feeding of the day, so it didn't make her sick—and to keep it very low key; lights off, no talking, just feed, change, back to bed.) Gradually, since she was sleeping less during the day, Haven started eating more—and wanted to go for longer and longer stretches of sleep at night. Of course, we aren't militant about this. Some nights, it's closer to 7:30, and when we travel, all bets are off. But we do our best to be as consistent as possible, and it really does work most of the time.

You might feel selfish at first, trying to get your baby on a schedule that lets you have 12 uninterrupted hours to yourself every night—*don't*. That big chunk of "you time" is actually just a side benefit. Babies and little kids crave routine and stability—plus all of the health benefits that come with eating at regular intervals and getting a good night's sleep. Babies learn self-soothing more quickly this way, which I think translates to having more confidence and self-reliance as they grow. Both of my girls are pretty independent, and I think a lot of that has to do with our strategy of letting them figure themselves out as much as possible.

Plus a happier, less-sleep-deprived mommy means happier kids, too! I had almost no baby blues with either of my kids, and I think the schedule was a big part of it; it helped me wrap my head around a day and a night. Which is not to knock cosleeping or less scheduled parenting whatsoever—again, this all about figuring out the best approach for you and your baby.

SAFE SLEEPING

While we're on the subject of sleep, here are a few important tips, via Dr. Alan Greene, on making sure your baby is sleeping in the safest space possible to reduce her risk of sudden infant death syndrome (SIDS).

❊ ALWAYS PLACE YOUR BABY ON HIS OR HER BACK on a firm, tight-fitting mattress in a crib that meets current safety standards.

❊ REMOVE PILLOWS, QUILTS, STUFFED TOYS, and other soft products from where your baby is sleeping.

❊ CONSIDER A SLEEPER, SLEEP SACK, or another alternative to bedding (with no other covering). If you do use a blanket, make sure it reaches only as far as the baby's chest so her head remains uncovered.

❊ NEVER LET YOUR BABY SLEEP ON A WATER BED, SOFA, SOFT MATTRESS, PILLOW, or other soft surface. Some playpens and portable cribs may have soft mattresses, so double-check.

❊ DON'T SMOKE during pregnancy or around the baby—exposure to smoking significantly increases a baby's risk of SIDS.

❊ KEEP THE ROOM TEMPERATURE COMFORTABLE for a lightly clothed adult.

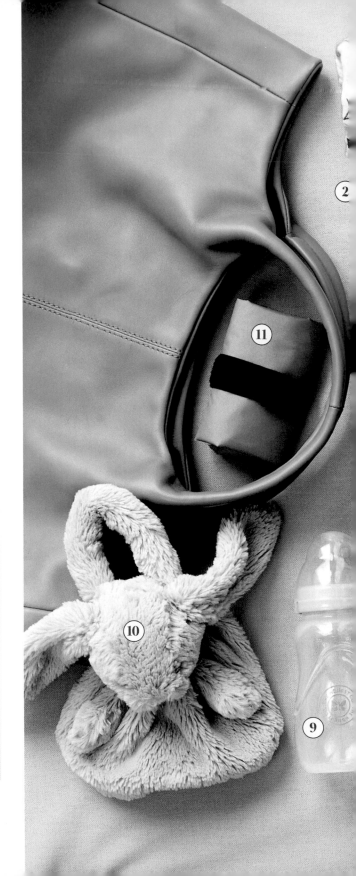

Anatomy of My Diaper Bag

One thing I've learned after having two kids is that you can never be too prepared. Kids get dirty, they get hungry, and they always need a change at the most inconvenient moment.

Don't feel like you need to cramp your style with an actual diaper bag—any oversized tote will do. Here's what I keep stashed in mine:

1. **A lightweight blanket.** For use in the car or stroller—when they're taking a nap or just get a little chilled.

2. **Diaper cream.** Make sure it's free of parabens and other nasty chemicals. Butt cream is also handy for minor scrapes.

3. **Hand sanitizer.** For disinfecting your hands after changing a diaper on the go—be sure it's made with natural ingredients.

4. **A clean outfit.** You never know when a diaper is going to leak, or the weather may change suddenly. Always carry a sun hat to protect baby's delicate skin.

5. **Eco-friendly doggie poop bags.** A great trick for wrapping dirty diapers if you're somewhere without a trashcan.

6. **Extra diapers, wipes, and changing pad.** You always need more than you think (particularly wipes, because kids touch absolutely *everything*).

7. **Pacifier.** Make sure it's BPA and PVC free; silicone pacifiers are safer than the yellow rubber kind. A strap keeps it from falling on the ground!

8. **Baby food, spoon, and bibs.** I always bring two meals' worth of food (if you take them out of the freezer before you leave, they'll defrost in your bag) and an extra bib.

9. **A bottle—or two.** Fortunately, all baby bottles are now required by law to be BPA free.

10. **A lovey or your kid's favorite soft toy.** You want to be prepared for a meltdown!

11. **An extra reusable bag.** Because shopping happens.

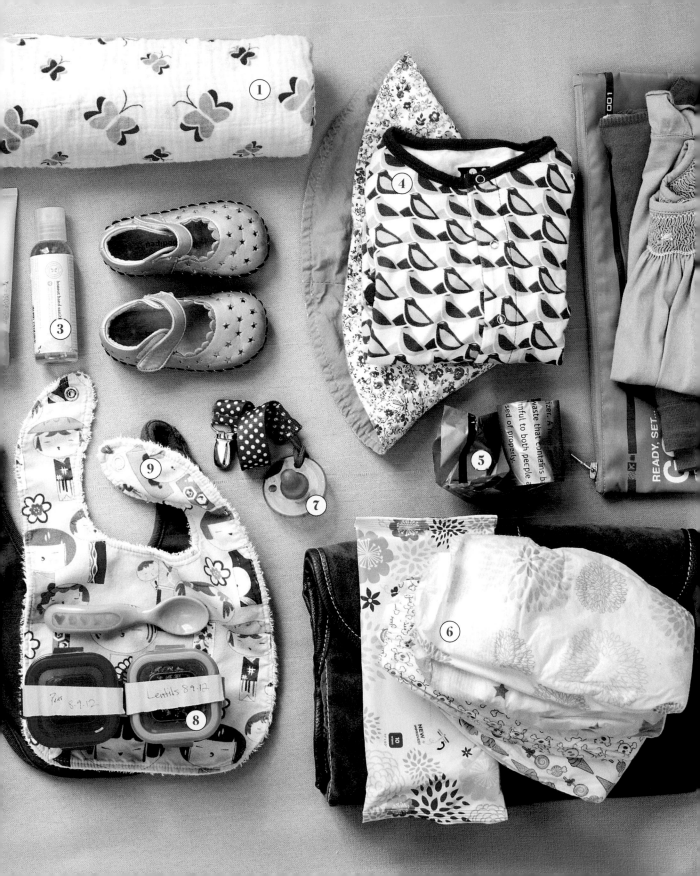

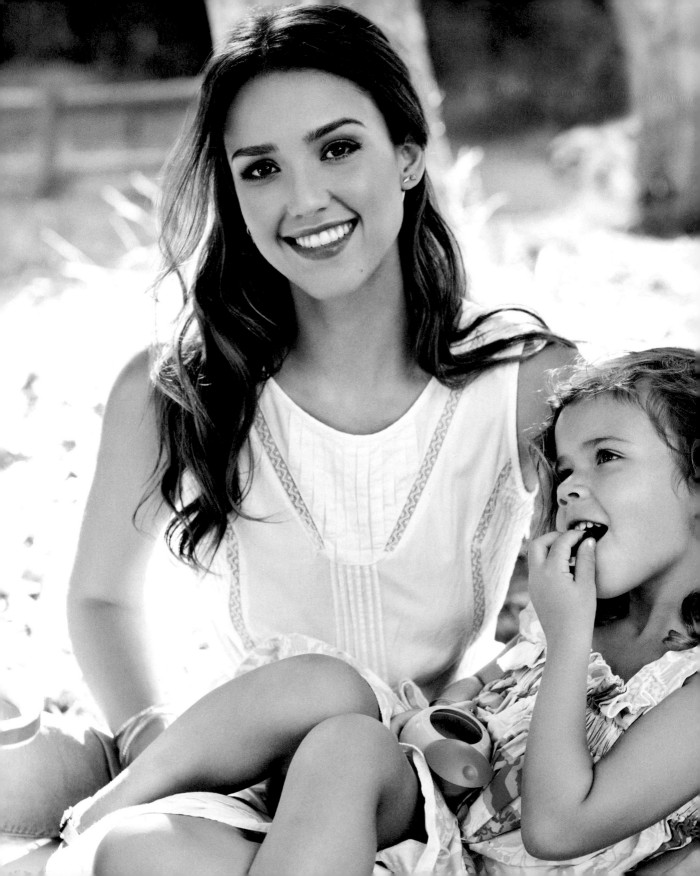

Honest Parenthood

THE ONE THING I've learned for sure about parenthood? That it all flies by faster than you want it to. When I look at Honor, it feels like just yesterday we were bringing home this tiny bundled-up baby from the hospital—and then I blinked and I was planning a mermaid-themed party for her 4th birthday! It's just the same with Haven. As I write this now, she's a squishy little sweetheart who drools, smiles, and blows raspberries at us all day long—but by the time this book is published and you're reading it, she'll be walking, talking, and who knows what.

Cash and I can't stop them from growing up (oh, how I wish!), but we can focus on being totally present and do what we can to enjoy each stage as it comes.

The Honest Routine

ONE THING I KNEW FOR SURE before I became a mom: I never wanted to be one of those women who look constantly strung out and exhausted, who never have time to change out of their sweatpants (see Chapter 4: Honest Style, lovelies!) and spend all their time griping about their husbands and lack of free time. I didn't even realize it when I first tried it out, but Kelly's Genius Sleep Schedule saved us from this in a huge way.

With the girls going to bed at 7:00 most nights, Cash and I know we're going to get a few hours of dedicated grown-up time on a regular basis—to have a glass of wine, see a movie, go to dinner, whatever. At this point, the routine is so ingrained that I can call a babysitter and make a 8:00 p.m. dinner reservation and feel entirely confident that we'll be at the restaurant on time and stress free. Carving out this alone time is especially important after almost 10 years of being together, too. Of course, we're often tired after a busy day, and it's easy to take each other for granted—but the routine reminds us that no, this is our time to be together. Even if all we do is collapse on the couch and watch bad reality TV (which . . . yeah, we do, a lot!), it feels good to be making our together time a priority.

Of course, the girls won't *always* go to bed at 7 o'clock—I'm pretty sure you can't convince a teenager to do that—and their daily schedules shift, too. Honor doesn't take naps anymore (except when we travel); and she has nursery school now. Soon Haven will have her own set of activities. But I plan to always keep meals and bedtimes as consistent as I can—I'm convinced that kids benefit from the structure. It's what has enabled us to take our girls all over the world—to Japan, Korea, the south of France, Mexico, New York, and so on—because it doesn't really matter where they are; we stick to the routine and they're happy. And it helps Cash and me juggle all of our work and other priorities around our two most important priorities, too.

TRAVELING WITH KIDS

People might think we're crazy, but it never occurred to me that becoming a mom could mean never getting on an airplane again. I have to travel for work. I don't want to be without my kids, and I'm fortunate that I can often bring the girls to work with me—so that means the entire family hits the road as needed! Of course, packing up two little ones does require a little more preparation and planning. Here are my best tips for family travel:

❋ STAY WARM. Airplanes are always freezing, and they never have enough blankets. I always bring my Nuddle so the girls and I can get cozy together.

❋ PACK REMINDERS OF HOME. When we travel from city to city and hotel to hotel, I think it's important to make life as homey as possible for the girls, so I always pack familiar things like Honor's favorite books, dress-up clothes, dollies, and the burp cloths she still snuggles for comfort, plus Haven's dolly and lovey and favorite teething toys. I also bring a collapsible storage bin (3 Sprouts makes cute ones) so we can keep it all neatly corralled in the hotel room.

❋ DIY YOUR FOOD. In my experience, kids won't touch airline food. LunchSkins reusable baggies are great for toting snacks like raw carrots, broccoli, and homemade granola mix. We bring Honor's meals in a stainless-steel bento-style ECOlunchbox (usually a sandwich, sliced fruit, and Honest Kids drinks) and pack Plum Organics baby food for Haven (homemade is too perishable, so it doesn't happen when we're on the road).

❋ ENTERTAINMENT IS KEY! Yes, we'll let Honor watch a movie or play games on the video monitor, smartphones, or tablet—they're all super helpful in getting through a flight. Make sure to keep these devices switched to airplane mode while kids are using them (even when you're not flying!), as that's supposed to decrease emitted radiation.

❋ GET THEM ON THEIR ROUTINE RIGHT AWAY. We do our best to adopt the time zone of wherever we're going as soon as we get on the plane. That means if we're landing in the afternoon, we'll try to have the girls sleep the first half of the flight; if we're landing in the morning, we hope they'll sleep the second half. Once we get to our destination, we switch things up from the usual schedule slightly—we've found the girls cope with jet lag better if they both go down for one big nap right after lunch until about 3:00 p.m. We'll usually have to wake them and keep them up until 7:00 p.m. the first day or two—but then they sleep through the night like champs.

> I feel so fortunate that I can often bring the girls on my work trips . . . but it's important to get them on their routine right away.

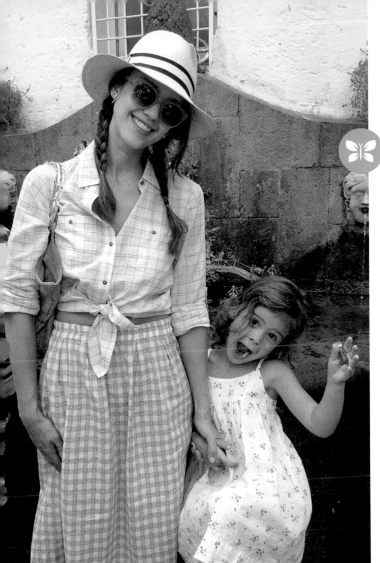

PACKING SECRETS

I always pack in outfits when I travel—and do the same for the kids. I check my schedule and the weather forecast, then I plan exactly what I'm going to wear each day and night and pack each whole outfit together in reusable nylon bags, which I label (I got these at Paris' Hotel Costes, but I love the Spacepak system from Flight 001). Then when I'm on the road, I just unzip that day's bag and boom, I'm good to go. No more stressing about what happens if the weather changes or panic attacks because you brought a skirt that doesn't go with any of your shoes.

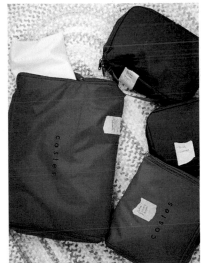

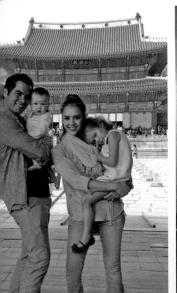

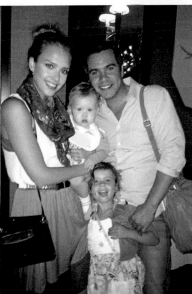

Combating Clinginess

HAVEN IS a very laid-back baby and generally happy to hang out with anyone. Honor was a whole other story. Maybe because she was my first baby, or maybe because that's just Honor, but she had a lot of attitude—and she went through a major phase of screaming if anybody but me or Cash picked her up. If you're dealing with that kind of clinginess, I feel your pain. It can be super un-fun and stressful. Here's what worked for me (with some advice from Dr. Greene):

Remember to be present. When you're alone with your baby, focus on your baby, *not* on multitasking like crazy around her. Save that for when you can tag team with her dad or someone else.

Make sure she spends time with other people. This can be so hard, I know—especially if there are tears at every departure. But having her dad or another responsible adult take your child for an hour or so each day will give you a little time to do the things you need to do (without her crying to be picked up) and help her build some resilience to being without you. I put Honor in situations with family and friends from the beginning.

Let her cry sometimes—it's really okay. Trust your maternal instincts on this one, because you're best able to distinguish between real distress and crocodile tears. If you'd rather stop what you're doing and pick her up, great. Otherwise, do what it takes to proceed with what you're doing. She will learn both that you love her intensely and that other people have needs, too.

Building Self-Esteem

SOMETIMES I HAVE TO STOP and marvel at how my girls are growing up so differently than I did. We try hard to keep their day-to-day life normal, but there's no question that they're growing up with more resources than my parents could offer. This means I'm super conscious of making sure they grow up strong and confident—but not spoiled. A big part of that is knowing how to use praise judiciously. I believe in rewarding hard work and good behavior—not just blindly praising kids for existing. So when I talk to Honor, I try to emphasize how proud I am of specific things she's done—like helping me cook dinner, being a good friend to a playmate, and practicing her reading during story time. Here are some tips from Dr. Greene on how to praise your kids in ways that will build their self-esteem:

Always join your child in celebrating his accomplishments. It doesn't matter if the event seems significant to you or not—you can be proud that he has achieved his own goals. Point out that he must be very proud of himself, and so are you.

Offer specific praise. This is especially important if your child has accomplished something (like a finger painting) but isn't really sure whether it's "good." Even if you have no idea what she drew, you can say, "I love how you expressed yourself" or "I like the colors you chose!"

Perhaps most crucial: Offer praise when she thinks she's failed. It's so important to let kids know that it's the effort that matters (trying to get to the potty on time or use the big slide at the park), not the results. Praise for positive character traits builds self-esteem more than praise for perceived accomplishments.

Honest Discussion: When You Go from One to Two . . .

WE ALWAYS KNEW we'd want more than one child—my brother and I fought like crazy growing up, but we were also best friends. And I've loved watching my mom friends add to their broods— seeing siblings love on each other is the sweetest thing ever. But we wanted to wait until Honor was out of her "baby" stage before expanding our family. This was for two reasons: First, we wanted Honor to get as much love and attention as humanly possible as a baby. Second, we couldn't imagine hauling twice the amount of baby gear everywhere we went. Having two kids in diapers would make any decision (going to the park, eating at a restaurant, family travel, playdates, etc.) way more challenging because of the amount of baby swag you would need to bring.

While I was pregnant with Haven, our main focus was how to help Honor prepare for the

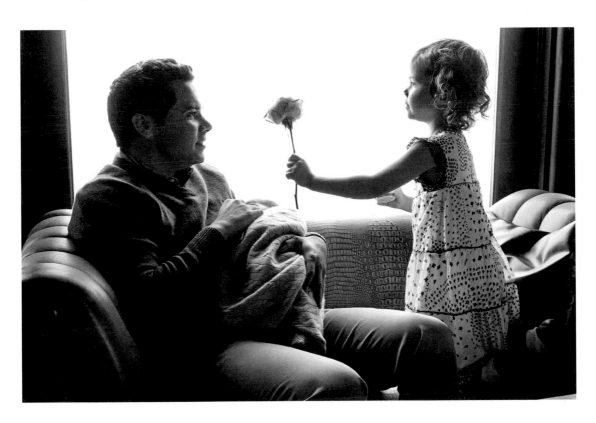

transition. We talked up how impressed we were by all of her newfound "big girl" skills—like how she got to use the toilet instead of diapers, could have dessert like cupcakes and ice cream, and play dress-up and use her swing set. By emphasizing all these awesome things that she could do, which the baby wouldn't be able to, we prevented a lot of the regression you often see in older siblings—she was all about being the big sister and having someone in the house who was younger and needed Honor to show her how to do things.

Meanwhile, my biggest concern was how on earth I'd love someone as much as we loved Honor—she was our everything! It just didn't seem like we could have the capacity to love even more. But as soon as cuddly, smiley, sweet-natured Haven arrived, that changed—all of our hearts burst open even more. Honor really can't stop herself from constantly loving on her little sister. It's just good that Haven is starting to get more mobile and vocal about objecting when all that affection gets to be a bit *too* much—as in, getting choked out by her affectionate big sister!

The best thing about having two kids, besides their sweet bond, is seeing how much of my irrational, overprotective new-mom behavior has evolved into a more easygoing, laid-back approach. I guess, in some ways, it helped that I did all that research the first time around with Honor—there wasn't as much to learn and figure out (and second-guess!) this time. But I'm also better at trusting *myself*. I know we got Honor through infancy

in one piece, so I feel confident that we could do it again with Haven. A little cough or bump on the head no longer feels like the end of the world. And *I've stopped holding myself to that unrealistic supermom standard*. When I make mistakes, I let it go and move on to more important things—like snuggling with my sweet girls.

The Honest Kid's Room

IT WAS REALLY FUN to transition Honor from her nursery to her "big girl room." We kept her in her crib until around age 3, but at that point, she was done—she screamed bloody murder and jumped right out! So we got her a trundle bed and talked about how now she could have sleepovers, and the transition went pretty smoothly. I think it also helped that the new baby was coming—Haven was getting a nursery but Honor was getting a real bed, and along with those changes, a big girl room was also an opportunity to help her learn to express herself and her sense of creativity even more and to foster her sense of independence.

Of course, when it comes to safe materials, the same principles hold for kids' rooms as for nurseries: Steer clear of toxin-emitting fiberboard furniture, wall-to-wall carpet, polyurethane-stuffed mattresses or pillows, and VOC-emitting paint. Their little bodies are still growing rapidly and they are more vulnerable than adults to all of these toxic exposures around the house.

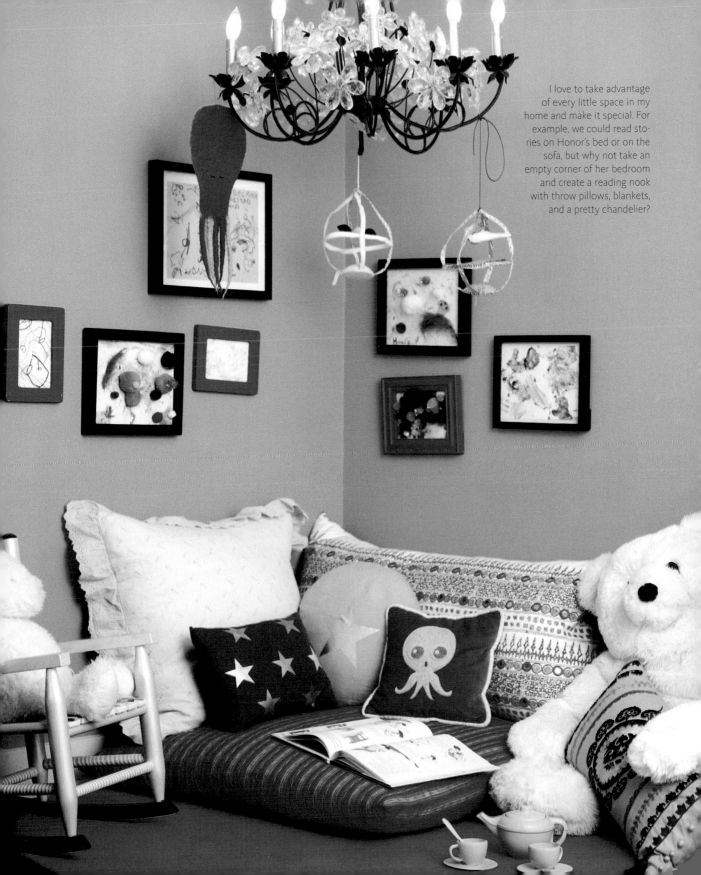

I love to take advantage of every little space in my home and make it special. For example, we could read stories on Honor's bed or on the sofa, but why not take an empty corner of her bedroom and create a reading nook with throw pillows, blankets, and a pretty chandelier?

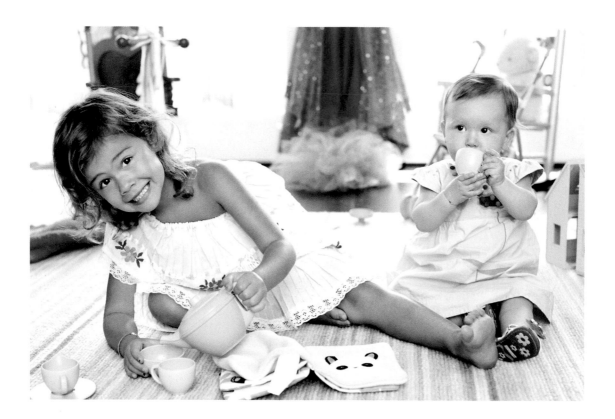

Make Playtime Safe

Shop for safer stuffed animals. Lots of the conventional teddy bears and bunnies are treated with flame retardants and stuffed with off-gassing foam filling. Your kid is going to sleep with her stuffed friend, so consider splurging on one made from organic, untreated cotton, hemp, or wool.

Opt for unfinished (or no-VOC paint) solid wood toys and PVC-free plastic toys. They are health-safe and release few, if any, harmful chemicals. For wood, natural finishes, like walnut and linseed oil, are gorgeous and safe. They do tend to be expensive—but they last for years and look great in your house, too!

You can search by product name, brand, or toy type to see if testing has revealed any toxic chemicals at HealthyStuff.org.

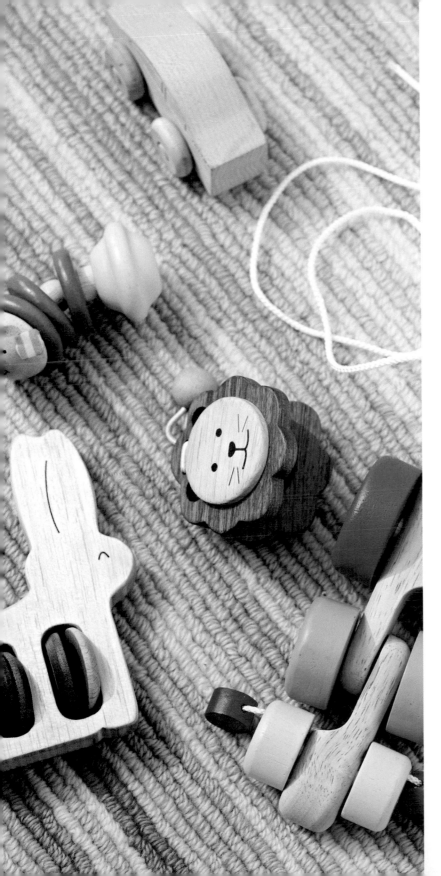

GET THE LEAD OUT OF THE TOY BOX

Just like with your walls and trim, you'll want to make sure that your children's toys and gear are lead free.

WHAT TO LOOK FOR:

✳ **If a metal or plastic toy has painted surfaces,** check the country of origin (usually stamped on the bottom). If it was made in Asia, where regulations are looser, you might want to reconsider the purchase.

✳ **Avoid antique toys.** The paint on vintage trucks and dolls is likely to be lead based, since laws prohibiting lead use didn't go into effect until 1978.

✳ **Check for recalls.** The Consumer Product Safety Commission makes an announcement whenever it recalls toys (or any consumer goods) for a safety reason; sign up at www.cpsc.gov to receive e-mail alerts.

✳ **Do a swab test.** Inexpensive lead testing kits are available at hardware stores; they aren't 100 percent accurate, but they are a good guide.

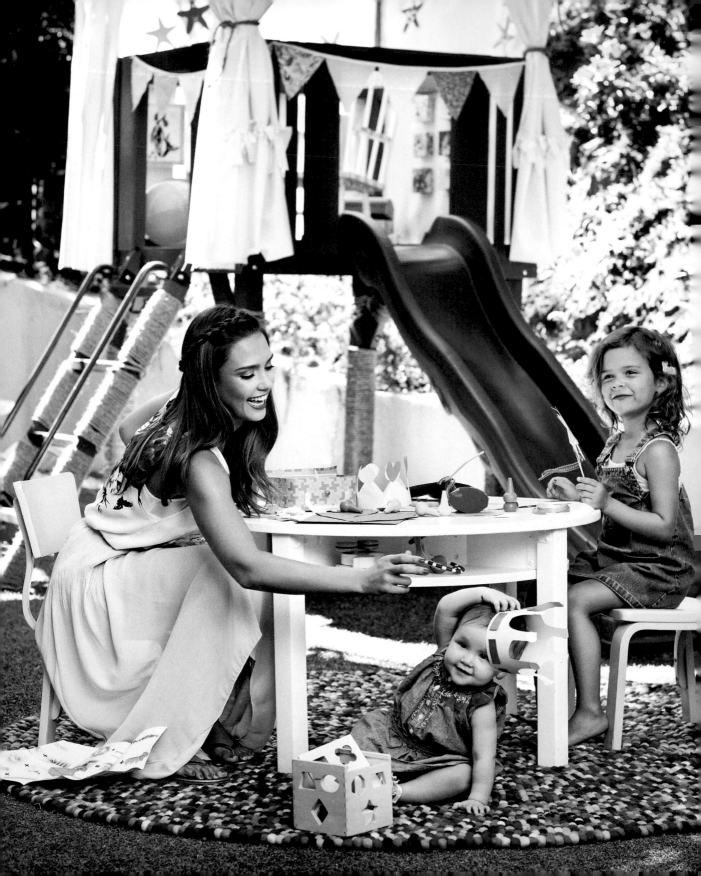

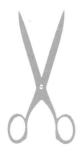

chapter 7

HONEST
inspiration

CREATE, PLAY,
LOVE, LAUGH—
HONESTLY!

THE FIRST SIX CHAPTERS OF THIS BOOK ARE YOUR practical guidebook for living the Honest Life. I've downloaded everything I figured out myself and learned from all of the experts I'm lucky enough to encounter and work with on a daily basis: environmental health gurus, doctors, nutritionists, toxicologists, cosmetic chemists, makeup artists, aestheticians, designers, stylists— and maybe most important of all, my own family members and fellow mom friends.

We've talked about my philosophies for Honest Eating, Honest Beauty, Honest Style, Honest Home, and Honest Parenting. I've packed in a ton of information, but I hope you haven't felt overwhelmed—these chapters are designed to be dog-eared, underlined, and referenced again and again. I promised no pop quizzes, and I wasn't kidding! You should keep this book handy and flip to a section whenever you have a question—like how to remove a carpet stain naturally (page 132) or make your own chicken stock (page 23).

Because Honest Living isn't only about staying organized with schedules and lists of ingredients. That's just how we keep our lives operating smoothly and ensure that our home—and primary environment—is a happy and healthy place to be. Honest Living is also about following your bliss, being creative, and thinking outside the box (or sometimes in and around it, as Honor loves to convert old boxes into play castles!). It's about finding the fun in the daily details of living, and taking every opportunity to share your love.

Some ways I express my creativity and show my family I love them are through the food I make and the way I've made our house a home—in a super-hands-on, project-oriented, far-from-perfect, thoroughly "us" style. So this chapter is a "how to" for some of my favorite Honest projects, many of which you've read about already. Some are fairly involved (refinishing a dresser). Others are quick-and-easy things you can do with the kids to foster a connection—and keep them entertained on a rainy day. What all of these projects have in common:

* They're **steeped in honest values**—healthy, safe, nontoxic, colorful, kid friendly!
* They'll **create opportunities to connect** with your kids, family, and friends.
* They'll **help you make memories**—whether that's of a beautiful day eating pizza and telling funny stories with your kids, or because you created a piece of furniture on its way to becoming an heirloom.
* Above all, they'll put a smile on your face.

I'm never one for following directions or recipes to a T—you know by now how much I love to ask questions and put my own spin on things. So don't be afraid to do the same. Consider this a collection of ideas and inspiration that you can use to jump-start your own thinking and to create your own vision for the Honest Life.

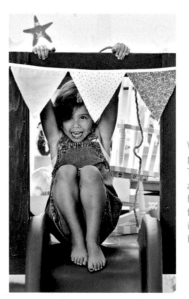

We love a good project in my house! To see how Honor and her friends helped me transform this play set into a pirate playhouse, see page 199.

ON FINDING BALANCE
(LET ME KNOW IF YOU SPOT SOME!)

Ah, yes: "balance." That elusive state in life where you're totally happy with the amount of time you get to spend with your kids, your spouse, your work . . . and don't forget about some nights out with friends and a little downtime for yourself! (I think we're also supposed to exercise regularly? Right!)

Yeah, I'm still working on this one. And to be honest, I'm not sure I'll ever have it down. I do feel fortunate that I'm in a position in my career where I don't have to work as much as I used to, and when I do, I can make sure that it's time worth spending away from my family, which means anything for The Honest Company (my third baby!) or film projects where I'm genuinely passionate about the material and excited to collaborate with the actors and filmmakers involved. But my schedule changes pretty often, depending on whether I'm shooting a film, working on a new product launch, or traveling—and whenever the daily routine shifts, there's a major ripple effect.

So like most working parents, Cash and I do the best we can during the week, although it can get a little crazy—I make sure to grab some time to talk to Honor about her day while we're eating breakfast, or I'll run home to do bath and bedtime with the girls before I need to be at an event. Our primary uninterrupted family time happens on weekends. That's when Cash and I step away from work—no e-mails, meetings, or texting—so Honor and Haven have our undivided attention. Cash makes breakfast, or we'll go out to brunch and to the park, and then usually all four of us just hang out at home, swimming and playing on the girls' swing set. It's so important to us not to be "half present," which can happen when you never turn work mode off completely. I learned that family-centered focus from my mom and dad. At some points during my childhood, they were holding down three jobs each, but my brother Josh and I never felt neglected, because when they were around, we were treated like we were the only things that mattered.

As for Cash and me, it's a never-ending, ever-evolving process—I believe that's known as "marriage"?—but keeping the girls on a regular schedule, with a 7:00 p.m. bedtime (see page 164!) has been a lifesaver.

That gives us a few hours to have dinner, talk about our days, watch TV together—or if it's a week where one of us is traveling or busy with work, that's when we can squeeze in some time with friends or have a night alone to take a bath, crack open a book, or (in my case) catch up on my favorite food, design, and mommy blogs.

I guess for me, balance isn't about treating your time like a pie chart and dividing it into equally sized slices for you, the kids, work, and so on. It's about the quality of how you spend your time, not the quantity—are you being present and focused on whatever you're doing while you're doing it? I truly believe that's how you can be the best version of yourself, whether you're in work mode, mom mode, or wife mode. When I know I'm giving my undivided attention in each of these areas, I don't feel so guilty about the time spent away from them.

Note I said not *so* guilty. This is a work in progress.

Honest Food

CHAPTER 1 of this book is full of quick recipes and easy meal ideas to keep your family well fed and to get dinner on the table in a hurry. But sometimes, I like to pull out all the stops for special-occasion eating—this can be for a literal special occasion (Honor's birthday or Thanksgiving!), or it can be one of those random Tuesday nights when I really need to catch up with my good friends.

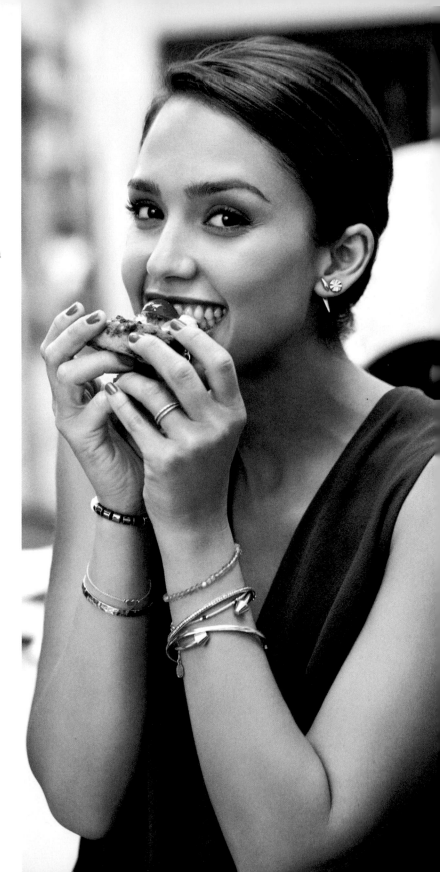

Make-Your-Own-Pizza Party

One of our favorite ways to entertain is to throw a pizza party. We have a pizza oven in our backyard, so one of our most fun Saturday projects is heating it up (it takes all day) and then going to town with lots of personal-size pizzas and toppings, which enable each guest to top his or her own. Kids love it, but you can also do very elegant topping combinations to please even the pickiest grown-up palate. No pizza oven? No worries. These recipes will work in your home oven, too.

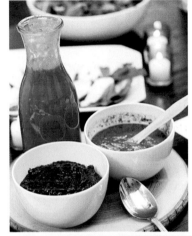

Makes 4 to 6 small pizzas

Materials

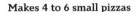

FOR DOUGH

1 packet instant yeast

2 cups warm water (about 115°F)

5 cups high-gluten organic bread flour, divided

2 tablespoons sea salt

Olive oil

FOR TOPPINGS

FOUR CHEESE: Mixture of shredded mozzarella, Parmesan, asiago, and goat cheese

VEGGIE MIX: Mushrooms, diced roasted red bell peppers, broccoli—with or without cheese; I also like to add some fresh basil or rosemary.

CLASSIC: Fresh tomato sauce with or without cheese, plus nitrate-free pepperoni

SPICY: Jalapeños, nitrate-free chorizo sausage, deep-fried sage leaves (trust me—out of this world!); awesome over the Four Cheese mix

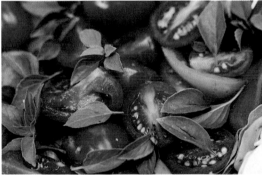

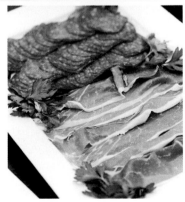

Experiment with your favorite combinations—here are some of mine!

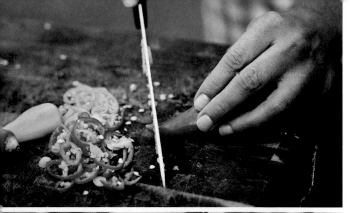

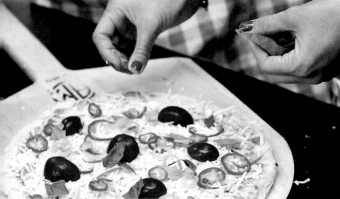

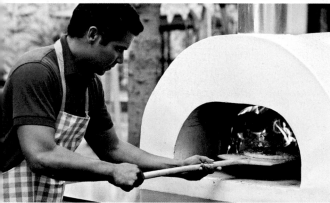

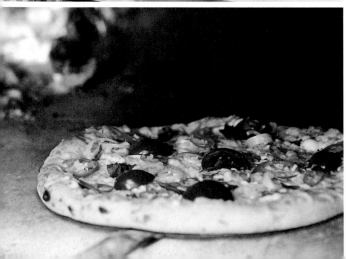

How-To

1. Mix the packet of instant yeast and then ½ cup of the flour in the warm water. Let it sit for 15 minutes until it all turns spongy or "proofs." (Once you start making dough regularly, save a little hunk from your last ball and mix it into the warm water at this stage for future pizza dough.)

2. When the yeast has proofed, add the remaining flour slowly, ½ cup at a time, mixing thoroughly with a wooden spoon as you go.

3. When all the flour has been mixed in, add the salt. At this point, the dough will be wet and tacky.

4. Knead the dough into a ball with one hand. Then move it to a floured cutting board or wood surface and knead it with two hands for 8 to 10 minutes.

5. Put the kneaded dough in a large bowl, coat it with olive oil, cover with plastic wrap, and stick it in the fridge for at least 8 hours and up to 30 hours.

6. If you're using a pizza oven, follow the manufacturer's instructions to heat it (you'll probably need to start early in the day). If you're using a regular oven, preheat it as hot as it will go (at least 450°F) about half an hour before you want to cook the pies.

7. One or 2 hours before cooking, remove the dough from the fridge and punch it down, then "scale it out," which means cutting and shaping it into round balls to make individual pizzas.

8. Place the balls gently in a big casserole dish or covered fiberglass pizza dough box and let the dough come to room temperature, then gently stretch and shape the balls into individual pies. Dust a pizza stone or an oiled baking sheet with cornmeal or flour to prevent the pies from sticking, then place the pies one at a time on the stone or sheet.

9. Cook plain pie dough for a minute to make it easier to handle, then add your toppings and bake about 15 minutes (less if pies are small), until the dough is golden and crispy and the cheese is melted.

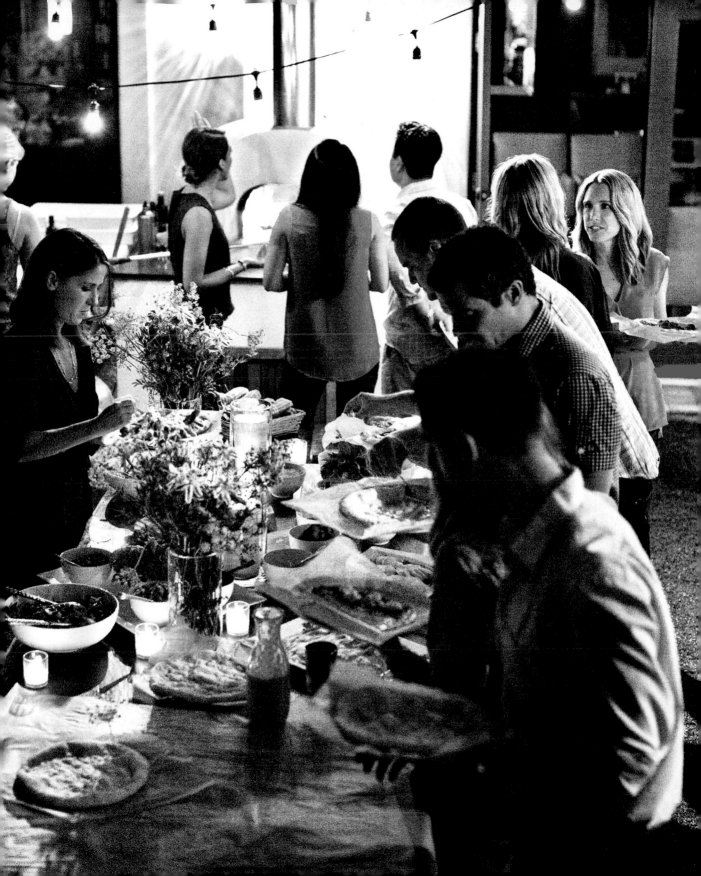

THE POST-7:00 P.M. DINNER PARTY

A roasted bird-centric meal looks impressive, but it comes together quickly. You can work it around the kids' bath time—get the chicken in the oven before you take them up, and it will be ready to come out by the time your first guests arrive. Rely on store-bought nuts, cheese, and olives for your apps—and ask friends to bring wine and dessert. Done!

Makes 6 to 8 servings

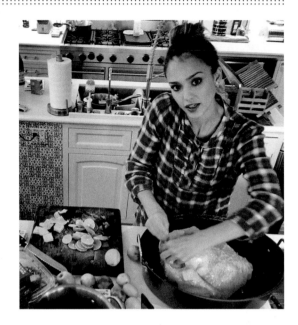

Materials

2 whole chickens (about 3 pounds each)

2 whole lemons

Seasonings of your choice: I like rosemary, garlic, olive oil, sea salt, and freshly ground black pepper

For a spicy version, add a jalapeno to the lemon in the cavity, then rub ground pepper, paprika, salt, and lemon pepper on the outside.

How-To

1. Preheat the oven to 450°F and place two cast-iron skillets or a casserole dish inside the oven to heat.

2. Season the birds. I like to put one or two sliced lemons inside the cavities and really season the heck out of the outside: Combine 4 teaspoons chopped rosemary, 4 cloves minced garlic, 2 tablespoon olive oil. Spread the mixture over the surface of the chickens, then sprinkle them with sea salt and pepper.

3. When the oven and the skillets are hot, carefully place the chickens breast sides up. Roast for 45 minutes, or until a meat thermometer registers 155°F in the thigh (you typically need about 15 minutes per pound). Remove from the oven and let rest about 15 minutes. Carve and serve.

SUPER SIDES

✳ **Kale Salad:** Thinly slice 2 bunches kale, as well as some red cabbage, carrots and Swiss chard. Toss with ½ cup olive oil and juice from 4 lemons and let sit for 30 minutes to soften tough leaves. Sprinkle with ½ cup slivered blanched almonds, salt and pepper.

✳ **Zucchini Salad:** Ribbon 2 to 3 pounds zucchini with a vegetable peeler. Dress with 3 tablespoons olive oil and juice from 1 or 2 lemons, plus sea salt and pepper. Top with ½ cup shaved Parmesan and ½ cup toasted pine nuts.

SWEET TREATS

My girls and I cannot get enough of homemade ice pops. They are a cinch to whip up, super delicious—and you get to skip the added sugar, high-fructose corn syrup, and other crap that comes in most of the store-bought kinds. Plus you can even sneak in some veggies—kids will totally gobble up anything that looks like an icy sweet! Here's how to make our favorites:

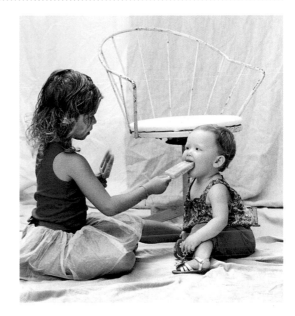

Makes 4 to 6 pops

Materials

Small paper cups or empty yogurt containers repurposed as ice-pop molds—or invest in reusable BPA-free molds from Tovolo (stars and rocket ship shapes!) or Kinderville

Ice-pop sticks (if you're DIYing)

Flavor combos—see ingredient lists, right

How-To

For all of these combinations, place the ingredients in a blender or food processor. Puree to a smoothielike consistency, then pour into molds and freeze for 1 to 3 hours. When you are ready to serve the pops, you'll find that the molds will slide off more easily if you run them under warm water for 30 seconds first. Enjoy!

STRAWBERRY LOVER'S ICE POPS

2 cups strawberries, stems removed

3 tablespoons honey

2 tablespoons lemon juice

2 tablespoons chopped basil leaves

RED, WHITE & BLUE POPS

Organic plain or vanilla yogurt

1 cup strawberries

1 cup blueberries

Organic honey to taste

Tip: Puree each kind of berry separately, then swirl them into the yogurt or pour into the molds in red, white, and blue layers for a fun design.

GO GREEN ICE POPS

3 bananas

2 cups fresh pineapple chunks

2 cups fresh spinach

1 cup water, milk of your choice, or 100% natural pineapple juice (depending on the creaminess or sweetness desired)

Honest Beauty

ONE WAY I offset some of the higher-priced products in my bathroom cabinets is by figuring out which kinds of products I don't have to buy—because I can make them myself right in my own kitchen. I grew up watching my grandmother and my mother do the same, so I wanted to share a few favorite recipes with you.

FACE Coffee Scrub

Stir 1 tablespoon finely ground coffee into ½ cup full-fat Greek yogurt with a squirt of lemon juice if you have oily skin or a tablespoon of coconut oil for dry skin. Then apply to your skin using a gentle, circular motion. Let dry and wash off.

I like to exfoliate with coffee grounds because they're high in antioxidants and the caffeine reduces puffiness. Finely ground oatmeal is a gentle alternative; baking soda also works if you're breaking out and need something a bit more aggressive.

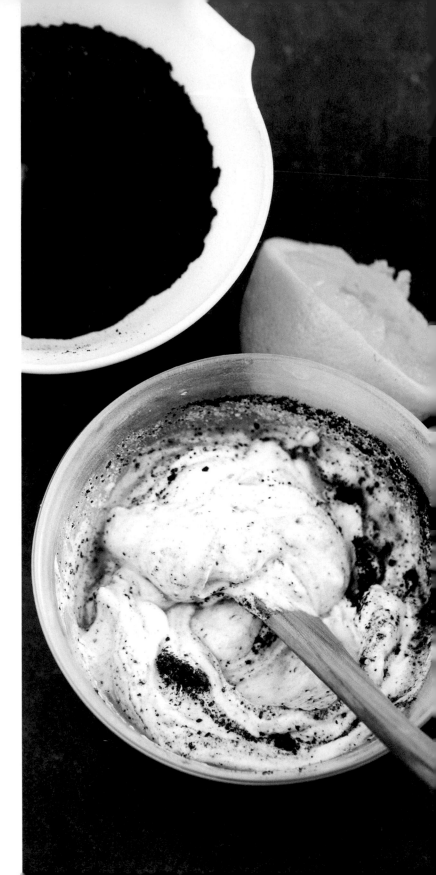

BODY Lavender Salt Bath

Mix a few drops of lavender and chamomile essential oils into a cup of Epsom salts and sprinkle them in your bath for a lovely, relaxing soak. If you need more of a pick-me-up, try a mixture of ginger, peppermint, and lemon.

::

VANILLA SUGAR SCRUB

Mix 1 part olive oil (or Honest Body Oil, or coconut oil!) and 2 parts sugar. I like to use raw cane sugar—brown sugar and sea salt are also nice, or try a combination to achieve your desired level of scrubbiness. Then add a few drops of vanilla extract (you can also use your favorite essential oil) so it smells yummy. Slather this on in the shower to exfoliate all over, then—gently!—slough it off with a washcloth.

ESSENTIAL OIL CHEST RUB

When my girls have allergies or a cold, I mix a couple of drops of eucalyptus, ginger, peppermint, and tea tree oil in with our Honest Healing Balm (you could use any balm or body oil) to make a salve that I rub on their chest and back as well as under the nose and on the bottoms of their feet.

HAIR Clarifying Apple Cider Rinse

Mix 1 or 2 tablespoons of apple cider vinegar into a cup of water, then pour it over your hair in the shower, comb through, and rinse out. This is great for getting rid of buildup, and it makes your hair crazy soft. You can experiment with adding a few drops of an essential oil to balance out the vinegar smell or follow up with a pretty-smelling conditioning treatment. In my experience, this rinse is best left for an around-the-house day when you don't mind smelling a little saladlike until your next shampoo.

::

AVOCADO & OLIVE OIL MASK

Mash up 2 avocados with a cup of olive oil. Apply this just to the ends of your hair—not to the roots or you'll be a grease ball! Wrap your hair in a towel or plastic bag and sit in the sun or under a hair dryer for 5 to 15 minutes; the heat will help all that moisturizing omega-3 fatty acid goodness penetrate more deeply. Rinse out (use cold water for extra shine) and your hair will be silky soft.

Honest Home

I HAVE SO MUCH FUN decorating our house—especially our girls' rooms, which I'm constantly tweaking and updating to suit their changing needs and tastes. I love projects that let kids interact with their rooms and add to it themselves so that they start to develop a sense of personal space.

This is great for teaching responsibility—because if you love your room, you're a little more likely to want to keep it tidy. At least, that's the hope! Maybe more important, it fosters kids' sense of their own identity and creativity: They realize that they have the power to invent their own little worlds within your bigger family world. That is so cool. Here are some ways I've infused our family's personality and spirit into the girls' rooms from day one.

One of the easiest and most impactful ways to transform the look of an old piece is with modern or whimsical hardware. Try vandykes.com or anthropologie.com for some fun options.

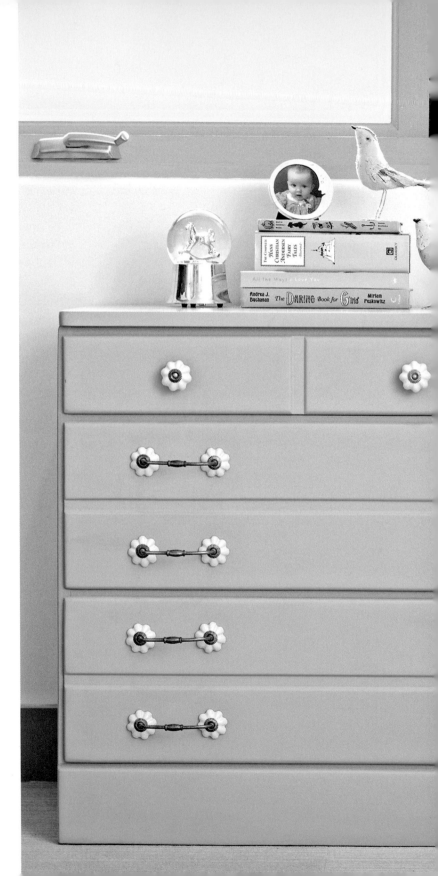

Refinished Flea Market Furniture

I found Haven's dresser and bookcase at the flea market. Originally, they didn't look anything like each other or like Honor's old changing table (which we were repurposing) or Haven's crib. A fresh coat of paint took care of all of that!

Pregnant and allergy-prone people should not be anywhere near this work. Always check a vintage piece for lead before you do any sanding (see page 154); if you get a positive result on your lead test, head straight for a professional refinisher. If you are doing the work yourself, work outside or in an extremely well-ventilated area.

Materials

Plenty of 100 grit sandpaper

Primer (oil based will be the most durable)

No-VOC latex paint

No-VOC, nontoxic water-based poly finisher like Safecoat Acrylacq

Don't be afraid of color on big pieces, especially for kids' rooms.

How-To

1. Thoroughly clean and assess the current surfaces of your piece. If they're painted, varnished, or sealed, you'll need to gently scuff the surfaces with the sandpaper (then wipe off the excess dust) so paint will adhere. If it's unfinished wood, you can probably skip the sanding part.

2. Apply a thin and even coat of nontoxic primer with a small foam roller or paintbrush. It won't look perfect, but as long as the finish isn't gloppy, you're good to go once the piece dries. (Check the recommended drying time on the primer can.)

3. Apply at least two coats of paint, again using a small foam roller or paintbrush. Keep each coat super thin and light—about the thickness of a piece of paper—and let the piece dry thoroughly between coats so you can see how the paint is adhering. I know it's a pain, but you'll be way happier in the long run if you do three or even four super-thin and even coats rather than one or two messy coats.

4. Optional: Brush on two thin and even coats of a poly finisher like Safecoat—again, making sure the paint is 100 percent dry before you start and letting each coat dry completely before moving on to the next. Applying a finisher will make your piece more durable, scratchproof, and easy to clean, plus it looks more "finished" and less "I painted this my own self!" But steer clear of the conventional polyurethane finishes—they are crazy toxic and will off-gas for ages.

5. Let your piece thoroughly dry (so that it finishes any pesky off-gassing, because even the greenest paints and finishes have some not-so-pleasant stuff in them!) on a back porch or other well-ventilated space for several days before you bring it in to its new home. Take lots of pictures and brag like heck.

MURAL WALL

I'm obsessed with the woodland mural we created in Haven's room—it makes the whole room feel like such a soothing sanctuary. Although the wall-decal trend has been hot for a while, I like that we made it three-dimensional by adding sweet little knit birds to perch on the tree branches. You can follow this idea literally or add your own touches to the decal of your choice—cloud decals with miniature toy airplanes? A garden of flower decals ornamented with fuzzy wiggly worms and pretty paper butterflies? Endless possibilities!

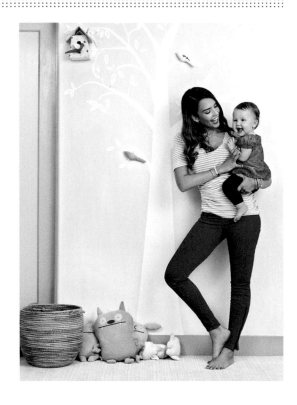

Materials

PVC-free wall decals of your choice (I like WeeDECOR, Love Mae, Pop & Lolli, and Chocovenyl on Etsy)

Bird ornaments (mine were from a mobile I scored off Etsy and then cut apart to use individually) or other accents

Tiny nails or thumbtacks

How-To

1. Decide how you want to arrange your decals on the wall—it helps to sketch this out on a piece of paper first or even lightly sketch it with a pencil on the wall. It took us forever to figure out how to evenly space the trees on either side of Haven's crib and make sure the branches were nicely arranged—don't skimp on this step. It's the difference between a wall that looks professional and one that looks, well, covered in stickers.

2. Follow the instructions that come with your decals for installation; don't forget to do any wall-prep steps to make sure you have as smooth and even a surface to work with as possible.

3. Use tiny nails or thumbtacks to add your 3-D ornaments wherever your heart desires. This is a great step to involve kids in—it's almost like decorating a Christmas tree!

FRAMED FABRIC AS ART

I found these happy vintage sheets on a trip to France years ago and had no idea what to do with them until we started on Haven's room and I realized—art! (I always pick up scraps or yardage of fabric I fall in love with and inevitably find something to use it for down the road.)

I think it's fun to mix frame sizes and shapes for a more eclectic effect.

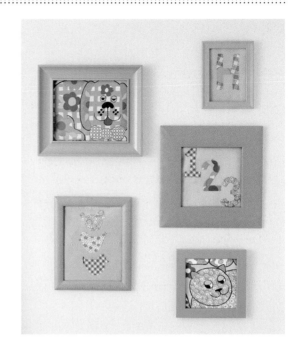

Materials

Frames (I pick these up from thrift stores or places like IKEA and Bed Bath & Beyond)

No-VOC latex paint (that color-coordinates with your fabric)

Fabric of your choice

How-To

1. Pop out the frame glass (so it doesn't get paint-y). Sand the frames if they have glossy surfaces; this will help the paint adhere. Using a small foam brush, paint the frames in colors that coordinate with your fabric, applying thin and even coats (you'll probably need two coats, especially if the frames are at all ornate).

2. While your frames are drying, measure the space inside your frames (you can usually use the glass you popped out as a template), then spread out your fabric and decide which section you'd like to frame. Use the glass template to trace that area, then cut it out with fabric scissors.

3. When the frames are completely dry, reassemble them, framing your fabric just as you would a regular photo or print. (It may help to stick the fabric to the piece of cardboard that comes in the back of the frame with a little double-sided tape so the fabric doesn't slide around.)

Honest Play

BEFORE I WAS A MOM, I thought of "playing" as just something kids did to kill time. But now I know playing is basically their job—it's how kids use their imaginations, expand their minds, and explore the world. We're always encouraging Honor to think outside the box when she plays and finding ways to sneak a little learning in, too. If we're drawing with chalk, we might draw a road and get Honor to tell us where she's going (and practice telling our left and right to get there!). If we're doing a craft project, I'll ask her to count up the glitter stars for me. Trust me . . . it doesn't feel like "education" or "work" when you're having this much fun.

Keep a stockpile of frames and paint on hand so you can add to this collection over time—it will be so cool to see how your little artist's talents and style evolve!

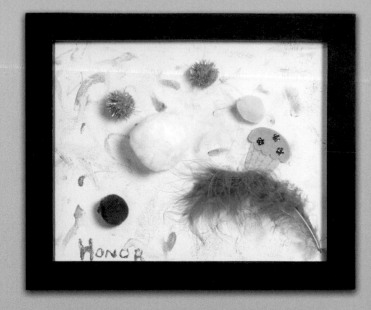
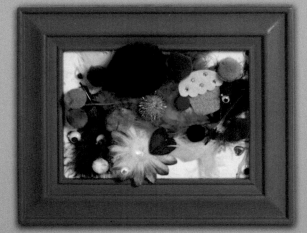
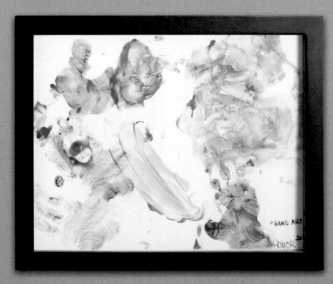

Artwork Displays

I absolutely love making art with Honor. It's such a fun way to talk to her about our imaginations and how completely limitless they are—that she really can be anything and go anywhere in her own mind. When we're painting or crafting together, I'm careful to compliment her creativity. My comments aren't along the lines of "I like how you stayed inside the lines," because to me, life is so not about staying inside the lines! It's "I love how many colors you used" or "I love how you decided to put feathers on this part—what were you thinking about when you did that?"

This project gives you a way to keep your little Picasso's treasures . . . without succumbing to kid art overload all over your house.

Materials

Art and collage supplies

Thrift-store frames

Nontoxic paint

How-To

1 Get your mini-Monet to work creating some masterpieces—finger painting, collage, whatever medium she loves. (Honor was really into feathers, so our artworks were a mix of finger paints with some feathers and other fun stuff glued on.) If your child's room has a specific color scheme, try to limit the art supplies to that palette. Otherwise, go wild!

2 Carefully remove and discard the glass from your thrift-store frames, then give them a fresh coat of paint—match your paint choices to your kid's room and/or her artwork creations.

3 Let everything dry, then slide the new masterpieces into their frames and group them on a wall of her room.

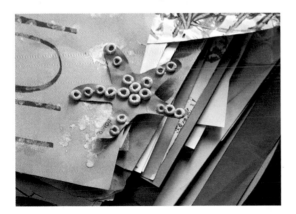

I love to store extra artwork by slipping pieces into three-ring binders (you could label one for every school year!) or rolling bigger pieces around reused wrapping paper tubes, which are easy to stash in the attic or a closet.

HOW TO FIND NONTOXIC ART SUPPLIES

This is such a bummer, but a lot of art and craft supplies (even those aimed at really little kids!) can contain hidden health hazards like lead and solvents. Companies aren't required by law to list toxic ingredients, only whether the product contains a serious hazard—indicated by statements like "fatal if swallowed." The good news: A nonprofit called the Art and Creative Materials Institute (ACMI) will grant its Approved Product (AP) seal to any product proved to contain no hazardous ingredients through testing by independent toxicologists. (If a product does contain something sketchy, it gets a CL, or Cautionary Label.) It's not fail-safe, but it's the best benchmark we have for now—so check for the AP and CL labels on any art supplies you buy for your kids. (I'm a big fan of Todd Oldham's Kid Made Modern line at Target!) Some other tips:

❊ AVOID ANY ART SUPPLIES THAT WARN AGAINST USE BY GRADE SIX AND UNDER. (California's Office of Environmental Health Hazard Assessment has a useful list at www.oehha.org; search "art hazards list.") Watercolors and water-based tempera paints are safer than anything oil or acrylic based.

❊ CHOOSE PRODUCTS LABELED "LOW ODOR," which means the markers, pens, or paint thinners have been formulated to produce fewer fumes. Bypass permanent or waterproof markers, which emit higher levels of toxic particles; scented markers are also a no-fly zone because they contain synthetic fragrances.

❊ IF A PRODUCT SAYS "DANGER," "WARNING," "CAUTION," steer clear.

❊ GET YOUR MINI-MONETS TO WASH UP WELL after they finish their art projects.

❊ LOOK FOR SOYBEAN- OR BEESWAX-BASED CRAYONS AND "NO DUST" CHALK—these may be safer than regular crayons and chalk, some of which tested positive for asbestos in a 2000 study.

❊ CHOOSE LIBRARY PASTE OR GLUE STICKS (Elmer's is a good brand) over liquid glues that can get on the skin and are more easily inhaled; definitely skip rubber cement, which contains a super-sketchy chemical called hexane.

❊ LOOK FOR BEESWAX-BASED PLAY DOUGH instead of conventional polymer clay, which contains PVCs softened by phthalates. (ACMI says the amount is too small to cause harm so it labels them "nontoxic," but FYI.)

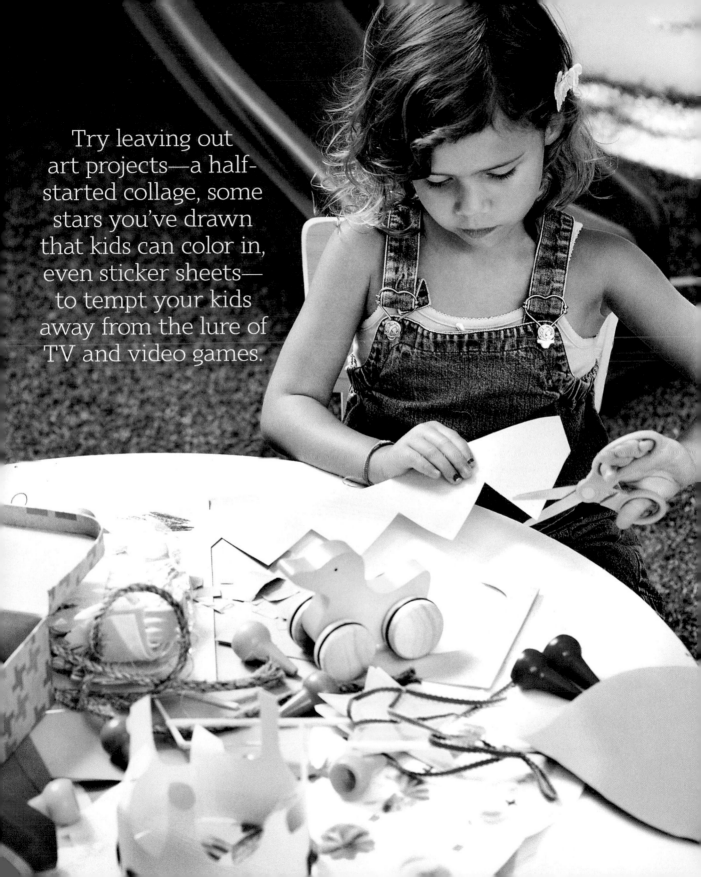

Try leaving out art projects—a half-started collage, some stars you've drawn that kids can color in, even sticker sheets— to tempt your kids away from the lure of TV and video games.

Honest Outdoors

WE GET THE GIRLS outdoors as much as possible, whether that means simply hanging out in our backyard, swimming and swinging, or heading to the park or a local nature trail. You can't teach your kids about being kind to the planet if you aren't out showing them the planet—plus going out to play is what being a kid is all about!

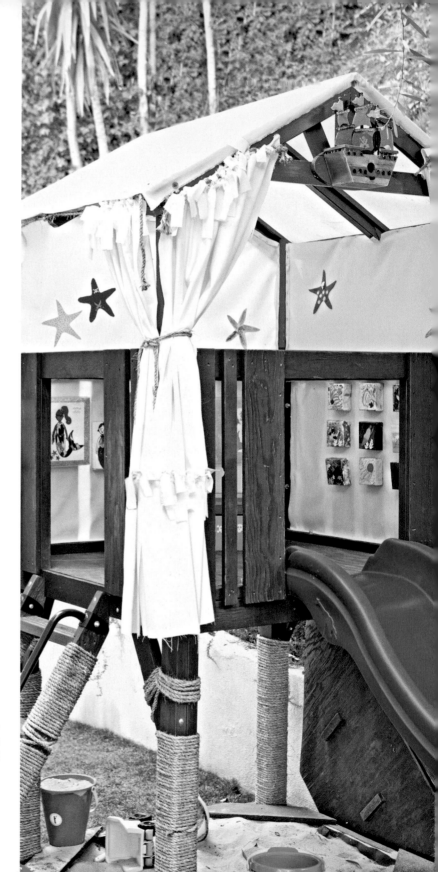

Wrap the ladder and legs of your playhouse in marine-quality rope for a fun nautical look!

Pirate Ship Playhouse

When Honor got big enough to start climbing, swinging, and sliding, we broke down and purchased one of those enormous play sets, complete with slide and playhouse, like so many parents do. I researched which brands were the most eco-conscious and went with a company called Play Well, which uses sustainably sourced redwood and environmentally friendly finishes. Then we had this big hulking play set in the backyard, which Honor and her friends loved . . . but I thought could be a little more stylish and more inspiring for their creativity. I started hunting for ideas on Pinterest and saw fabulous handmade versions, but I knew it would be way too wasteful to dump the play set we already had. Instead, I brainstormed some easy ways we could dress it up. Honor loves mermaids and pirates, so I went with a nautical theme and got her and both her cousins involved in the fun.

How-To

1. We pulled off the play set's original green awning. Using screws and a staple gun, we replaced the awning with white fabric that was reminiscent of a ship's sails.

2. Next, we wrapped the legs of the playhouse and the sides of the ladder in rope for a nautical touch. Just tie off the ends—no glue required.

3. Meanwhile, the kids got to work painting the wood pirate ships and mini–framed canvases we'd bought. We limited the color palette slightly, to keep things bright and under-the-sea themed (aquas, purples, pinks—Honor's favorites!), but otherwise basically let them go wild.

4. Once the masterpieces had dried, we coated everything with the poly finish and let that cure.

5. Last, we screwed four pirate ships to the top of the swing set and one to the top of the playhouse, then hung the mermaid-themed mini- canvases inside.

Materials

Sunbrella or other outdoor-appropriate fabric

Lots and lots of marine-quality rope

Plain wood pirate ships (you can find these on Etsy or in craft stores)

Mini–framed canvases

Nontoxic craft paint

No-VOC poly finisher—for this project we used Vermont Natural Coatings PolyWhey Exterior Wood Finish because we knew the pirate ships had to withstand the stormy seas or at least life outdoors in Los Angeles!

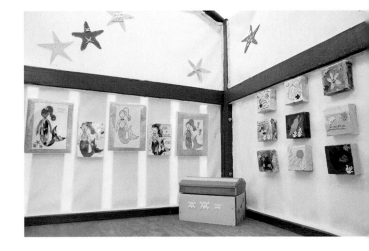

WALL GARDEN

Most of our backyard is covered in eco-friendly turf because in California, water restrictions make keeping a lawn unsustainable. So we don't have a lot of space to properly garden, but I still wanted a way to teach Honor about how plants grow and how you have to nurture and care for them with water and sunlight. Enter the wall garden! You can fit it anywhere you have a sunny spot. It's very low maintenance, and it looks fantastic. We put an herb-filled one by the kitchen—I love stepping out to snip some fresh herbs when I'm cooking!—and filled another with begonias and succulents to decorate our outdoor dining area.

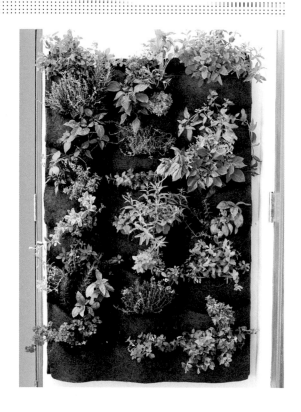

Materials

Vertical planters (I used Florafelt planters, but you can also repurpose rain gutters, wood pallets, vintage boxes, and all sorts of other things to make your own planters)

Organic potting soil

Seeds or plants of your choice (I mixed herbs in one and succulents in another)

How-To

1. Hang your planter on the wall and fill each pocket or planting space with a small amount of organic potting soil.

2. Add your plants or seeds and water well.

3. Water regularly; during hot weather, most plants need an inch of water per week from you or from the sky. Depending on what you've planted, you may need to add a small amount of organic fertilizer and compost to keep things happy. For more gardening tips and ideas, visit organicgardening.com.

Honor loves to pick a few sprigs of oregano or basil when we need it!

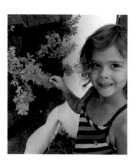

WANT MORE INSPIRATION?

Every day on The Honest Company blog, our team gets busy posting healthy recipes, arts and crafts projects, easy entertaining ideas, outdoor adventures, and other fun activities for you and your kids. Check us out at **blog.honest.com** and join our community! Here's a sampling:

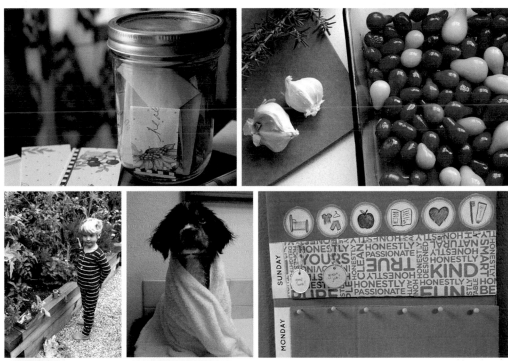

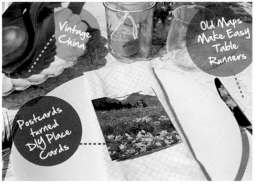

Our latest DIY projects, clockwise from top left: a daily gratitude jar; healthy pasta recipes; a creative chore chart; outdoor entertaining ideas; an edible container garden; and make-your-own nontoxic pet cleaner.

epilogue

Now on to the Rest of Your Honest Life

While you've finished the book, your Honest Life is just beginning. I hope you feel inspired to live a healthier and more sustainable lifestyle that is true to you. One where you can:

Eat (organic) meat

Wear makeup and hair products that perform

Use (eco-friendly) disposable diapers

Enjoy nontoxic items beyond the cream and the beige

. . . all the while, never sacrificing quality, performance, style, or fun.

IN FACT, I feel like we're at the start of an Honest Revolution where we are redefining the whole idea of "being green" and working to change the world into a place where we aren't constantly faced with a series of trade-offs. (Shampoo that washes your hair *or* is carcinogen free? Paint that comes in the colors you want *or* smells like toxic soup?) Instead, we get a series of trade-ups: ways to make life easier and better, while also being healthy and doing good for the planet.

People thought manufacturing eco-diapers in cute patterns and creating effective nontoxic products would be impossible. But it wasn't—we did it!—and neither is this. Honest Living is so simple that once you start doing it, you'll wonder why life wasn't always this way. Food tastes better because it's fresher and more flavorful. You have more energy because you're getting all the nutrients you need and free of all the bad stuff. Your skin clears up, and your natural beauty shines through. Getting dressed (you and the kids) becomes fun again because your closet is streamlined and you've honed your own personal sense of style. And every space in your home is a healthy, organized reflection of who you are, what you love, and how you want to live.

Friends, this is just the beginning.

Because the more automatic your Honest Living habits become, the more benefits you accrue. It's about the little stuff—like fewer squabbles in the morning over what to wear because you figured it out the night before . . . which

means more time to giggle and play mermaids and pirates with your kids (okay, maybe that's just what we do at my house). And it's about peace of mind because you can stop worrying about the health and safety ramifications of every meal you serve or products you purchase. Now, your family gets to enjoy that delicious dinner or awesome new toy—guilt free.

What can you do to make today amazing?

Actually, living guilt free is a huge part of the Honest Life. Because you know you're doing the best you can, you're letting yourself off the hook for the rest. We all are—me included.

"Perfect" is the enemy of good, and it's also the enemy of honest, because there's no such thing as the perfect wife, friend, mom, or sustainable and nontoxic environment. So let's reject those labels and standards and recognize that some weeks we're patching it together the best we can—but we don't judge ourselves. I'm not saying that living the Honest Life will keep you in some happy bubble where you never, ever sweat the small stuff. But if you cut yourself some slack and stop expecting yourself to be perfect all the time, then at least a bad day is just one bad day and nothing more.

Now that you've read the book, started making your own changes, and are living the life, your next step is a big one: taking what you've figured out about the Honest Life and sharing it with your family and friends, especially other parents. Not in a preachy way, but because you know it might make their lives a little bit easier, more fun, and healthier, too.

I hope you'll keep in touch and share with me what you're learning and making in your Honest Life. **Go to Honest.com and join our forums to trade tips and recipes, post questions—really, to share anything that's on your mind!** These types of communities were indispensable to me as a mom-to-be and brand-new mom and still are to this day. I'm excited for everyone living the Honest Life to come together and create an inspired Honest Community.

When you're talking to people about the lifestyle changes you've been making, keep it positive! It's so much better to promote what you love than to bash what you hate.

10 Essentials for an Honest Life

If you have all of these on hand (or on speed dial), you'll be more than prepared for any little dramas the day may bring.

1. WHOLE FOODS AT EVERY MEAL. That means vegetables, fruits, whole grains, beans (legumes), and lean meat—all organic, when you can manage it.

2. SOMETHING SWEET, whether that's dark chocolate or a homemade fruit pop (see page 187).

3. NONTOXIC CLEANSER, SHAMPOO, CONDITIONER, AND LOTION. To keep your skin clean and hydrated, without the nasty stuff.

4. MASCARA, LIP GLOSS, CONCEALER, AND A CLEAN TINTED MOISTURIZER WITH SPF. To pull off your 10-Minute Face.

5. SCARVES. My go-to layering piece that pulls together any outfit, hides stains, and can be endlessly customized (color! pattern! size!) to suit your style.

6. A GREAT NONTOXIC ALL-PURPOSE CLEANER. To keep your house clean—but also healthy.

7. AN INSPIRATION BOOK OR FILE. To track all your design ideas for your home.

8. A WELL-PACKED DIAPER BAG. Don't forget the change of clothes! (See page 166.)

9. "ME" TIME. Changing your life one nontoxic carpet tile at a time—while juggling your busy mom and work schedule—isn't always easy. Make sure you leave time to recharge, whether that's a glass of wine with dinner or a rocking GNO (Girl's Night Out). A happier mom = a happier family. Honestly.

10. AMAZING FRIENDS. Sharing inspiration, finding community, and loving a healthy life together is what this is all about.

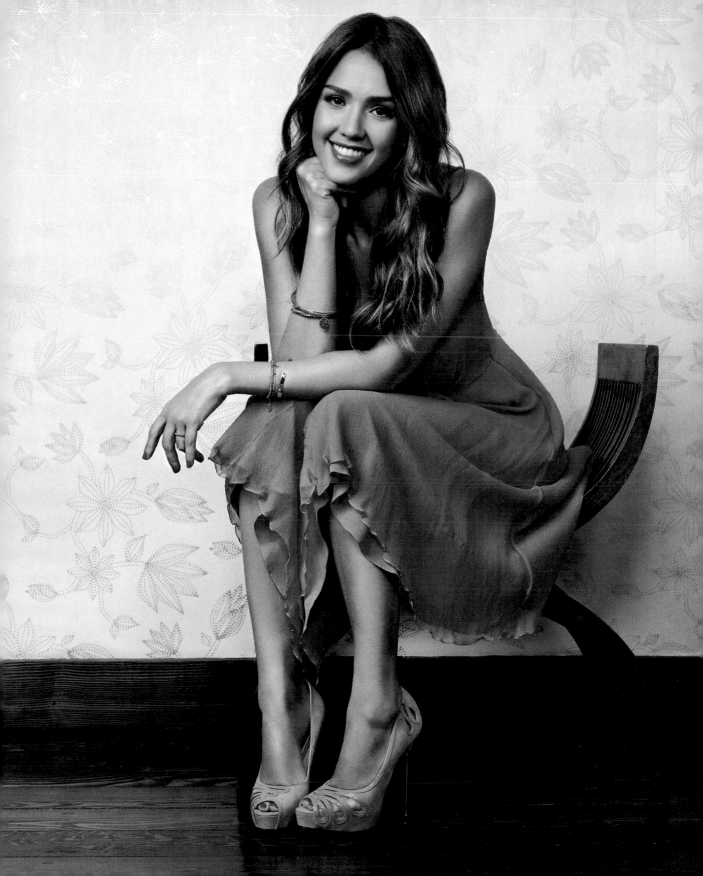

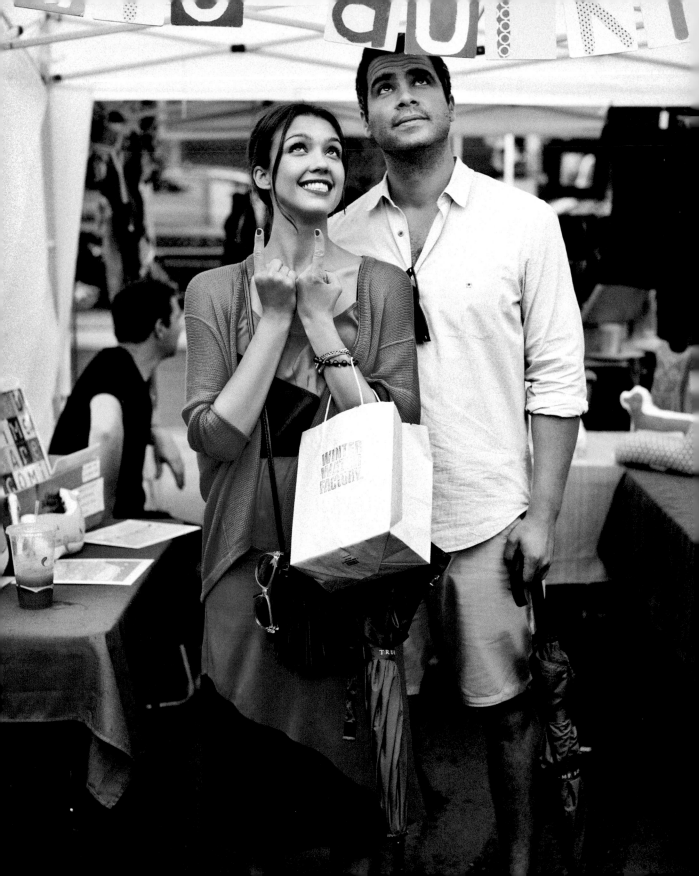

the HONEST
details

RESOURCES,
SHOPPING GUIDES,
AND ALL THE INFO
FIT FOR FINE PRINT

REMEMBER HOW I KEEP SAYING NO POP QUIZZES? THIS IS why! I've pulled together many of the resources you'll need for your Honest Life—all in one place. So just flip here the next time you want to know which low-mercury seafood to grill or the best design blogs to consult before your home renovation. I've got you covered.

207

Food Cooking & Shopping Guides

USE THESE CHARTS WHEN YOU'RE PLANNING MEALS OR AT THE GROCERY STORE TO MAKE SURE YOU'RE FEEDING YOUR FAMILY THE CLEANEST, TASTIEST, MOST HONEST MEALS POSSIBLE.

12 FOODS TO BUY ORGANIC
(and 15 to Stress Less About)

You know all about why you should buy certified organic when you can (a reminder: pesticides have been linked to everything from cancer to autism). But since it's sort of impossible to find (or afford) organic produce all the time, you can rely on the Environmental Working Group's guide to the "Dirty Dozen" to make sure you're at least doing it for the fruits and vegetables grown with the highest pesticide levels (and you can stress less about the produce on their "Clean 15" list).

Dirty Dozen Plus (Highest in pesticides; buy these organic!)	Clean 15 (Lowest in pesticides)
* Apples	* Onions
* Celery	* Sweet corn
* Sweet bell peppers	* Pineapples
* Peaches	* Avocado
* Strawberries	* Cabbage
* Nectarines (imported)	* Sweet peas
* Grapes	* Asparagus
* Spinach	* Mangoes
* Lettuce	* Eggplant
* Cucumbers	* Kiwifruit
* Blueberries (domestic)	* Cantaloupe (domestic)
* Potatoes	* Sweet potatoes
* Green beans	* Grapefruit
* Kale/greens	* Watermelon
	* Mushrooms

Source: Environmental Working Group, 2012

A GUIDE TO COOKING GRAINS

As I mentioned earlier, I love to cook a big pot of grains on the weekend: It's a great habit to get into, whatever your grain of choice, and especially if you like some of the slower-cooking whole grains like wheat berries and brown rice. All you really need is a pot, some water, and your stovetop. They all keep well for days in the fridge.

Grains that have their bran layers intact—whole grain barley, wheat, rye, kamut, and spelt— should be soaked overnight to shorten their cooking time. If you don't soak, the cooking time will be longer by an hour or more. Also, most grains benefit from a standing time of about 10 minutes, with the pot cover still on, after they've been cooked.

1 cup dry grain	Water (cups)	Approximate cooking time	Cooked yield (cups)
AMARANTH	3	20–25 minutes	2½
BARLEY, pearled	3	55 minutes	3
BUCKWHEAT GROATS	2	15 minutes	2½
CORNMEAL	4	25 minutes	3
FARRO, unhulled	3	2 hours	3⅔
FARRO, semipearled	3	30 minutes	3
KAMUT	3	2 hours	2⅔
MILLET	3	45 minutes	3½
OATS, rolled	3	15 minutes	3½
OATS, steel-cut	3	30–40 minutes	3½
QUINOA	2	12–15 minutes	3½
RICE, black	2	30 minutes	3
RICE, brown	2	35–45 minutes	3
RICE, red	2	20 minutes	3
RICE, white	2	20 minutes	3
RICE, wild	3	1 hour	4
SPELT	3	2 hours	2⅔
WHEAT BERRIES	3	2 hours	2⅔
WHEAT, bulgur	2	15–20 minutes	2½
WHEAT, cracked	2	25 minutes	2⅓

Source: The Rodale Whole Foods Cookbook

MORE TIPS FOR COOKING GRAINS:

❉ Use a large, heavy-bottomed pan to avoid possible scorching.

❉ To attain distinct, separate cooked grains, add 1 tablespoon of vegetable oil or butter to the cooking water. Bring the water to a boil, then add the uncooked grains.

❉ For a creamier grain (nice for breakfast porridge), combine the recommended cups of water with your uncooked grain and bring the mixture to a boil; then cover and cook.

❉ Don't overstir—it makes grains gummy—and use a fork.

❉ Cooked grains can sit happily in a covered pot off the heat until you need them. They will hold heat for quite a while.

A GUIDE TO COOKING BEANS, PEAS, AND LENTILS

If you want to reap all the savings and health benefits of beans, buying them dried is the way to go. Don't be intimidated—you really can't overcook them. Just like you do with your whole grains, you can make a pot on the weekend and keep it in the fridge to use all week as the foundation for many meals. All you need is a pound of dried beans (any kind!), rinsed, and salt and pepper.

Always sort through dry beans to remove any small stones or debris, then rinse well. The cooking times here are for beans that have been presoaked overnight (except lentils and split peas, which need no presoaking). Use the water amounts as general guidelines, but to be safe, make sure the beans are covered by 1 to 2 inches of water. You'll know your beans are ready when they are firm but tender and not mealy. (For a simple test, spoon out a few beans and blow on them—if the skins burst, they are sufficiently cooked.)

1 cup dried beans	Water (cups)	Approximate cooking time	Cooked yield (cups)
ADZUKI	4	45–50 minutes	2½
ANASAZI	4	1½ hours	2½
BLACK (turtle)	4	45–60 minutes	2½
CANNELLINI	4	1½ hours	2½
CHICKPEAS (garbanzos)	4	2 hours	3¼
CRANBERRY	4	45–60 minutes	2½
FAVA	4	45–60 minutes	2½
FLAGEOLETS	4	45–60 minutes	2¾
KIDNEY	3	1½ hours	2½
LENTILS, green or brown	4	30 minutes	2¾
LENTILS, red	3	20 minutes	2½
LENTILS, small (beluga, pardina, French)	3	25 minutes	2½
LIMA	4	45–60 minutes	2½
LIMA (baby)	4	45–50 minutes	2½
MUNG	4	1½ hours	2½
PEAS, BLACK-EYED	4	1 hour	2½
PEAS, split (green or yellow)	3	35–40 minutes	2¼
PEAS, whole	4	1 hour	2½
PEAS, pigeon	4	1 hour	2½
PINTO	3	1½ hours	2
RED	4	45–60 minutes	2½
SOYBEANS	5	3 hours	2¾
WHITE (great Northern, marrow, navy, pea)	4	45–60 minutes	2½–3

Source: The Rodale Whole Foods Cookbook

THE SMART SEAFOOD SELECTOR

Seafood is such an amazing form of lean protein: It's low in saturated fat and high in omega-3 fatty acids, which are insanely good for your health. But some fish are really bad for you—thanks to ocean pollution, some species are high in mercury and toxic chemicals.

But don't let confusion keep you from eating fish. The amazing team of marine ecologists and other scientists at the Environmental Defense Fund put together this Smart Seafood Selector chart; learn more at edf.org/oceans. **Any fish name in bold means it's a good source of heart-healthy omega-3s and low in contaminants.** Make these your go-to fish!

FISH	BEST	OKAY	AVOID
ARCTIC CHAR	**Farmed**		
CATFISH	US	Basa/swai/tra	
CAVIAR/STURGEON		US (farmed)	Imported or wild
CLAMS	Farmed	Wild	
COD	Pacific (Alaska longline)	Atlantic (nontrawl), Pacific (US trawl)	Atlantic (trawl), Pacific (imported)
CRAB	Dungeness, stone	Blue, king (US), snow	King (imported)
CRAWFISH	US		Imported
FLOUNDER/SOLE		Pacific, summer	Atlantic (all other)
GROUPER		Black and red (US Gulf of Mexico)	All other
HADDOCK	Hook and line	All other	
HALIBUT	Pacific	Greenland turbot	Atlantic
LOBSTER	Spiny (US)	American/Maine, spiny (Bahamas)	Spiny (Brazil)
MACKEREL, ATLANTIC	**Canada**	**US**	
MAHIMAHI	US Atlantic (pole/troll)	US (other), imported (pole/troll)	Imported (longline)
ORANGE ROUGHY			All
OYSTERS	**Farmed**	**Wild**	
POLLOCK		US (wild)	
ROCKFISH		Pacific (hook and line)	Pacific (trawl)

FISH	BEST	OKAY	AVOID
SABLEFISH/ BLACK COD	**Alaska, Canada**	California, Oregon, Washington	
SALMON	**Alaska (wild), canned (sockeye, pink)**	California, Oregon, Washington (wild)	Atlantic or farmed
SARDINES	**US**		Mediterranean
SCALLOPS	Farmed (off-bottom)	Farmed (on-bottom), sea	
SEABASS	White (Pacific)		Chilean
SHARK			All
SHRIMP	Pink (Oregon), spot prawns (Canada)	US or Canada (all other)	Imported
SNAPPER		Gray, lane, mutton, yellowtail (US)	Red, imported, vermilion
SQUID	Longfin (US)	All other	
SWORDFISH		US	Imported
TILAPIA	US	Central & South America	Asia
TROUT	**Rainbow (farmed)**		
TUNA, ALBACORE	**Canada or US (pole/troll)**	Hawaii (longline)	Imported longline, canned white
TUNA, BIGEYE, YELLOWFIN	US Atlantic (pole/troll)	Imported (pole/troll) or US (longline)	Imported (longline)
TUNA, BLUEFIN			All
TUNA, SKIPJACK	Pole/troll	US (longline)	Canned light

Source: Environmental Defense Fund

To Learn More

I ALWAYS SAY THAT I'M NO EXPERT—
I'M JUST A MOM FIGURING OUT WHAT'S
BEST FOR MY FAMILY. BUT THERE ARE
PLENTY OF TRUSTWORTHY EXPERTS
OUT THERE WHOM I TURN TO AGAIN
AND AGAIN FOR RELIABLE, UNBIASED
INFORMATION. HERE'S MY GO-TO LIST.

Change Makers

BABY2BABY
baby2baby.org

CAMPAIGN FOR
SAFE COSMETICS
safecosmetics.org

ENVIRONMENTAL
DEFENSE FUND
edf.org

ENVIRONMENTAL
WORKING GROUP
ewg.org

EVERY MOTHER
COUNTS
everymothercounts.org

GATES FOUNDATION
gatesfoundation.org

HEALTHY CHILD
HEALTHY WORLD
healthychild.org

NATURAL RESOURCES
DEFENSE COUNCIL
nrdc.org

ONE CAMPAIGN
one.org

OUR TIME
ourtime.org

SAFER CHEMICALS,
HEALTHY FAMILIES
saferchemicals.org

WOMEN'S VOICES FOR
THE EARTH
womensvoices.org

Government

CENTERS FOR
DISEASE CONTROL
AND PREVENTION
cdc.gov

CONSUMER
PRODUCT SAFETY
COMMISSION
cpsc.gov

ENVIRONMENTAL
PROTECTION AGENCY
epa.gov

FOOD & DRUG
ADMINISTRATION
fda.gov/Cosmetics/

NATIONAL ORGANIC
PROGRAM
ams.usda.gov/nop

USDA NUTRIENT
DATABASE
ndb.nal.usda.gov/ndb/
foods/list

Health

AMERICAN ACADEMY
OF ALLERGY, ASTHMA &
IMMUNOLOGY
aaaai.org

AMERICAN ACADEMY
OF DERMATOLOGY
aad.org

CLIFFORD BASSETT, MD
nyc-allergist.com

CHILDREN'S
ENVIRONMENTAL
HEALTH CENTER
AT MOUNT SINAI
SCHOOL OF MEDICINE
Philip J. Landrigan, MD,
director; cehcenter.org

JAY GORDON, MD
drjaygordon.com

ALAN GREENE, MD
drgreene.com

MAYO CLINIC
mayoclinic.com/health/

News Sources

THE ATLANTIC WIRE
theatlantic.com,
@TheAtlanticWire

BABBLE
babble.com,
@BabbleEditors

CNN
cnn.com, @cnn

HUFFINGTON POST
huffingtonpost.com,
@huffingtonpost

NEWSWEEK
newsweek.com,
@newsweek

NEW YORK TIMES
nytimes.com, @nytimes

PARENTING
parenting.com,
@parenting

POLITICO
politico.com, @politico

RODALE
Rodale.com,
@RodaleNews

TIME
time.com,
@Time and @TIMEIdeas

TREEHUGGER
treehugger.com,
@treehugger

WALL STREET JOURNAL
wsj.com, @WSJ

WIRED
wired.com, @wired

Nonprofit Databases

BUILDING GREEN
buildinggreen.com

THE ECOLOGY CENTER
& HEALTHY STUFF
healthystuff.org

HEALTHY BUILDING
NETWORK
healthybuilding.net

LOCAL HARVEST
localharvest.org

NATURAL RESOURCES
DEFENSE COUNCIL'S
SMARTER LIVING
PROGRAM
nrdc.org/living

PESTICIDE ACTION
NETWORK (PAN)
PESTICIDE DATABASE
pesticideinfo.org

SKIN DEEP COSMETICS
DATABASE
run by the Environmental
Working Group;
ewg.org/skindeep/

SUSTAINABLE TABLE
sustainabletable.org

On My Bookshelf

BORN TO BE BRAD
Brad Goreski
(HarperCollins, 2012)

DOMINO: THE BOOK
OF DECORATING
Deborah Needleman
(Simon & Schuster, 2008)

THE ESSENTIAL
GREEN YOU
Deirdre Imus
(Simon & Schuster, 2009)

HEALTHY CHILD
HEALTHY WORLD
Christopher Gavigan
(Plume, 2009)

LISTENING TO
YOUR BABY: A NEW
APPROACH TO
PARENTING YOUR
NEWBORN
Jay Gordon, MD
(Perigree Trade, 2002)

NO MORE DIRTY
LOOKS: THE TRUTH
ABOUT YOUR BEAUTY
PRODUCTS AND THE
ULTIMATE GUIDE TO
SAFE AND CLEAN
COSMETICS
Siobhan O'Connor &
Alexandra Spunt
(Da Capo, 2010)

NOT JUST A PRETTY
FACE: THE UGLY
SIDE OF THE BEAUTY
INDUSTRY
Stacy Malkan
(New Society Publishers,
2007)

THE ORGANIC BABY &
TODDLER BOOK: EASY
RECIPES FOR NATURAL
FOODS
Lizzie Vann & Daphne
Razazan
(Dorling Kindersley, 2001)

RAISING BABY GREEN
Alan Greene, MD
(Jossey-Bass, 2007)

RECIPES FROM AN
ITALIAN SUMMER
Editors of Phaidon Press
(Phaidon, 2010)

THE RODALE WHOLE
FOODS COOKBOOK
(Rodale Inc., 2009)

WHAT TO WEAR
WHERE
Hillary Kerr &
Katherine Power,
(Abrams Image, 2011)

AND OF COURSE . . .

THE HONEST COMPANY
We post tons of news you can use plus fun ideas
for projects and recipes on our Honest Blog;
blog.honest.com, @Honest.

Get Inspired

HERE'S WHERE I TURN WHEN I
NEED PRACTICAL TIPS OR A BURST
OF CREATIVITY.

Magazines

ARCHITECTURAL DIGEST
The international design authority and bible for beautiful architecture— a classic for a reason.
architecturaldigest.com

ELLE DÉCOR
The bible for design. I'll always pick up the international editions when I'm in airports, too.
elledecor.com

DO IT YOURSELF
This magazine is published by Better Homes & Gardens (they also do a whole series of special issues on say, kitchens or bathrooms, throughout the year) and is such a great primer for just about anything you want to DIY!
diyadvice.com

DWELL
All about modern design. Basically, if *Milk* and *Dwell* had a baby, that would be my design aesthetic in a nutshell.
dwell.com

HOUSE BEAUTIFUL
Also must-have plane reading, and the Web site has lots of helpful resources.
housebeautiful.com

LONNY
An online magazine inspired by the original *Domino*.
lonny.com

MILK
Incredible French mag that focuses on children's design and fashion.
milkmagazine.net

MONOCLE
Focusing on global affairs, business, culture, and design, *Monocle's* mission is to keep an eye on the world.
monocle.com

Design Blogs

79 IDEAS
79ideas.org

APARTMENT THERAPY
apartmenttherapy.com

DÉCOR BY COLOR
decorbycolor.com

DESIGN MILK
design-milk.com

DESIGN*SPONGE
designsponge.com

DESIRE TO INSPIRE
desiretoinspire.net

DOOR SIXTEEN
doorsixteen.com

ECOSALON
ecosalon.com

EMILY HENDERSON
stylebyemilyhenderson.com

HOUZZ
houzz.com

PAPERNSTITCH
papernstitchblog.com

REMODELISTA
remodelista.com

RE-NEST
apartmenttherapy.com

YOUNG HOUSE LOVE
younghouselove.com

Design-Savvy—and Eco-Inspired—Mom Blogs

A CUP OF JO
joannagoddard.blogspot.com

DESIGN MOM
designmom.com

ECOKAREN
ecokaren.com

GIRL'S GONE CHILD
girlsgonechild.net

LITTLE GREEN NOTEBOOK
littlegreennotebook.blogspot.com

PURE MAMAS
puremamas.squarespace.com

SALT & NECTAR
saltandnectar.com

THINGS WE MAKE
amypalanjian.com

Food Blogs

101 COOKBOOKS
101cookbooks.com

THE CHALKBOARD
thechalkboardmag.com

CHOCOLATE & ZUCCHINI
chocolateandzucchini.com

COOKIE + KATE
cookieandkate.com

HOMERUNBALLERINA
homerunballerina.com

MY LITTLE FABRIC
mylittlefabric.com

PIONEER WOMAN
thepioneerwoman.com

SMITTEN KITCHEN
smittenkitchen.com

WEELICIOUS
weelicious.com

Fashion Blogs

BLEACH BLACK
bleachblack.com

BRYAN BOY
bryanboy.com

THE COVETEUR
thecoveteur.com

DEREK BLASBERG
derekblasberg.com

MAN REPELLER
manrepeller.com

NASTY GAL
blog.nastygal.com

REFINERY29
refinery29.com

WHO WHAT WEAR
whowhatwear.com

Lifestyle Blogs

EJECT
kellyoxford.tumblr.com

HELLOGIGGLES
hellogiggles.com

RIP + TAN
ripplustan.com

KID BRANDS GOING PVC FREE

There has been such a great consumer backlash against PVC in kids' products—and manufacturers are listening! These brands have pledged to remove PVC and phthalates and many are already phthalate free (although it's always a good idea to double-check).

BRIO	LEGO	TINY LOVE
GERBER	LITTLE TIKES	
IKEA	SASSY	

Start Shopping

HERE'S WHERE YOU'LL FIND EVERY BRAND OR PRODUCT MENTIONED IN THIS BOOK—PLUS SOME OF MY FAVORITE STORES (BOTH BRICK AND MORTAR AND ONLINE!) FOR STYLISH, HEALTHY, HONEST FINDS.

Boutiques

10 CORSO COMO
A store in Milan that's always super curated. They also have an impressive eco-section with bags, books, and gadgets!
10corsocomo.com

ER BUTLER & CO
Officially, this is a New York City hardware store where I found knobs for my pizza oven . . . but they also create the most amazing window displays I've ever seen.
erbutler.com

GREEN DEPOT
Awesome resource for all kinds of green building and home supplies, from countertops to cleaning products. *Love.*
greendepot.com

JENNI KAYNE
I love her West Hollywood boutique, where I can always find fabulously chic day pieces, modern and unique staples, and the best collection of accessories—I practically live in the D'Orsay flats from her store.
jennikayne.com

MERCI
One of my favorite Parisian shops—located in an airy loft where you move from room to room (filled with cozy reading nooks and a tea lounge), browsing among haute vintage fashions and furniture or one-of-a-kind creations by young French designers. All profits go to a children's charity in Madagascar.
merci-merci.com

OPENING CEREMONY
This West Hollywood concept store is in Charlie Chaplin's former dance studio, and every brand has its own shop-in-the-store.
openingceremony.us

SATINE
Owner Jeannie Lee's private label collection is amazing because it's a fashionable, modern twist on classics—like the perfect little black dress or the best oversize T-shirt. And everything is limited edition so you don't have to worry about every girl on the block stealing your style.
Satineboutique.com

SERENDIPITY
The most beautiful, inspired children's store in France. I love how they'll juxtapose graffiti art with say, handmade birdhouses—or use all-natural linens but dye them fluorescent colors.
serendipity.fr

WUHAO
I discovered this boutique on a trip to Beijing—it's in the home of the last emperor's wife—think very traditional Chinese architecture and fitted tiny rooms, with gorgeous clothing and home and children's goods.
wuhaoonline.com

Baby & Kids

3 SPROUTS
3sprouts.com

ADEN + ANAIS
adenandanais.com

APPLE PARK
applepark.com

ARGINGTON
argington.com

**ART AND CREATIVE
MATERIALS INSTITUTE**
acminet.org

BABYCCINO
babyccinokids.com/shop

DWELL BABY
dwellstudio.com

ECOLUNCHBOX
ecolunchboxes.com

ERGOBABY
store.ergobaby.com

ETSY
etsy.com

GARNET HILL
garnethill.com

HANNA ANDERSSON
hannaandersson.com

**THE HONEST
COMPANY**
honest.com

LITTLE BEAN
littlebeanshop.com

**LITTLE FASHION
GALLERY**
littlefashiongallery/en/

LOVE MAE
lovemae.com.au

LUNCHSKINS
lunchskins.com

NUDDLE
Nuddleblanket.com

POP & LOLLI
popandlolli.com

TARGET
Target.com

WALMART
walmart.com

WEEDECOR
weedecor.com

Beauty

100% PURE
100percentpure.com

ALBA BOTANICA
albabotanica.com

BEAUTYBLENDER
beautyblender.net

**BURT'S BEES
NATURAL SOLUTIONS**
burtsbees.com

CELLCEUTICALS
cellceuticalskincare.com

CHOCOLATE SUN
chocolatesun.com

DERMELECT ME
dermelect.com

DIORSHOW
dior.com/mascara

**DR. BRONNER'S
MAGIC SOAP**
drbronner.com

DR. HAUSCHKA
drhauschka.com

ECOTOOLS
ecotools.com

FUTURENATURAL
futurenatural.com

HERBAN COWBOY
herbancowboy.com

HONORE DES PRES
honoredespres.com

HOPSCOTCH KIDS
hopscotchkids.com

**HOURGLASS
COSMETICS**
hourglasscosmetics.com

JANE IREDALE
janeiredale.com

**JOHN MASTERS
ORGANICS**
johnmasters.com

**KOH GEN DO
COSMETICS**
kohgendocosmetics.com

KORRES
korresusa.com

L'OREAL
loreal.com

PANGEA ORGANICS
pangeaorganics.com

PARISSA
parissa.com

PRITI NYC
pritinyc.com

**RESURFACE BY
SHANI DARDEN**
shanidarden.com

RMS BEAUTY
rmsbeauty.com

SCOTCH NATURALS
scotchnaturals.com

SEPHORA
sephora.com

SHOBHA
myshobha.com

SHU UEMURA
shuuemura-usa.com

**SPIRIT BEAUTY
LOUNGE**
spiritbeautylounge.com

SUKI SKINCARE
sukiskincare.com

TARTE
tartecosmetics.com

TATA HARPER
tataharperskincare.com

ZOYA NATURAL
zoya.com

Fashion

AZZEDINE ALAIA
alaia.fr

BROOK&LYN
brookandlyn.com

BROOKS BROTHERS
brooksbrothers.com

C&C CALIFORNIA
candccalifornia.com

CELINE
celine.com

CHANEL
chanel.com

CHEAP MONDAY
cheapmonday.com

DIANE VON
FURSTENBERG
dvf.com

DOLCE & GABBANA
dolcegabbana.com

EARNEST SEWN
earnestsewn.com

ELIZABETH AND JAMES
elizabethandjames.us

ELLE MACPHERSON
INTIMATES
ellemacphersonintimates.
com

FLIGHT 001
flight001.com

FREDERICK'S OF
HOLLYWOOD
fredericks.com

GAP
gap.com

GIVENCHY
givenchy.com

H&M
hm.com

J BRAND
jbrandjeans.com

J.CREW
jcrew.com

KATE SPADE
katespade.com

LEVI'S
levi.com

L.L.BEAN
llbean.com

LNA
lnaclothing.com

NARCISO RODRIGUEZ
narcisorodriguez.com

PRADA
prada.com

PROENZA SCHOULER
proenzaschouler.com

RALPH LAUREN
ralphlauren.com

ROGER VIVIER
rogervivier.com

SEVEN FOR ALL
MANKIND
7forallmankind.com

SIMONE
simonecollection.com

SPANX
spanx.com

SVPPLY
svpply.com

TARGET
target.com

THEORY
theory.com

TOMS
toms.com

TOPSHOP
topshop.com

TORY BURCH
toryburch.com

Food

ANNIE'S ORGANIC
(MAC & CHEESE)
annies.com

BALL MASON JARS
canningfresh.com

EDEN ORGANIC
(CANNED BEANS)
edenfoods.com

EVOLUTION FRESH
(JUICES)
evolutionfresh.com

GLUTINO (PRETZELS
AND PIZZA CRUST)
glutino.com

GREEN & BLACK'S OR-
GANIC (CHOCOLATE)
greenandblacks.com

HONEST KIDS (JUICES)
honesttea.com/kids

KINDERVILLE
kinder-ville.com

KING ARTHUR
(GLUTEN-FREE
PANCAKES MIX)
kingarthurflour.com

LIGHTLIFE SMART
DOGS
lightlife.com

MELISSA'S SOYRIZO
melissas.com

PLUM ORGANICS
(BABY FOOD)
plumorganics.com

PYREX
pyrex.com

REED'S ORIGINAL
(SODAS)
reedsinc.com

SODASTREAM
sodastreamusa.com

TOVOLO
tovolo.com

VAN'S (WAFFLES)
vansfoods.com

WEAN GREEN
weangreen.com

Home

ANTHROPOLOGIE
Anthropologie.com

CAPEL RUGS USA
capelrugs.com

FLOR
flor.com

GAIAM
gaiam.com

GARNET HILL
garnethill.com

GRAHAM & BROWN
WALLPAPER
grahambrown.com

GREEN DEPOT
greendepot.com

THE HONEST
COMPANY
honest.com

ICESTONE COUNTERS
icestoneusa.com

MYTHIC PAINT
mythicpaint.com

NATUREPEDIC
naturepedic.com

PHILLIP JEFFRIES
WALI PAPER
phillipjeffries.com

PRISTINE PLANET
pristineplanet.com

RESTORATION
HARDWARE
restorationhardware.com

ROCK CANDY LIFE
rockcandylife.com

SAFECOAT ACRYLACQ
afmsafecoat.com

SIMPLY ORGANIC
simplyorganic.com

SUNDANCE CATALOG
sundancecatalog.com

URBAN OUTFITTERS
urbanoutfitters.com

VAN DYKES
vandykes.com

VERMONT NATURAL
COATINGS
vermontnaturalcoatings.
com

VINTAGE WOOD
FLOOR COMPANY
vintagewoodfloors.com

WEST ELM
westelm.com

Outdoors

FLORAFELT
florafelt.com

PLAY WELL
play-well.com

Vintage

CRAIGSLIST
craigslist.com

EBAY
ebay.com

ETSY
etsy.com

TINI (THIS IS NOT IKEA)
thisisnotikea.com

Dishonest Ingredients

YOU'VE SEEN THESE THROUGHOUT THE BOOK, BUT I'VE LISTED THEM ALL HERE SO YOU CAN REFER TO THEM EASILY. HERE'S YOUR MASTER GUIDE TO THE TOXIC CHEMICALS TO AVOID THROUGHOUT YOUR HOME AND LIFE (ESPECIALLY WHEN YOU'RE EXPECTING OR HAVE LITTLE ONES).

Pronunciation Guide

There's no pressure to memorize this list of confusing-sounding chemicals and other sciencey terms . . . but if you want to sound authoritative when you're talking to friends and family about your new Honest Life, trotting out a couple of these will do the trick.

BISPHENOL A (BPA)
"bis-PHEEN-al A"

DIETHYLENE GLYCOL
"DI-ethel-leen GLI-col"

FORMALDEHYDE
"for-MAL-de-HIDE"

HYDROQUINONE
"HIGH-dro-quin-ohn"

MONOSODIUM GLUTAMATE (MSG)
"mono-SEW-dee-um GLOO-ta-mate"

PARABENS
"PARE-a-bins"

PERFLUORINATED COMPOUNDS (PFCS)
"PER-FLER-in-ate-ed"

PHTHALATES
"THAL-ates"

TRICLOSAN
"TRIK-lo-san"

TRIETHANOLAMINE (TEA) AND DIETHA-NOLAMINE (DEA)
"TRI-eth-anol-a-meen" and "DIE-eth-anol-a-meen"

TOLUENE
"TOL-loo-een"

THE COMPLETE LIST OF DISHONEST INGREDIENTS

BE AWARE THAT THIS STUFF . . .	COULD CONTAIN THIS TOXIN . . .	WHY IT'S SKETCHY	WHAT TO DO ABOUT IT
Beef, pork, lamb, and poultry	**Antibiotics,** which are fed to livestock in mass quantities to prevent the spread of disease on cramped factory farms.	When we have to use so many antibiotics as a preventive measure to raise healthy food, we wind up not having enough robust antibiotics to treat ourselves when we get sick because bacteria evolve so rapidly—a growing problem known as antibiotic resistance.	* Look for the words "no antibiotics added" whenever you buy meat or poultry products, to make sure your dinner wasn't raised on medication. For more information, see Chapter 1.
Canned goods, cash register receipts, plastic water bottles, and any other plastic labeled #7	**Bisphenol A (BPA),** a plasticizer that makes polycarbonate plastic clear and hard.	BPA is an endocrine disruptor, which means it messes with healthy hormonal development. It's associated with infertility, obesity, metabolic disorders, thyroid problems, and low birth weight.	* Avoid fast food and canned goods. * Say "no receipt, thanks" at the cash register. * Cut back on bottled water (it's also less regulated than tap, so may be more contaminated in general) and avoid any other #7 plastic containers. * Don't microwave in plastic; when it heats up, BPA can leach into your food.
Laundry detergent, stain removers, bleach (duh)	**Chlorine bleach,** the stuff used to make whites whiter and kill bacteria.	When the active ingredient in bleach reacts with water, it forms a group of nasty, cancer-causing by-products called dioxins. Bleach is harmful if inhaled and powerfully irritating to eyes, noses, and throats. It also wears your clothes out faster!	* Pretreat stains with a paste of baking soda and white vinegar, which have natural antiseptic properties. * Look for "oxy" stain removers made from sodium percarbonate (a solid form of hydrogen peroxide bonded with natural soda ash) and sodium carbonate. * If you must bleach, make sure the label says "nonchlorinated."
Nonstick cookware, stain-resistant fabric, foam cushions, mattresses, anything "flame resistant," carpeting, pizza boxes, fast-food containers, conventional cleaning products, paints, roof treatment, floor protectant	**Flame retardants like perfluorinated compounds (PFCs), brominated flame retardants (BFRs), and halogenated flame retardants (HFRs),** coating used to reduce flammability of textiles and other goods.	PFCs, BFRs, and HFRs are endocrine disruptors, which means they interfere with hormonal development and can lead to reproductive and developmental disorders. They are also associated with liver, pancreatic, testicular, and breast cancer.	* Replace any old, scratched nonstick cookware with cast iron or stainless steel. * Don't buy fabrics that advertise as being water repellant, flame resistant, or stain resistant, and don't use products designed to increase a fabric's stain resistance (like Scotchgard). * Skip the fast food and take-out pizza. * Switch to nontoxic cleaning products (see page 132). * Use nontoxic paints, treatments, and carpeting if you're remodeling (see page 114). * Invest in nontoxic mattresses and pillows (see page 116).

BE AWARE THAT THIS STUFF . . .	COULD CONTAIN THIS TOXIN	WHY IT'S SKETCHY	WHAT TO DO ABOUT IT
Nail polish, polish remover, eyelash glue, Brazilian blowout and other keratin hair-straightening treatments, mattresses, foam cushions, kitchen cabinets, carpeting, particleboard furniture	**Formaldehyde,** a preservative and/or by-product released from other preservatives	Formaldehyde can cause cancer after chronic, long-term exposure, plus it can cause more immediate allergic reactions, rashes, asthma, nosebleeds, and other respiratory issues.	* Skip the mani-pedis until after your pregnancy, or DIY at home with "three-free polish" (see page 76). Maybe get a massage instead! * Do not get any kind of keratin hair-straightening treatment, period. * Shop for safer mattresses and other furnishings (see pages 116–18). * Let new furniture, carpets, and other home goods off-gas in an open garage or on the back porch for several days before you bring them inside, then run a fan and leave windows open for another few days. * Look for used furniture and cabinets if you're upgrading—they're more likely to have finished off-gassing.
Beauty products, cleaning supplies, scented candles, scented cat litter—and just about anything else with a fragrance (Even "unscented" is technically a scent!)	**Fragrance,** parfum, dyes, and synthetic musks; all perfume components	Fragrances can contain phthalates (see below) or just about anything else—product manufacturers don't have to tell you what's in their fragrance formulas because they're considered "trade secrets." That means you have no idea what you're being exposed to when you use a fragrance-containing product.	* Look for "fragrance free" on the label of every personal care product and cleaning product you buy. * For extra insurance, only buy brands that specifically denote themselves as "phthalate free." * Avoid using candles of any kind until after your pregnancy.
Any food (especially processed) made with canola oil, soybeans, or corn.	**Genetically modified organisms (GMOs),** which are added to food crops that have been engineered to be stronger and more pest resistant.	The reason GMO food crops are more pest resistant is usually because a toxic chemical pesticide has been bred right into the grain! The US government and biotech companies say GMO foods are safe, but they've been banned throughout Europe.	* Choose organic whenever you can (even snack foods) because GMO ingredients are not allowed. * Support brands that advertise being GMO free. (For more on this issue, see Chapter 1.)
Skin lighteners, moisturizers, hair dyes, anti-aging creams	**Hydroquinone,** a skin and hair lightener	Can cause cancer and affect your immune system and reproductive health. Also associated with developmental problems when little kids are exposed. All-around bad news.	* Choose cleaner cosmetics and personal care products; see Chapters 2 and 3. * Skip any skin lightening treatments and hair dye while pregnant.
Drinking water; anything made from vinyl (PVC)—children's toys, shower curtains, backpacks, raincoats, umbrellas, pacifiers, teething rings, etc. Lead has also been found in children's face paint, lipstick, the paint on metal toys and jewelry. Mercury and lead have both been found in batteries, lightbulbs, and microwaves. Mercury also accumulates in fish and has been found in some mascaras.	**Lead, mercury,** and other **heavy metals** used as stabilizers or preservatives.	There is no safe level of lead exposure for babies and children: Lead is a known neurotoxin and can play a role in the development of learning delays, autism, and other neurological problems. Mercury is a known neurotoxin that can also cause allergic reactions or skin irritation, plus it's easy to absorb through your skin and it accumulates in your body.	* If you live in a home built before 1978, have your water and painted surfaces tested for lead (see page 154). Use filters, replace pipes, and have paint sealed (by pros!) if appropriate. * Run your cold water for a minute every morning to flush out any lead that may have accumulated in the pipes overnight. * Steer clear of vinyl or painted toys, jewelry, and other gear that was made in China or other parts of Asia—these were the most likely to test positive for lead during investigations over the past few years. * When you eat seafood, be sure to choose kinds low in mercury (see page 211).

BE AWARE THAT THIS STUFF . . .	COULD CONTAIN THIS TOXIN . . .	WHY IT'S SKETCHY	WHAT TO DO ABOUT IT
Bathroom corners, dank basements, and fridges or under kitchen sinks.	**Mold,** the microscopic spores that can build up in damp, humid environments	A mold infestation can trigger asthma and allergies, or, in more concentrated doses, dizziness and flulike symptoms.	* Keep moisture under control with good ventilation. Any mold growth that covers an area larger than 10 square feet, or has spread inside the ducts of your central air system, should be handled by a professional, according to the Environmental Protection Agency. * Scrub the mold off of hard surfaces with a mixture of detergent and hot water, then fix the source of the water damage. (Throw out infested porous materials like carpets or ceiling tiles.) * Visit www.epa.gov/mold for more information on handling mold in your home.
Laundry detergent	**Optical brighteners,** certain types of dyes that absorb UV light to make your whites whiter and your clothes brighter (by removing yellow tones)	Optical brighteners bind irreversibly to the skin and may cause rashes and allergic reactions; they may also be hormone disruptors, and we just don't know whether they're safe to use over long periods of time. One bummer: They're definitely toxic to fish.	* Choose cleaner nontoxic laundry products (see Chapter 5).
Any water-based personal care product or cosmetic like shampoo, conditioner, cleanser, shower gel, lotion, you name it	**Parabens,** a group of preservatives	We can absorb parabens through our skin, blood, and digestive system, and they've even been found inside breast tumors and, thus, linked to cancer. They may also be toxic to our reproductive, immune, and nervous systems and can cause skin rashes.	* Check labels and choose cleaner personal care products (see Chapters 2 and 3).
Newly dry-cleaned clothes	**Perchloroethylene (PERC),** a colorless, nonflammable liquid that's used as the major ingredient in most dry-cleaning formulas.	PERC off-gasses when it's exposed to air, which means we can breathe it in. Short-term exposure can cause dizziness, fatigue, sweating, and headaches. Long-term exposure may cause liver and kidney damage, memory loss, and cancer.	* Handwash or use the gentle cycle on your washing machine instead of dry-cleaning whenever possible. (It's cheaper, too!) * When you do dry-clean, ask them to take your clothes out of the bag before you bring them home. * Let newly dry-cleaned clothes air out on your porch or in the garage for a day before you hang them in your closet.

THE COMPLETE LIST OF DISHONEST INGREDIENTS—*CONTINUED*

BE AWARE THAT THIS STUFF . . .	COULD CONTAIN THIS TOXIN . . .	WHY IT'S SKETCHY	WHAT TO DO ABOUT IT
Foundations, lipsticks, lip balms, mascara, many other color cosmetics	**Petrochemicals** including **mineral oil, petroleum jelly, propylene glycol,** and **paraffin,** all of which are used as moisturizers (Avoid any products with *petroleum* or *liquid paraffin* on the label.)	Using a lot of petroleum-filled products can make you break out because they work by blocking your pores. Long-term, we don't totally understand what petrochemicals in personal care products might do to your health, but petroleum distillates may cause cancer—and anyway, this stuff is used in paint, antifreeze, and—hello—gasoline.	* Look for water-based moisturizers and cosmetics made with plant oils like jojoba, shea, and coconut.
Some nail polishes; anything vinyl (shower curtains, raincoats, backpacks); anything that lists "fragrance" on the ingredient label, like cleaning supplies, laundry detergent, scented candles, etc.	**Phthalates,** a group of chemicals used as plasticizers or fragrance components	Twenty years of research suggests that phthalates can mess with our hormones and damage our reproductive health, so it's especially critical for pregnant women, babies, and young children to steer clear.	* Look for nonvinyl alternatives whenever you're purchasing a traditionally vinyl item (shower curtain, raincoat, etc.). * Only use "fragrance-free" cleaning supplies and personal care products. * Skip the mani-pedis or DIY at home with three-free polish.
Cigarettes, candles, gas stoves, incense	**Scents and smoke** released from cigarettes, candles, and other sources	Tobacco smoke components, including nicotine, can quickly cross the placenta and lead to birth defects and low birth-weight babies. Any kind of smoke releases particles that can cause respiratory problems and may pose other risks for pregnant women.	* Don't smoke (duh). * Don't let anyone smoke around you or anywhere in your home—even if you're not there. Tobacco smoke particles can linger in curtains and carpets for days. * Steer clear of candles and incense. * Always crack a window and use the range hood when you use a gas stove. * Get your chimney cleaned seasonally
Children's bubble bath, regular shampoo, soap, shower gel, hair relaxers	Sudsing agents like **sodium lauryl** or **laureth sulfate, "PEG,"** and ingredients that include the terms **"xynol," "ceteareath,"** and **"oleth."**	They make things foamy—but when they undergo a manufacturing process called "ethoxylation," they create a toxic by-product chemical called **1,4-dioxane,** which easily penetrates our skin and may cause cancer and birth defects. It may also be toxic to our kidneys, neurological system, and respiratory system.	* Choose cleaner personal care products; see Chapter 2.
Hot dogs, bacon, other cured meats, some smoked fish	**Sodium nitrates** (meat preservatives)	Can trigger migraines, may be linked to cancer.	* Skip smoked and cured meats during your pregnancy (your doctor has probably already told you avoid the deli counter!) or, when you do indulge, choose only *nitrate-free* bacon.

BE AWARE THAT THIS STUFF . . .	COULD CONTAIN THIS TOXIN . . .	WHY IT'S SKETCHY	WHAT TO DO ABOUT IT
Concealer, mascara, sunless tanning lotion	**Triethanolamine (TEA)** and **diethanolamine (DEA)**, both types of proteins used to adjust the pH level of a product or as a wetting agent.	When TEA is combined with certain preservatives, it can create cancer-causing compounds called nitrosamines.	* Check product labels.
Nail polish, adhesives, painting supplies, ink, fuel	**Toluene** (a clear, odorless solvent)	At high levels of exposure, toluene is toxic to your kidneys and liver and may also damage reproductive health, so pregnant women need to avoid it.	* Skip the mani-pedis or DIY at home with three-free polish. * Don't do any remodeling or craft projects involving heavy use of adhesives or paint. * Don't pump your own gas if you're pregnant—always pull up to the full-service pump. (Toluene is just the beginning of the list of toxins in gasoline that aren't fetus friendly!)
Antibacterial soap, hand sanitizer, toothpaste, deodorants, plus some special "mold-resistant" or "antibacterial" fabrics and plastics	**Triclosan** and **triclocarban**, both antimicrobial agents	This stuff gets absorbed and piles up in our bodies, where it may disrupt our hormones. And because we use so damn much of it, it's also helping create dangerous bacteria that are resistant to antibiotics. In 2005, the FDA found no evidence that antibacterial soaps are in any way superior to good old soap and water. So stick with that.	* Check product labels. * Use regular soap and water to wash your hands. * Use alcohol-based sanitizers when necessary.
Paints, cleaning supplies, pesticides, building materials, furnishings—you name it!	**Volatile organic compounds (VOCs):** a general umbrella term for a wide variety of chemicals that release fumes and gases from household supplies and building materials	Some VOCs can cause serious health issues ranging from respiratory illness to cancer, while others have no affect on our health whatsoever. Unfortunately, the US Environmental Protection Agency doesn't know much yet about what health effects occur from the levels of VOCs usually found in homes—although they do know that indoor levels are typically much higher than outdoor.	* Don't do any painting or home renovation projects yourself during your pregnancy—and make sure whoever is doing the work only uses no-VOC paint and other products. * Only use nontoxic cleaning supplies (see Chapter 5). * Invest in nontoxic carpets and other furnishings whenever you're buying new (see page 114), or buy used—older pieces will have had more time to finish off-gassing.

Notes

BOY, YOU REALLY *DO* WANT TO KNOW THE DETAILS! HERE'S HOW I RESEARCHED THIS BOOK, CHAPTER BY CHAPTER.

introduction

ON THE TOXIC SUBSTANCES CONTROL ACT

SAFER CHEMICALS, HEALTHY FAMILIES
A national effort to protect families from toxic chemicals. I've testified on their behalf in Washington, DC, and find their Web site to be an indispensable source of information.
www.saferchemicals.org/resources/tsca.html

CAMPAIGN FOR SAFE COSMETICS
A coalition of environmental health and women's issue nonprofits working to make personal care products and cosmetics safer.
www.safecosmetics.org

ON DIETHYLENE GLYCOL AND FANCY BABY DETERGENT

ENVIRONMENTAL WORKING GROUP'S SKIN DEEP DATABASE
www.ewg.org/skindeep/ingredient/701959/DIETHYLENE_GLYCOL/

ON GOVERNMENT RECALL POWER

CONSUMER PRODUCT SAFETY COMMISSION
www.cpsc.gov/businfo/8002.pdf

FOOD & DRUG ADMINISTRATION (FDA)
www.safecosmetics.org/downloads/FDA-regulatory-shortcomings_Cosmetics_Jul2010.pdf

ON BABIES' VULNERABILITY TO TOXIC CHEMICALS

PHILIP J. LANDRIGAN, MD
(phone interviews)

ENVIROMENTAL PROTECTION AGENCY (EPA)
www.rodale.com/chemical-regulation

www.epa.gov/opptintr/existingchemicals/pubs/sect6.html

ON BANNED CHEMICALS

FDA VS. EU
http://safecosmetics.org/article.php?id=346

ON TSCA REFORM

SAFER CHEMICALS, HEALTHY FAMILIES

chapter 1
HONEST food

ON PINK SLIME IN BEEF

PER THE MAYO CLINIC
www.mayoclinic.com/health/meat-news/MY02058

USDA DEFENSE OF PINK SLIME
http://blogs.usda.gov/2012/03/22/setting-the-record-straight-on-beef/

PINK SLIME LAWSUIT
www.rodale.com/pink-slime-lawsuit

ON INDUSTRIALIZATION OF FOOD AND LINKS TO HEALTH RISKS

JAY GORDON, MD
(Phone interview and op-ed)
www.dailynews.com/opinions/ci_20893697/jay-gordon-disneys-junk-food-ad-ban-doesnt

DAVID WALLINGA, MD
for the Institute for
Agriculture & Trade Policy,
Exporting Obesity Report
(April 2012).
www.iatp.org/documents/
exporting-obesity

ON "HEALTH HALOS"

PIERRE CHANDON AND
BRIAN WANSINK
"The Biasing Health Halos of
Fast Food Restaurant Health
Claims: Lower Calorie Esti-
mates and Higher Side-Dish
Consumption Intentions,"
*Journal of Consumer
Research* 34, no. 3 (October
2007), pages 301–14.
http://foodpsychology.cornell.
edu/outreach/health-halos.html

ON COW'S MILK AND
FOOD ALLERGIES

AMERICAN ACADEMY
OF ALLERGY, ASTHMA &
IMMUNOLOGY
Food Allergy Overview.
www.aaaai.org/conditions-and-
treatments/allergies/food-
allergies.aspx

NATIONAL INSTITUTE
OF ALLERGY &
INFECTIOUS DISEASES
Understanding Food
Allergy—Milk.
www.niaid.nih.gov/topics/
foodAllergy/understanding/
Pages/milkAllergy.aspx

ON CERTIFIED
ORGANIC STANDARDS

UNITED STATES
DEPARTMENT OF
AGRICULTURE (USDA)
Agricultural Marketing
Service, National Organic
Program.
www.ams.usda.gov/AMSv1.0/
ams.fetchTemplateData.do?tem
plate=TemplateN&navID=Organ
icStandardslinkNOPConsumers
&rightNav1=OrganicStandardsli
nkNOPConsumers&topNav=&le
ftNav=NationalOrganicProgram
&page=NOPOrganicStandards&
resultType=&acct=nopgeninfo

ON THE DIRTY DOZEN

ENVIRONMENTAL
WORKING GROUP'S
DIRTY DOZEN PLUS
AND CLEAN 15
http://ewg.org/dirty-dozen

ON BUYING FROM
FARMERS

LOCAL HARVEST
Farmers' Markets
www.localharvest.org/farmers-
markets/

COMMUNITY SUPPORTED
AGRICULTURE
www.localharvest.org/csa/

RODALE INSTITUTE
Farm Locator.
www.rodaleinstitute.org/farm_
locator

ON SEASONAL
PRODUCE

NATURAL RESOURCES
DEFENSE COUNCIL
Smarter Living—Eat Local.
www.simplesteps.org/eat-local/
state/california

ON GMOS

CHRISTOPHER GAVIGAN
Healthy Child, Healthy World,
page 83.

ON PESTICIDES' LINK
TO AUTISM AND
LEARNING
DISABILITIES

PHILIP J. LANDRIGAN,
LINDA BIRNBAUM,
AND LUCA LAMBERTINI
"A Research Strategy to
Discover Environmental
Causes of Autism and
Neurodevelopmental
Disabilities." *Environmental
Health Perspectives* 120:7
(July 2012).
http://library.constantcontact.
com/download/get/file/
1102175172120-212/Autism_
editorial_final.pdf

ROBYN O'BRIEN
"Top Chemicals Most
Likely to Cause Autism
and Learning Disabilities."
Inspired Bites Blog for
Prevention Magazine, 2012.
http://blogs.prevention.com/
inspired-bites/2012/04/25/top-
10-chemicals-most-likely-to-cause-
autism-and-learning-disabilities/

ON WHOLE GRAINS

*THE RODALE WHOLE
FOODS COOKBOOK*,
pages 446–47.

USDA NUTRIENT
DATABASE
(fiber Information)
http://ndb.nal.usda.gov/ndb/
foods/list

VIRGINIA SOLE-SMITH
"Milling Around: Mix Up
Carbs and Add Nutrients to
Your Diet with Tasty Pasta
Alternatives," *Runner's World*
(January 2007), pages 54–55.
http://virginiasolesmith.com/
wp-content/uploads/2012/01/
RW_Grains.pdf

CHEF SHOP
(nutritional information)
http://chefshop.com/Farro-
Emmer-Organic-Wholegrain-
Wash—P6425.aspx

MARK BITTMAN
The Food Matters Cookbook,
pages 269–70.

SUZANNE HAMLIN
"Farro, Italy's Rustic Staple:
The Little Grain That Could,"
New York Times (June 11, 1997).
www.nytimes.com/1997/06/11/
garden/farro-italy-s-rustic-staple-
the-little-grain-that-could.html

ON "EXTRA LEAN" AND
"LEAN" CUTS OF BEEF

MAYO CLINIC
"Cuts of Beef: A Guide to
the Leanest Selections."
www.mayoclinic.com/health/
cuts-of-beef/MY01387

ON DIOXINS

CHRISTOPHER GAVIGAN
Healthy Child, Healthy World,
pages 16–17.

ON GRASS-FED BEEF

DEIRDRE IMUS
The Essential Green You,
pages 19–20.

ON ORGANIC CHICKEN

CENTER FOR SCIENCE
IN THE PUBLIC INTEREST
The Antibiotic Resistance
Project.
www.cspinet.org/ar/ar_
livestockuse.html

INSTITUTE FOR
AGRICULTURE & TRADE
POLICY
Buying Better Chicken
Guide.
www.iatp.org/files/Buying%20
Better%20Chicken042011.pdf

BEN LILLISTON AND
INSTITUTE FOR
AGRICULTURE & TRADE
POLICY
"The War on Antibiotics"
(July 2010).
www.iatp.org/documents/
the-war-on-antibiotics-without-
strict-new-regulations-us-beef-
poultry-and-pork-production-

ON EGGS

THE HUMANE SOCIETY:
AN HSUS REPORT
The Welfare of Animals in
the Egg Industry.
www.humanesociety.org/assets/
pdfs/farm/welfare_egg.pdf

ON ANTIBIOTICS
IN FOOD

DAVID WALLINGA, MD
for the Institute for Agriculture & Trade Policy:
www.iatp.org/blog/201209/
the-invisible-epidemic-giving-
voice-to-the-faceless-victims-of-
antibiotic-overuse

"Poultry on Antibiotics Hazards to Human Health" Report (December 2002) www.iatp.org/files/Poultry_on_Antibiotics_Hazards_to_Human_Health.pdf

ON BUYING CERTIFIED HUMANE

HUMANE FARM ANIMAL CARE Certified Humane Label. http://certifiedhumane.org/

ON HEALTHY CANNED BEANS

EDEN ORGANIC http://edenfoods.com/about/environment.php

HARVARD SCHOOL OF PUBLIC HEALTH SALT REDUCTION STRATEGIES (TIP #23) http://hsph.harvard.edu/nutrition source/salt/

ON SEAFOOD

TIMOTHY FITZGERALD senior scientist at the Environmental Defense Fund. http://apps.edf.org/documents/1980_pocket_seafood_selector.pdf http://apps.edf.org/page.cfm?tagID=29796

ON DAIRY

JAY GORDON, MD (Phone interview)

ON WHEN TO INTRODUCE FOODS TO BABIES

JAY GORDON, MD. (Phone and e-mail interviews.)

ON HEATING FOOD IN PLASTIC

KATHLEEN SCHULER, MPH Institute for Agriculture and Trade Policy

SMART PLASTICS GUIDE iatp.org/files/421_2_102202.pdf

ON ASPARTAME

CENTER FOR SCIENCE IN THE PUBLIC INTEREST Chemical Cuisine: A Guide to Food Additives http://cspinet.org/nah/05_08/chem_cuisine.pdf

ON HIGH-FRUCTOSE CORN SYRUP

See "On Aspartame"

ON TRANS FAT

See "On Aspartame"

ON ARTIFICIAL COLORS

See "On Aspartame"

ON SODIUM NITRATES

See "On Aspartame"

ON MSG

See "On Aspartame"

ON SPLENDA

MARIAN NESTLE, PHD "The latest Splenda in rats study" foodpolitics.com/2008/09/the-latest-splenda-rat-study-oops/

ON AGAVE

MARIAN NESTLE, PHD "Stevia and other natural sweeteners—are they?" foodpolitics.com/2012/05/stevia-and-other-natural-sweeteners/

chapter 2
HONEST clean

ON TOXINS IN BATH PRODUCTS

HONEST COMPANY RESEARCH www.honest.com/whats-inside/baby-bath-products

ON THE NUMBER OF PERSONAL CARE PRODUCTS WE USE DAILY

ENVIRONMENTAL WORKING GROUP RESEARCH www.ewg.org/skindeep/faq/

ON LIAR LABELS

HYPOALLERGENIC

KIERA BUTLER "Do Hypoallergenic Products Really Cause Fewer Allergies?" *Mother Jones* (2010). http://www.motherjones.com/blue-marble/2010/09/hypoallergenic-cosmetic-fda

FOOD & DRUG ADMINISTRATION Cosmetic Labeling & Label Claims—Hypoallergenic. www.fda.gov/Cosmetics/CosmeticLabelingLabelClaims/LabelClaimsandExpirationDating/ucm2005203.htm

NATURAL

ALEXANDRA GORMAN director of science and research, Women's Voices for the Earth. (E-mail exchange with Virginia Sole-Smith, September 22, 2011)

ORGANIC

FOOD & DRUG ADMINISTRATION Product Ingredients & Safety—Organic. www.fda.gov/Cosmetics/ProductandIngredientSafety/ProductInformation/ucm203078.htm

UNITED STATES DEPARTMENT OF AGRICULTURE National Organic Program, "Cosmetics, Body Care Products and Personal Care Products." www.ams.usda.gov/AMSv1.0/getfile?dDocName=STELPRDC5068442

UNSCENTED

CAMPAIGN FOR SAFE COSMETICS Fragrance Research Summary Page. http://safecosmetics.org/article.php?id=222

ON CHOOSING SAFER PRODUCTS

ENVIRONMENTAL WORKING GROUP'S SKIN DEEP DATABASE www.cosmeticsdatabase.com

SIOBHAN O'CONNOR AND ALEXANDRA SPUNT *No More Dirty Looks: The Truth about Your Beauty Products and the Ultimate Guide to Safe and Clean Cosmetics* www.nomoredirtylooks.com

ON THE TOP CHEMICALS OF CONCERN IN PERSONAL CARE PRODUCTS

ENVIRONMENTAL WORKING GROUP Shopper's Guide to Safe Cosmetics. http://static.ewg.org/skindeep/pdf/EWG_cosmeticsguide.pdf

FORMALDEHYDE

CAMPAIGN FOR SAFE COSMETICS Formaldehyde & Formaldehyde-Releasing Preservatives Research Summary Page. http://safecosmetics.org/article.php?id=599

INTERNATIONAL AGENCY FOR RESEARCH ON CANCER "IARC classifies formaldehyde as carcinogenic to humans," press release, June 15, 2004. www.iarc.fr/en/Media-Centre/IARC-Press-Releases/Archives-2006-2004/2004/IARC-classifies-formaldehyde-as-carcinogenic-to-humans.

J. N. MOENNICH,
D. M. HANNA, AND
S. E. JACOB
"Formaldehyde-releasing
preservative in baby and
cosmetic products,"
*Journal of the Dermatology
Nurses' Association* 1 (2009),
pages 211–14.

SCIENTIFIC COMMITTEE
ON COSMETIC
PRODUCTS AND
NONFOOD PRODUCTS
Opinion concerning a clari-
fication on the formaldehyde
and para-formaldehyde entry
in Directive 76/768/EEC on
cosmetic products. Opinion:
European Commission, 2002.
http://ec.europa.eu/food/fs/sc/
sccp/out187_en.pdf.

U.S. DEPARTMENT OF
HEALTH AND HUMAN
SERVICES, PUBLIC
HEALTH SERVICE,
NATIONAL TOXICOLOGY
PROGRAM
"Formaldehyde (Gas) CAS
No. 50-00-0: Reasonably
anticipated to be a human
carcinogen." Eleventh
Report on Carcinogens,
December 2002.
http://ntp.niehs.nih.gov/ntp/roc/
eleventh/profiles/s089form.pdf.

FRAGRANCE

CAMPAIGN FOR
SAFE COSMETICS
"Not So Sexy: The Health
Risks of Secret Chemicals
in Fragrance," 2010 report.
http://safecosmetics.org/article.
php?id=644

CAMPAIGN FOR
SAFE COSMETICS
Fragrance Research
Summary Page.
http://safecosmetics.org/article.
php?id=222

PARABENS

CAMPAIGN FOR
SAFE COSMETICS
Parabens Research
Summary Page.
http://safecosmetics.org/article.
php?id=291

P. D. DAUBRE,
A. ALJARRAH,
W. R. MILLER,
N. G. COLDHAM,
M. J. SAUER, AND
G. S. POPE
"Concentrations of parabens
in human breast tumours,"
Journal of Applied Toxicology
24 (2004), pages 5–13.

J. GRAY
"State of the Evidence:
The Connection between
Breast Cancer and
the Environment," San
Francisco, CA: The Breast
Cancer Fund, 2008.

PETROCHEMICALS

CHRISTOPHER GAVIGAN
*Healthy Child, Healthy
World,* pages 111–12.

PHTHALATES

CAMPAIGN FOR
SAFE COSMETICS
Phthalates Research
Summary Page.
http://safecosmetics.org/article.
php?id=290

B. C. BLOUNT, M. J. SILVA,
S. P. CAUDILL,
L. L. NEEDHAM,
J. L. PIRKLE, E. J. SAMPSON,
G. W. LUCIER, R. J. JACKON,
AND J. W. BROCK
"Levels of Seven Urinary
Phthalate Metabolites in a
Human Reference Popula-
tion," *Environmental Health
Perspectives* 108 (2000),
pages 979–82.
www.ehponline.org/members/
2000/108p972-982blount/
blount.pdf

CHRISTOPHER GAVIGAN
*Healthy Child, Healthy
World,* page 106.

J. HOULIHAN, C. BRODY,
AND B. SCHWAN
"Not Too Pretty: Phthalates,
Beauty Products and the
FDA," 2002.
www.safecosmetics.org/down-
loads/NotTooPretty_report.pdf

STACY MALKAN
*Not Just a Pretty Face:
The Ugly Side of the Beauty
Industry,* page 17.

SLS AND "PEG"

CAMPAIGN FOR
SAFE COSMETICS
1,4-Dioxane Research
Summary Page.
http://safecosmetics.org/article.
php?id=288

ENVIRONMENTAL
PROTECTION AGENCY
1,4-Dioxane (CASRN 123-
91-1), Integrated Risk
Information System, 2003.
www.epa.gov/NCEA/iris/subst/
0326.htm

ENVIRONMENTAL
WORKING GROUP
Impurities of Concern in
Personal Care Products, 2007.
www.cosmeticsdatabase.com/
research/impurities.php.

NATIONAL TOXICOLOGY
PROGRAM
Report on Carcinogens,
11th edition; U.S. Depart-
ment of Health and Human
Services, Public Health
Service, National Toxicology
Program, January 2005.
http://ntp.niehs.nih.gov/ntp/roc/
eleventh/profiles/s080diox.pdf

OFFICE OF
ENVIRONMENTAL
HEALTH HAZARD
ASSESSMENT (OEHAA)
State of California Environmental Protection Agency,
Chemicals known to the
state to cause cancer or
reproductive toxicity, 2004.
http://oehha.ca.gov/prop65/
prop65_list/files/41604list.html

ORGANIC CONSUMERS
ASSOCIATION
Results of Testing for
1,4-Dioxane.
www.organicconsumers.org/
bodycare/DioxaneResults08.cfm

TRICLOSAN AND
TRICLOCARBAN

http://safecosmetics.org/article.
php?id=718

TRIETHANOLAMINE
(TEA) AND
DIETHANOLAMINE (DEA)

CAMPAIGN FOR
SAFE COSMETICS
TEA & DEA Research
Summary Page.
http://safecosmetics.org/article.
php?id=293

L. ZORRILLA, ET AL.
"The effects of Triclosan on
Puberty and Thyroid Hor-
mones in Male Wistar Rats,"
Toxicological Sciences 107,
no. 1 (2009), pages 56–64.

AHN, ET AL
"In Vitro Biologic Activities
of the Antimicrobials
Triclocarban, Its Analogs,
and Triclosan in Bioassay
Screens: Receptor-Based
Bioassay Screens," Environmental Health Perspectives
116, no. 9 (2008), pages
1203–10.

SCCS (SCIENTIFIC COMMITTEE ON CONSUMER SAFETY) Preliminary opinion on triclosan antimicrobial resistance,European Commission, Brussels, March 23, 2010.

ON FLUORIDE IN TOOTHPASTE

CHRISTOPHER GAVIGAN
Healthy Child, Healthy World, page 122.

PHILIP J. LANDRIGAN, MD
www.mountsinai.org/patient-care/health-library/diseases-and-conditions/tooth-decay
www.mountsinai.org/patient-care/health-library/diseases-and-conditions/teething

ON RETINOL AND REPRODUCTIVE DEFECTS

PHILIP J. LANDRIGAN, MD
(E-mail exchange with Alexandra Postman)

PESTICIDES ACTION NETWORK DATABASE
Toxicity Information for Retinoic Acid.
www.pesticideinfo.org/Detail_Chemical.jsp?Rec_Id=PC42142#Toxicity

UNIVERSITY OF MARYLAND MEDICAL CENTER
www.umm.edu/altmed/articles/vitamin-a-000331.htm

ON SUNSCREENS

ENVIRONMENTAL WORKING GROUP
Quick Tips for a Good Sunscreen, 2012.
http://breakingnews.ewg.org/2012sunscreen/top-sun-safety-tips/

PHILIP J. LANDRIGAN, MD
www.mountsinai.org/patient-care/service-areas/cancer/cancer-services/skin-cancer/prevention-tips
www.mssm.edu/static_files/MSSM/Files/Research/Programs/Pediatric%20Environmental%20Health%20Specialty%20Unit/Sunscreen_2011.pdf

ON DEODORANT

SIOBHAN O'CONNOR AND ALEXANDRA SPUNT
"What's So Bad about Antiperspirant?" *GOOD.*
www.good.is/post/what/

ON NATURAL WOUND AND BRUISE HEALING

JENNIFER PIRTIE
"Medicine Cabinet Make-over." *Whole Living,* no. 4 (September 2005).
www.wholeliving.com/134288/medicine-cabinet-makeover

ON BRAZILIAN BLOWOUT

WOMEN'S VOICES FOR THE EARTH
Brazilian Blowout information page
Womensvoices.org/campaigns/brazilian-blowout/

ON TALC IN BABY POWDER

ENVIRONMENTAL WORKING GROUP
Talc Information Page.
www.ewg.org/guides/substances/5917

ON BETTER BATH TOYS

KATHLEEN SCHULER, MPH
Institute for Agriculture and Trade Policy

SMART PLASTICS GUIDE
iatp.org/files/421_2_102202.pdf

chapter 3
HONEST beauty

ON CHEMICALS IN COSMETICS

CADMIUM AND OTHER HEAVY METALS

ENVIRONMENTAL DEFENCE CANADA
"Heavy Metal Hazard: The Health Risks of Heavy Metals in Makeup."
http://environmentaldefence.ca/reports/heavy-metal-hazard-health-risks-hidden-heavy-metals-in-face-makeup

DENISE MANN
"Can Heavy Metals in Food, Cosmetics Spur Breast Cancer Risk?" *Health Day* (April 2012).
http://consumer.healthday.com/Article.asp?AID=664026

HYDROQUINONE

ENVIRONMENTAL WORKING GROUP SKIN DEEP DATABASE.
Hydroquinone Toxicity Information Page.
www.ewg.org/skindeep/ingredient/703041/HYDROQUINONE/

WOMEN'S VOICES FOR THE EARTH
15 Toxic Trespassers.
www.womensvoices.org/avoid-toxic-chemicals/15-toxic-trespassers/

"Not So Pretty Toxic Products Marketed to Black Women" (2011).
www.womensvoices.org/wp-content/uploads/2011/08/Products_Marketed_to_Black_Women.pdf

LEAD

CAMPAIGN FOR SAFE COSMETICS
Letter to the office of Linda Katz, director of the FDA Office on Cosmetics and Colors (2012)
http://safecosmetics.org/article.php?id=951

FOOD & DRUG ADMINISTRATION
Lead in Lipstick Questions & Answers.
www.fda.gov/Cosmetics/ProductandIngredientSafety/ProductInformation/ucm137224.htm#expanalyses

WOMEN'S VOICES FOR THE EARTH
15 Toxic Trespassers.
www.womensvoices.org/avoid-toxic-chemicals/15-toxic-trespassers/

"A Poison Kiss: The Problem of Lead in Lipstick" (2007).
www.womensvoices.org/wp-content/uploads/2010/06/PoisonKiss1.pdf

MERCURY

ENVIRONMENTAL WORKING GROUP SKIN DEEP DATABASE.
Mercury Toxicity Information Page.
www.ewg.org/skindeep/ingredient/703866/MERCURY/

FOOD & DRUG ADMINISTRATION
Cosmetic Ingredients Prohibited & Restricted by FDA Regulations.
www.fda.gov/Cosmetics/ProductandIngredientSafety/SelectedCosmeticIngredients/ucm127406.htm

ALEXANDRA GORMAN
director of science and research, Women's Voices for the Earth.
www.womensvoices.org/science/ask-alex/chemicals-in-cosmetics/

TEA AND DEA

ENVIRONMENTAL WORKING GROUP SKIN DEEP DATABASE
ewg.org/skindeep/

TOLUENE

ENVIRONMENTAL WORKING GROUP SKIN DEEP DATABASE. Toluene Toxicity Information Page.
www.ewg.org/skindeep/ingredient/706577/TOLUENE/

WOMEN'S VOICES FOR THE EARTH
"Glossed Over: Health Hazards Associated with Toxic Exposure in Nail Salons," Report 2010.
www.womensvoices.org/wp-content/uploads/2010/06/Glossed_Over.pdf

ON NAIL POLISH AND THE "TOXIC TRIO"

CALIFORNIA HEALTH NAIL SALON COLLABORATIVE
"Understanding the Toxic Trio" (2010).
www.cahealthynailsalons.org/wp-content/uploads/2010/07/Toxic_Trio_EN_March2012.pdf

VIRGINIA SOLE-SMITH
"Toxins Found in 'Toxin-Free' Nail Polish: Another Reason Beauty Industry Regulations Need a Make-over," Slate—XXFactor Blog (April 2012).
www.slate.com/blogs/xx_factor/2012/04/13/toxic_nail_polish_lies_found_on_beauty_industry_labels.html

WOMEN'S VOICES FOR THE EARTH
"Glossed Over: Health Hazards Associated with Toxic Exposure in Nail Salons," Report 2010.
www.womensvoices.org/wp-content/uploads/2010/06/Glossed_Over.pdf

ON ACRYLIC NAILS AND NAIL SALON SAFETY

CALIFORNIA HEALTHY NAIL SALONS COLLABORATIVE
"Toxic Beauty No More! Health and Safety of Vietnamese Nail Salon Workers in Southern California," 2011.
www.cahealthynailsalons.org/wp-content/uploads/2011/08/Nail-Salon-Report-2011.short_.english.pdf

ENVIRONMENTAL PROTECTION AGENCY
"Protecting the Health of Nail Salon Workers," 2007.
www.epa.gov/dfe/pubs/projects/salon/nailsalonguide.pdf

METHYL METHACRYLATE (MMA)
www.epa.gov/iris/subst/1000.htm

WOMEN'S VOICES FOR THE EARTH
"Glossed Over: Health Hazards Associated with Toxic Exposure in Nail Salons," Report 2010.
www.womensvoices.org/wp-content/uploads/2010/06/Glossed_Over.pdf

ON KERATIN HAIR STRAIGHTENERS

OREGON OSHA
"'Keratin-Based' Hair Smoothing Products and the Presence of Formaldehyde," Final Report 2010.
www.orosha.org/pdf/Final_Hair_Smoothing_Report.pdf

VIRGINIA SOLE-SMITH
"Hair Salons Still Putting Workers' Health at Risk with Brazilian Blowout," The Investigative Fund Blog, 2012.
www.theinvestigativefund.org/blog/1620/hair_salons_still_putting_workers%27_health_at_risk_with_brazilian_blowout/

WOMEN'S VOICES FOR THE EARTH
"The Blow Up on Blowouts," Fact Sheet for Consumers and Stylists.
www.womensvoices.org/campaigns/brazilian-blowout/the-blow-up-on-blowouts/

www.womensvoices.org/wp-content/uploads/2011/04/Hair-Straighteners.pdf

Brazilian Blowout Information Page
www.womensvoices.org/campaigns/brazilian-blowout/

ON TANNING BEDS

AMERICAN ACADEMY OF DERMATOLOGY
"2011 Indoor Tanning: Teen and Young Adult Women" Survey.
www.aad.org/stories-and-news/news-releases/new-survey-finds-tanning-salons-are-not-warning-teens-and-young-women-about-the-dangers-of-tanning-beds/

www.aad.org/media-resources/stats-and-facts/prevention-and-care/indoor-tanning

SKIN CANCER FOUNDATION
Tanning Information Page.
www.skincancer.org/healthy-lifestyle/tanning

ON SUNLESS TANNERS

ENVIRONMENTAL WORKING GROUP SKIN DEEP DATABASE. Dihydroxyacetone Toxicity Information Page.
www.ewg.org/skindeep/ingredient/70191/DIHYDROXYACETONE/

SIOBHAN O'CONNOR
"Are Sunless Tanners Safe? Making Sense of the New Research about DHA," No More Dirty Looks.
http://nomoredirtylooks.com/2012/06/are-any-self-tanners-actually-safe-making-sense-of-the-new-research-about-dha/

SKIN CANCER FOUNDATION
"Can Sunless Tanners Cause Skin Cancer?"
www.skincancer.org/skin-cancer-information/ask-the-experts/can-sunless-tanners-cause-cancer

ALEXANDRA SPUNT
"Eat Your Veggies to Look Beautiful." No More Dirty Looks.
http://nomoredirtylooks.com/2011/01/eat-your-veggies-to-look-beautiful/

ON GEL NAILS

WOMEN'S VOICES FOR THE EARTH
"Glossed Over: Health Hazards Associated with Toxic Exposure in Nail Salons," Report 2010.
www.womensvoices.org/wp-content/uploads/2010/06/Glossed_Over.pdf

ON HAIR DYE

ENVIRONMENTAL WORKING GROUP SKIN DEEP DATABASE. Ammonium Persulfate Toxicity Information Page.
www.cosmeticsdatabase.com/ingredient/700378/AMMONIUM_PERSULFATE/

Phenylenediamine Toxicity Information Page
http://www.cosmeticsdatabase.com/ingredient/704389/P-PHENYLENEDIAMINE/

W. UTER, H. LESSMANN, J. GEIER, AND A. SCHNUCH
"Contact allergy to hairdressing allergens in female hairdressers and clients—current data from the IVDK, 2003-2006," Journal of the German Society of Dermatology 5, no. 11 (November 5, 2007), pages 993–1001.
www.ncbi.nlm.nih.gov/pubmed/17976140

chapter 4
HONEST style

ON AMERICANS RATE OF PURCHASE AND DISCARD WITH CLOTHING
DEIRDRE IMUS
The Essential Green You, page 163.

ON PERC IN DRY CLEANING
ENVIRONMENTAL PROTECTION AGENCY
Frequently Asked Questions about Dry Cleaning.
www.epa.gov/dfe/pubs/garment/ctsa/factsheet/ctsafaq.htm

NATURAL RESOURCES DEFENSE COUNCIL
Smarter Living Index: Perchloroethylene (Tetrachloroethylene, PERC, PCE).
www.nrdc.org/living/chemicalindex/perc.asp

KATY SHERLACH, ET AL.
"Quantification of perchloroethylene residues in dry-cleaned fabrics,"
Journal of Environmental Toxicology & Chemistry (September 2011).
http://onlinelibrary.wiley.com/doi/10.1002/etc.665/abstract

UNITED STATES DEPARTMENT OF LABOR OCCUPATIONAL SAFETY & HEALTH ADMINISTRATION
Reducing Worker Exposure to PERC in Dry Cleaning.
www.osha.gov/dsg/guidance/perc.html

ON FLAME RETARDANTS AND KIDS' PAJAMAS
CHRISTOPHER GAVIGAN
Healthy Child, Healthy World, page 138.

chapter 5
HONEST home

ON BABIES AND CHILDREN HAVING MORE DIRECT ROUTES OF CHEMICAL EXPOSURE
PHILIP J. LANDRIGAN, MD
(E-mail exchange and phone interviews with Virginia Sole-Smith)

HOUSEHOLD ITEMS OFF-GAS CHEMICALS
PHILIP J. LANDRIGAN, MD
(E-mail exchange and phone interviews with Virginia Sole-Smith)

RICHARD DENISON, PHD
senior scientist with the Environmental Defense Fund.
(Phone interviews with Virginia Sole-Smith)

Are there secret chemicals in your house? Health Case for Reforming the Toxic Substances Control Act Chart
www.healthreport.saferchemicals.org

ON IMPORTANCE OF ALLERGEN-PROOF MATTRESS AND PILLOW COVERS
CHRISTOPHER GAVIGAN
(Conversation with Jessica Alba)

CLIFFORD BASSETT, MD
(Interview with Virginia Sole-Smith)
www.allergyreliefnyc.com/

ON HEALTH RISKS OF MATTRESSES AND CUSHIONS
DASHKA SLATER
"How Dangerous Is Your Couch?" *New York Times Magazine,* September 2012.
www.nytimes.com/2012/09/09/magazine/arlene-blums-crusade-against-household-toxins.html?pagewanted=all&_r=0

ARLENE BLUM, ET AL.
"Novel and High Volume Use Flame Retardants in US Couches Reflective of the 2005 PentaBDE Phase Out," *Environmental Science & Technology,* November 28, 2012
http://pubs.acs.org/doi/abs/10.1021/es303471d

ON CHEMICALS OFF-GASSING BUT DISSIPATING AFTER FIRST 5 YEARS OF A FURNITURE'S LIFE
CHRISTOPHER GAVIGAN
(Conversation with Jessica Alba)

JEFFREY SIEGEL, PHD
professor of civil engineering and indoor air quality researcher, University of Texas at Austin
(Interview with Virginia Sole-Smith)

ON CHECKING VINTAGE FURNITURE FOR LEAD PAINT
COUNTRY LIVING MAGAZINE
"Lead Paint on Antique Furniture Q&A."
www.countryliving.com/antiques/expert-advice/lead-paint-antique-furniture

ON LEAD PAINT
CHRISTOPHER GAVIGAN
Healthy Child, Healthy World, pages 225–26.

ENVIRONMENTAL PROTECTION AGENCY
epa.gov/lead/pubs/renovaterightbrochure.pdf

ON SIGNS OF QUALITY VINTAGE FURNITURE
J. D. ROTH
"How to Buy Quality Furniture." GetRichSlowly.org.
www.getrichslowly.org/blog/2012/06/13/how-to-buy-quality-furniture/

ON INDOOR AIR POLLUTION
ENVIRONMENTAL PROTECTION AGENCY
epa.gov/region1/communities/indoorair.html

ON THIRD PARTY ECO-CERTIFICATIONS
GREENGUARD
greenguard.org

FOREST STEWARDSHIP COUNCIL
fsc.org.healthybuilding.net

HEALTHY BUILDING NETWORK
healthybuilding.net

ON ASBESTOS
ENVIRONMENTAL PROTECTION AGENCY
epa.gov/asbestos

ON COMMON CHEMICALS IN FURNITURE AND HOME GOODS
BISPHENOL A

PHILIP J. LANDRIGAN, MD
Mount Sinai Pediatric Environmental Health Specialty Units BPA Fact Sheet.
www.mountsinai.org/static_files/MSMC/Files/Patient%20Care/Children/Childrens%20Environmental%20Health%20Center/BPA_Patient_Factsheet.pdf

SAFER CHEMICALS, HEALTHY FAMILIES COALITION
Congressional Action Needed on a Chemical of High Concern: Bisphenol A (BPA)
www.saferchemicals.org/resources/bpa.html

PERFLUORINATED COMPOUNDS (PFCs), BROMINATED FLAME RETARDANTS (BFRs), AND HALOGENATED FLAME RETARDANTS (HFRs)

HEALTHY BUILDING NETWORK
Screening the Toxics Out of Building Materials Fact Sheet.
www.healthybuilding.net/pdf/Healthy_Building_Material_Resources.pdf

POLYVINYL CHLORIDE/VINYL (PVC)

HEALTHY BUILDING NETWORK
PVC Alternatives.
www.healthybuilding.net/pvc/alternatives.html.

PHILIP J. LANDRIGAN, MD
Raising Healthy Children: Dr. Landrigan Answers Back-to-School Questions.
www.mountsinai.org/static_files/MSMC/Files/Patient%20Care/Children/Childrens%20Environmental%20Health%20Center/Fact%20Sheet%20-%20Back%20to%20School%20QA.pdf

SAFER CHEMICALS HEALTHY FAMILIES COALITION
Chemicals of Concern.
www.saferchemicals.org/resources/EPA-and-SCHF-Chemicals-of-Concern.html

VOLATILE ORGANIC COMPOUNDS (VOCs)

HEALTHY BUILDING NETWORK
Target Materials: Worst in Class Chemicals.
www.healthybuilding.net/target_materials.html

TOXIC CHEMICALS IN BUILDING MATERIALS
www.healthybuilding.net/healthcare/Toxic%20Chemicals%20in%20Building%20Materials.pdf

ON LETTING NEW FURNITURE, PAINT, ETC., BREATHE FOR SEVERAL DAYS TO OFF-GAS

JEFFREY SIEGEL, PHD
professor of civil engineering and indoor air quality researcher, University of Texas at Austin. (Interview with Virginia Sole-Smith)

ON THE HYGIENE HYPOTHESIS

S. F. BLOOMFIELD, ET AL.
"Too clean or not too clean? The Hygiene Hypothesis and Home Hygiene," *Journal of Clinical & Experimental Allergy* 36, no. 4 (April 2006), pages 402–5.
www.ncbi.nlm.nih.gov/pmc/articles/PMC1448690/

UNIVERSITY OF MICHIGAN HEALTH SYSTEM
"The Hygiene Hypothesis: Are Cleanlier Lifestyles Causing More Allergies for Kids?" *ScienceDaily*, September 9, 2007.
www.sciencedaily.com/releases/2007/09/070905174501.htm

ON THE IMPORTANCE OF OPENING WINDOWS

JEFFREY SIEGEL, PHD
(Interview with Virginia Sole-Smith)

ON TAKING SHOES OFF INDOORS

JEFFREY SIEGEL, PHD
(Interview with Virginia Sole-Smith)

ON TRACKING LEAD INDOORS

ENVIRONMENTAL PROTECTION AGENCY
"Natural Human Exposure Assessment Survey: Dust Sampling Work Plan"
http://cfpub.epa.gov/si/si_public_record_report.cfm?dirEntryId=17184

ON CLEANING FLOORS AND CARPETS

CHRISTOPHER GAVIGAN
Healthy Child, Healthy World, page 54.

ON SCREEN DUST

CNET NEWS
"Is the dust on your computer toxic?" June 2004
http://news.cnet.com/2100-1041_3-5225799.html

CLEAN PRODUCTION REPORT
"Sick of Dust" March 2005
cleanproduction.org/library/Dust%20Report.pdf

ON VACUUMING AND ALLERGIES

JEFFREY SIEGEL, PHD
(Interview with Virginia Sole-Smith)

CLIFFORD BASSETT, MD
(Interview with Virginia Sole-Smith)

ON MAKING YOUR OWN ALL-PURPOSE CLEANER

RODALE.COM/NATURAL-CLEANING-RECIPES

ON SEALING YOUR GROUT

JOHN PETERSIK
"How to Seal Grout," YoungHouseLove.com (2010).
www.younghouselove.com/2010/06/how-to-seal-grout/

ON DEALING WITH DUST

CLIFFORD BASSETT, MD
(Interview with Virginia Sole-Smith.)

ON GETTING KIDS TO PITCH IN

CHRISTOPHER GAVIGAN
Healthy Child, Healthy World, page 50.

ON DEALING WITH MOLD

CONSUMER PRODUCT SAFETY COMMISSION
The Inside Story: A Guide to Indoor Air Quality. CPSC Document #450.
www.cpsc.gov/cpscpub/pubs/450.html#Intro
www.cpsc.gov/cpscpub/pubs/450.html#Look6
www.cpsc.gov/cpscpub/pubs/450.html#Look3

ENVIRONMENTAL PROTECTION AGENCY
http://epa.gov/mold/moldbasics.html
http://epa.gov/mold/moldcleanup.html
http://epa.gov/mold/cleanupguidelines.html

JEFFREY SIEGEL, PHD
(Interview with Virginia Sole-Smith)

ON DEALING WITH SCENTS AND SMOKE

CHRISTOPHER GAVIGAN
Healthy Child, Healthy World, page 189.

JEFFREY SIEGEL, PHD
(Interview with Virginia Sole-Smith)

ON NATURAL
AIR FRESHENERS
RODALE.COM
"6 Weird All Natural Air Fresheners."
www.rodale.com/natural-air-fresheners?cm_mmc=TheDailyFixNL-_-922540-_-05222012-_-6_weird_all_natural_air_fresheners_title

ON PLANTS THAT
CLEAR AIR INDOORS
CLIFFORD BASSETT, MD
(Interview with Virginia Sole-Smith)

ON LAUNDRY
CHEMICALS
CHLORINE BLEACH
CENTERS FOR
DISEASE CONTROL
www.bt.cdc.gov/agent/chlorine/basics/facts.asp

ENVIRONMENTAL
PROTECTION AGENCY
www.epa.gov/kidshometour/products/bleach.htm

THE HONEST COMPANY
www.honest.com/whats-inside/cleaners

NATURAL RESOURCES
DEFENSE COUNCIL
Smarter Living, Chemical Index: Dioxins.
www.nrdc.org/living/chemicalindex/dioxins.asp

OPTICAL BRIGHTENERS
PROTECT KITTERY WATER
Spruce Creek Watershed Improvement Project, Optical Brighteners Fact Sheet.
www.protectkitterywaters.org/pledge/PKW_Optical_Brighteners_Factsheet.pdf

SEVENTH GENERATION
Just Say No to the Glow.
www.seventhgeneration.com/learn/video/no-glow

chapter 6
HONEST
baby

ON MY FEELINGS
ABOUT PARENTHOOD
JESSICA ALBA
"Jessica's Diary of a Spy Mom—Take 1!" *iVillage CelebVillage Blog* (2011).
www.ivillage.com/jessica-alba-spy-kids-blog/1-a-370157

JESSICA ALBA
"Jessica's Diary of a Spy Mom—Take 3!" *iVillage CelebVillage Blog* (2011).
www.ivillage.com/jessica-alba-spy-kids-blog-3/1-a-371374

JESSICA ALBA
"Jessica's Diary of a Spy Mom—Take 4!" *iVillage CelebVillage Blog* (2011).
www.ivillage.com/jessica-alba-spy-kids-blog-4/1-a-371863

JESSICA ALBA
"Why I'm Not Stressed about Losing the Baby Weight," *iVillage,* Video Interview (April 2012).
www.ivillage.com/jessica-alba-im-not-stressed-about-losing-baby-weight/1-h-374214

JESSICA ALBA
"How I Adjusted to Life with Baby No. 2," *iVillage CelebVillage Blog* (April 2012).
www.ivillage.com/jessica-alba-having-daughter-haven/1-a-444087

JESSICA ALBA
"My Secret to Keeping My Marriage Alive after Two Kids," *iVillage CelebVillage Blog* (May 2012).
http://www.ivillage.com/jessica-alba-marriage-after-two-kids/1-a-448696

ON THE DANGERS OF
SMOKE TO PREGNANT
WOMEN
CHRISTOPHER GAVIGAN
Healthy Child, Healthy World, pages 24.

ON NOT PUMPING
YOUR OWN GAS
CHRISTOPHER GAVIGAN
Healthy Child, Healthy World, pages 25.

ON REMODELING
SAFELY DURING
PREGNANCY
CHRISTOPHER GAVIGAN
Healthy Child, Healthy World, pages 28.

ON LEAD PAINT
CHRISTOPHER GAVIGAN
Healthy Child, Healthy World, pages 225–26.

ON BUYING USED
AND VINTAGE
FURNITURE FOR THE
NURSERY
CHRISTOPHER GAVIGAN
Healthy Child, Healthy World, pages 32.

ON PINPOINTING
TOXIC SMELLS IN
BABY PRODUCTS
CHRISTOPHER GAVIGAN
Healthy Child, Healthy World, pages 32.

ON TROUBLE-
SHOOTING
BREASTFEEDING
ISSUES
ALAN GREENE, MD
"Steps to Take Before Giving Up on Breast Feeding" (2008).
www.drgreene.com/article/steps-take-giving-breast-feeding?tid=280

ON ECO-HEALTH
ISSUES WITH DIAPERS
KIERA BUTLER
"A Brief History of the Disposable Diaper," *Mother Jones* (May/June 2008).
www.motherjones.com/environment/2008/04/brief-history-disposable-diaper

ENVIRONMENTAL
PROTECTION AGENCY
"Municipal Solid Waste in the United States: 2009 Facts and Figures," page 81 (amount in landfills).
www.epa.gov/wastes/nonhaz/municipal/pubs/msw2009rpt.pdf

THE HONEST COMPANY
What's Inside: Diapers.
www.honest.com/whats-inside/diapers

ON SAFE SLEEPING
ALAN GREENE, MD
"Safe Bedding to Help Prevent SIDS" (2008).
www.drgreene.com/article/safe-bedding-help-prevent-sids?tid=279

ON TRAVELING
WITH KIDS
RED TRICYCLE
"Unzipped: Jessica Alba's Can't-Live-Without Summer Travel Gear."
www.redtri.com/jessica-alba-travel-gear

ON BUILDING SELF-ESTEEM

ALAN GREENE, MD
"A Parent's Guide to Praise" (2008).
www.drgreene.com/article/parent%E2%80%99s-guide-praise?tid=1545

ON SAFER PLASTIC BATH TOYS

VIRGINIA SOLE-SMITH
"Staying Safe in a Toxic World." *Parents* (August 2010), pages 170–76.

ON SAFER KIDS TOYS, STUFFED ANIMALS AND OTHER GEAR

CHRISTOPHER GAVIGAN
Healthy Child, Healthy World, pages 131–32.

ON PAINTING FURNITURE

SHERRY PETERSIK
"How to Paint Furniture," YoungHouseLove.com (2009).
www.younghouselove.com/2009/02/how-to-paint-furniture/

ON FINDING NONTOXIC ART SUPPLIES

CHRISTOPHER GAVIGAN
Healthy Child, Healthy World, pages 141–43.

SAFER CHEMICALS, HEALTHY FAMILIES COALITION
"Nontoxic Art Supplies," Blog (February 2012).
http://blog.saferchemicals.org/2012/02/non-toxic-art-supplies.html

chapter 7
HONEST inspiration

ON FINDING BALANCE

JESSICA ALBA
"Jessica's Diary of a Spy Mom—Take 2!" *iVillage CelebVillage Blog.* (2011).
www.ivillage.com/jessica-alba-spy-kids-blog-2/1-a-371215

ON HOMEMADE ICE POPS

THE HONEST COMPANY
"Cool Down with Homemade Popsicles," Honest Blog: Honest Kitchen (July 2012).
http://blog.honest.com/cool-down-with-homemade-ice-pops/

acknowledgments

THE INSPIRATION BEHIND this book has been years in the making. During that time, I've been supported and encouraged by many people to follow my dreams. It's in honor of them and their love that I've written *The Honest Life*, as I hope it similarly inspires others to follow their hearts and achieve the impossible. And, while there's not enough space to thank everyone, I wish to personally express my gratitude for the following people whose contributions and help were essential to creating this book.

Thank you Mom and Dad for everything. It's through the values you instilled in me—having a good work ethic, giving everything 200 percent, never giving up, and always believing in myself—that I was able to write this book. To my brother, Joshua: It's thanks to you that I learned to share everything. And Nikki, you are everything—for your patience, love for our family, and for creating order out of all the chaos.

To my husband and daughters, you are the inspiration for all that I do. Cash, you push me to be thoughtful and curious while always giving me perspective and keeping me grounded. I'm so grateful that you were a sounding board and voice of reason throughout the creation of this book (and for letting me sleep in after long nights of writing). Honor and Haven, you are the reason I wrote it. Thank you for choosing me as your mommy—you're my life.

Lindsey Hanson and Sarah Reisert, thank you for being the rock stars that you are—I am so grateful to the both of you for your honest feedback, thorough constructive criticism, and literary prowess.

Christopher Gavigan, Brian Lee, and Sean

Kane—without you, The Honest Company would still be just a dream. Words don't describe how rewarding it is to create a company with like-minded partners who really want to change the world and the way people do business. I also want to give a big shout out to the entire Honest family for your passion, hard work, long hours, focus, and creativity to fulfill our dream to re-define the "family brand" and create something that's better for all families, everywhere.

My journey as a mother and entrepreneur—and this book—would not have been possible without the expertise, knowledge, and dedicated activism of Dr. Phil Landrigan, Dr. Jay Gordon, Dr. Alan Greene, Christopher Gavigan, and everyone at Safer Chemicals Healthy Families and Healthy Child Healthy World. Thank you for actively educating and pushing for a better environment for our children to grow up in.

My besties! Lauren Andersen—from our teen years to now, we've been through thick and thin—I love you gurrrl! Kelly Sawyer Patricof—your work and lifestyle have inspired who I am as a mom today and your friendship means more than you know. Thank you for sharing your creativity and know-how in this book and keeping me sane throughout the entire publication process. Hillary Kerr and Katherine Power—no one knows how to make high-fashion wearable and functional like you ladies—it's a true talent that I admire, appreciate, and aspire to. Ramona Braganza—I met you when I was 17; gosh, time has flown by. . . . but whenever I need to get into shape, a shoulder to lean on or just a good laugh, I'm glad that I can still call on you.

Justin Coit, I can't say this enough—you take the most beautiful photos ever, and you're so gracious and lovely. I love and appreciate you as a friend and your talent as a photographer. Nick Onken, your images similarly gave this book color, bringing it to life. Speaking of color . . . Brad Goreski, Thomas, and Hannah—you added style and punch to the book. Fiona Stiles, you helped me perfect my 10-minute face (all moms will thank you, too). Scott Horne and Jeanne Kelley, thank you for propping and styling so beautifully. And Kellan Hori, you were just as much a translator as chef, because you transformed my culinary creations into usable recipes. Like all busy moms know, it takes a village—and it's no exception when creating a book.

I'm grateful to Virginia Sole-Smith for helping to bring clarity to the research and shape to the story. And thank you to the Rodale team for your enthusiasm and work in getting this book published. Alex Postman, Dave Zinczenko, Marc Adelman, Steve Perrine, Kara Plikaitis, George Karabotsos, Nancy N. Bailey, Liz Krenos, Aly Mostel—your efforts behind the scenes helped me cross the finish line.

Thanks to all for your collaborative spirit and making *The Honest Life* a truly inspired and authentic take on living naturally.

Index

Underscored page references indicate sidebars and tables. **Boldface** references indicate photographs and illustrations.